Injury & Trauma Sourcebook

Learning Disabilities Sourcebook, 4th Edition

Leukemia Sourcebook

Liver Disorders Sourcebook

Medical Tests Sourcebook, 4th Edition

Men's Health Concerns Sourcebook, 4th Edition

Mental Health Disorders Sourcebook, 5th Edition

Mental Retardation Sourcebook

Movement Disorders Sourcebook, 2nd Edition

Multiple Sclerosis Sourcebook

Muscular Dystrophy Sourcebook

Obesity Sourcebook

Osteoporosis Sourcebook

Pain Sourcebook, 3rd Edition

Pediatric Cancer Sourcebook

Physical & Mental Issues in Aging Sourcebook

Podiatry Sourcebook, 2nd Edition

Pregnancy & Birth Sourcebook, 3rd Edition

Prostate & Urological Disorders Sourcebook

Prostate Cancer Sourcebook

Rehabilitation Sourcebook

Respiratory Disorders Sourcebook, 2nd Edition

Sexually Transmitted Diseases Sourcebook, 5th Edition

Sleep Disorders Sourcebook, 3rd Edition

Smoking Concerns Sourcebook

Sports Injuries Sourcebook, 4th Edition

Stress-Related Disorders Sourcebook, 3rd Edition

Stroke Sourcebook, 2nd Edition

Surgery Sourcebook, 2nd Edition

Thyroid Disorders Sourcebook

Transplantation Sourcebook

Traveler's Health Sourcebook

Urinary Tract & Kidney Diseases & Disorders Sourcebook, 2nd Edition

Vegetarian Sourcebook

Women's Health Concerns Sourcebook, 3rd Edition

Workplace Health & Safety Sourcebook

Worldwide Health Sourcebook

Teen Health Series

Abuse & Violence Information for Teens

Accident & Safety Information for Teens

Alcohol Information for Teens, 2nd Edition

Allergy Information for Teens

Asthma Information for Teens, 2nd Edition

Body Information for Teens

Cancer Information for Teens, 2nd Edition

Complementary & Alternative Medicine Information for Teens

Diabetes Information for Teens, 2nd Edition

Diet Information for Teens, 3rd Edition

Drug Information for Teens, 3rd Edition

Eating Disorders Information for Teens, 2nd Edition

Fitness Information for Teens, 3rd Edition

Learning Disabilities Information for Teens

Mental Health Information for Teens, 3rd Edition

Pregnancy Information for Teens, 2nd Edition

Sexual Health Information for Teens, 3rd Edition

Skin Health Information for Teens, 2nd Edition

Sleep Information for Teens

Sports Injuries Information for Teens, 3rd Edition

Stress Information for Teens

Suicide Information for Teens, 2nd Edition

Tobacco Information for Teens, 2nd Edition

Breast Cancer
SOURCEBOOK

Fourth Edition

Health Reference Series

Fourth Edition

Breast Cancer
SOURCEBOOK

Basic Consumer Health Information about the Prevalence, Risk Factors, and Symptoms of Breast Cancer, Including Ductal and Lobular Carcinoma in Situ, Invasive Carcinoma, Inflammatory Breast Cancer, and Breast Cancer in Men and Pregnant Women

Along with Facts about Benign Breast Changes, Breast Cancer Screening and Diagnostic Tests, Treatments Such as Surgery, Radiation Therapy, Chemotherapy, and Hormonal and Biologic Therapies, Tips on Managing Treatment Side Effects and Complications, a Glossary of Terms, and a Directory of Resources for Additional Help and Information

Edited by
Amy L. Sutton

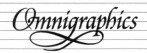

Omnigraphics

155 W. Congress, Suite 200, Detroit, MI 48226

Bibliographic Note
Because this page cannot legibly accommodate all the copyright notices, the Bibliographic
Note portion of the Preface constitutes an extension of the copyright notice.

Edited by Amy L. Sutton

Health Reference Series

Karen Bellenir, *Managing Editor*
David A. Cooke, MD, FACP, *Medical Consultant*
Elizabeth Collins, *Research and Permissions Coordinator*
Cherry Edwards, *Permissions Assistant*
EdIndex, Services for Publishers, *Indexers*

* * *

Omnigraphics, Inc.

Matthew P. Barbour, *Senior Vice President*
Kevin M. Hayes, *Operations Manager*

* * *

Peter E. Ruffner, *Publisher*

Copyright © 2012 Omnigraphics, Inc.

ISBN 978-0-7808-1279-6

E-ISBN 978-0-7808-1280-2

Library of Congress Cataloging-in-Publication Data

Breast cancer sourcebook : basic consumer health information about the
prevalence, risk factors, and symptoms of breast cancer ... / edited by Amy
L. Sutton. -- 4th ed.
    p. cm. -- (Health reference series)
  Includes bibliographical references and index.
  Summary: "Provides basic consumer health information on risk factors,
prevention, symptoms, diagnosis, and treatment of various types of breast
cancer, along with facts about coping during and after treatment. Includes
index, glossary of related terms and directory of resources"-- Provided by
publisher.
  ISBN 978-0-7808-1279-6 (hardcover : alk. paper) 1.
Breast--Cancer--Popular works. I. Sutton, Amy L.
  RC280.B8B6887 2012
  616.99'449--dc23
                                                                2012016023

This book is printed on acid-free paper meeting the ANSI Z39.48 Standard. The infinity
symbol that appears above indicates that the paper in this book meets that standard.

Printed in the United States

Table of Contents

Visit www.healthreferenceseries.com to view *A Contents Guide to the Health Reference Series*, a listing of more than 16,000 topics and the volumes in which they are covered.

Part III: Risk Factors, Symptoms, and Prevention of Breast Cancer

Part V: Breast Cancer Treatments

Part VI: Managing Side Effects and Complications of Breast Cancer Treatment

Part VII: Living with Breast Cancer

Preface

About This Book

Breast cancer is one of the most commonly diagnosed cancers in women, and an estimated one in eight U.S. women will eventually develop an invasive form of this disease. Although breast cancer still claims the lives of nearly 40,000 women annually, there has been progress in the battle against it. Thanks to treatment advances, earlier detection and screening techniques, and increased awareness of symptoms, the number of deaths attributable to breast cancer each year has declined since 1990. Furthermore, in 2010, there were more than 2.5 million breast cancer survivors living in the United States.

Breast Cancer Sourcebook, Fourth Edition, provides updated information about breast cancer and its causes, risk factors, diagnosis, and treatment. Readers will learn about the types of breast cancer, including ductal carcinoma in situ, lobular carcinoma in situ, invasive carcinoma, and inflammatory breast cancer, as well as common breast cancer treatment complications, such as pain, fatigue, lymphedema, hair loss, and sexuality and fertility issues. Information on preventive therapies, nutrition and exercise recommendations, and tips on living with cancer are also included, along with a glossary of related terms and a directory of organizations that offer additional information to breast cancer patients and their families.

How to Use This Book

This book is divided into parts and chapters. Parts focus on broad areas of interest. Chapters are devoted to single topics within a part.

Part I: Introduction to Breast Cancer identifies the parts of the breasts and lymphatic system, discusses common changes in the breast that pose no threat to health, and offers general information about breast cancer in men and women. It also examines the link between estrogen and the development of breast and ovarian cancer and offers statistical information on the prevalence of breast cancer in the United States.

Part II: Types of Breast Cancer identifies the most common types of breast cancer, including ductal carcinoma in situ (DCIS), lobular carcinoma in situ (LCIS), invasive carcinoma of the breast, medullary breast carcinoma, inflammatory breast cancer, Paget disease of the nipple, and triple-negative breast cancer.

Part III: Risk Factors, Symptoms, and Prevention of Breast Cancer provides information about hereditary and non-hereditary factors that increase the risk of developing breast cancer, including age, family health history, exposure to radiation, alcohol consumption, use of hormone replacement therapy, reproductive risk factors, and obesity. Genetic counseling for breast cancer risk is discussed, along with information about preventing breast cancer in people who are susceptible. The part also provides information about preventive mastectomy and oophorectomy.

Part IV: Screening, Diagnosis, and Stages of Breast Cancer identifies tests and procedures used to screen, diagnose, and stage breast cancer, including breast examinations, mammograms, and breast biopsies. Information about other breast imaging procedures, including breast magnetic resonance imaging, scintimammography, thermogram, and breast ultrasound, is also included.

Part V: Breast Cancer Treatments discusses how to find a treatment facility or doctor and offers information about considerations to make before undergoing breast cancer treatment. Surgical treatments for breast cancer, such as mastectomy, lumpectomy, and breast reconstruction, are discussed, and facts about radiation therapy, chemotherapy, hormone therapy, biologic therapies, and complementary and alternative medicine treatments for breast cancer are provided. The part also includes a discussion of the treatment of breast cancer in pregnant women, men, and patients with recurrent breast cancer.

Part VI: Managing Side Effects and Complications of Breast Cancer Treatment describes fatigue, infection, lymphedema, pain, sexual and fertility issues, and hair loss associated with breast cancer treatment. Information about complementary and alternative therapies that may relieve physical discomfort or emotional anxiety is also provided.

Part VII: Living with Breast Cancer discusses strategies for coping with the difficult emotions produced by a breast cancer diagnosis and offers information about talking to family members and friends about cancer. In addition, the part identifies nutrition and exercise recommendations after cancer treatment, tips for dealing with cancer in the workplace, information on purchasing breast prostheses and post-mastectomy bras, and suggestions for caregivers of breast cancer patients.

Part VIII: Additional Help and Information provides a glossary of important terms related to breast cancer and a directory of organizations that offer information and financial assistance to people with breast cancer.

Bibliographic Note

This volume contains documents and excerpts from publications issued by the following U.S. government agencies: Agency for Healthcare Research and Quality (AHRQ); Centers for Disease Control and Prevention (CDC); National Cancer Institute (NCI); National Center for Complementary and Alternative Medicine (NCCAM); National Institutes of Health (NIH) Clinical Center; U.S. Department of Health and Human Services (HHS); U.S. Department of Labor (DOL); U.S. Equal Employment Opportunity Commission (EEOC); and the U.S. Food and Drug Administration (FDA).

In addition, this volume contains copyrighted documents from the following organizations: A.D.A.M., Inc.; American Association for Clinical Chemistry; American Institute for Cancer Research; American Society for Radiation Oncology; Breast Cancer Care; California Pacific Medical Center; Cancer Care, Inc.; Caring, Inc.; Cleveland Clinic Foundation; College of American Pathologists; Imaginis Corporation; Living Beyond Breast Cancer; National Academy of Sciences; Simms/Mann–UCLA Center for Integrative Oncology; University of Illinois Board of Trustees; and the University of Texas MD Anderson Cancer Center.

Full citation information is provided on the first page of each chapter or section. Every effort has been made to secure all necessary rights to reprint the copyrighted material. If any omissions have been made, please contact Omnigraphics to make corrections for future editions.

Acknowledgements

Thanks go to the many organizations, agencies, and individuals who have contributed materials for this *Sourcebook* and to medical consultant Dr. David Cooke and prepress service provider WhimsyInk. Special thanks go to managing editor Karen Bellenir and research and permissions coordinator Liz Collins for their help and support.

About the Health Reference Series

The *Health Reference Series* is designed to provide basic medical information for patients, families, caregivers, and the general public. Each volume takes a particular topic and provides comprehensive coverage. This is especially important for people who may be dealing with a newly diagnosed disease or a chronic disorder in themselves or in a family member. People looking for preventive guidance, information about disease warning signs, medical statistics, and risk factors for health problems will also find answers to their questions in the *Health Reference Series*. The *Series*, however, is not intended to serve as a tool for diagnosing illness, in prescribing treatments, or as a substitute for the physician/patient relationship. All people concerned about medical symptoms or the possibility of disease are encouraged to seek professional care from an appropriate health care provider.

A Note about Spelling and Style

Health Reference Series editors use *Stedman's Medical Dictionary* as an authority for questions related to the spelling of medical terms and the *Chicago Manual of Style* for questions related to grammatical structures, punctuation, and other editorial concerns. Consistent adherence is not always possible, however, because the individual volumes within the *Series* include many documents from a wide variety of different producers and copyright holders, and the editor's primary goal is to present material from each source as accurately as is possible following the terms specified by each document's producer. This sometimes means that information in different chapters or sections may follow other guidelines and alternate spelling authorities. For example, occasionally a copyright holder may require that eponymous terms be shown in possessive forms (Crohn's disease *vs.* Crohn disease) or that British spelling norms be retained (leukaemia *vs.* leukemia).

Locating Information within the Health Reference Series

The *Health Reference Series* contains a wealth of information about a wide variety of medical topics. Ensuring easy access to all the fact sheets, research reports, in-depth discussions, and other material contained within the individual books of the *Series* remains one of our highest priorities. As the *Series* continues to grow in size and scope, however, locating the precise information needed by a reader may become more challenging.

A Contents Guide to the Health Reference Series was developed to direct readers to the specific volumes that address their concerns. It presents an extensive list of diseases, treatments, and other topics of general interest compiled from the Tables of Contents and major index headings. To access *A Contents Guide to the Health Reference Series*, visit www.healthreferenceseries.com.

Medical Consultant

Medical consultation services are provided to the *Health Reference Series* editors by David A. Cooke, MD, FACP. Dr. Cooke is a graduate of Brandeis University, and he received his M.D. degree from the University of Michigan. He completed residency training at the University of Wisconsin Hospital and Clinics. He is board-certified in Internal Medicine. Dr. Cooke currently works as part of the University of Michigan Health System and practices in Ann Arbor, MI. In his free time, he enjoys writing, science fiction, and spending time with his family.

Our Advisory Board

We would like to thank the following board members for providing guidance to the development of this *Series*:

- Dr. Lynda Baker, Associate Professor of Library and Information Science, Wayne State University, Detroit, MI

- Nancy Bulgarelli, William Beaumont Hospital Library, Royal Oak, MI

- Karen Imarisio, Bloomfield Township Public Library, Bloomfield Township, MI

- Karen Morgan, Mardigian Library, University of Michigan-Dearborn, Dearborn, MI

- Rosemary Orlando, St. Clair Shores Public Library, St. Clair Shores, MI

Health Reference Series Update Policy

The inaugural book in the *Health Reference Series* was the first edition of *Cancer Sourcebook* published in 1989. Since then, the *Series* has been enthusiastically received by librarians and in the medical community. In order to maintain the standard of providing high-quality health information for the layperson the editorial staff at Omnigraphics felt it was necessary to implement a policy of updating volumes when warranted.

Medical researchers have been making tremendous strides, and it is the purpose of the *Health Reference Series* to stay current with the most recent advances. Each decision to update a volume is made on an individual basis. Some of the considerations include how much new information is available and the feedback we receive from people who use the books. If there is a topic you would like to see added to the update list, or an area of medical concern you feel has not been adequately addressed, please write to:

Editor
Health Reference Series
Omnigraphics, Inc.
155 W. Congress, Suite 200
Detroit, MI 48226
E-mail: editorial@omnigraphics.com

Part One

Introduction to Breast Cancer

Chapter 1

Breast and Lymphatic System Basics: Understanding Breast Health

You may be reading this text because you, or your health care provider, found a breast lump or other breast change. Keep in mind that breast changes are very common. Most breast changes are not cancer. But it is very important to get the follow-up tests that your health care provider asks you to.

Many breast changes are changes in how your breast or nipple looks or feels. You may notice a lump or firmness in your breast or under your arm. Or perhaps the size or shape of your breast has changed. Your nipple may be pointing or facing inward (inverted) or feeling tender. The skin on your breast, areola, or nipple may be scaly, red, or swollen. You may have nipple discharge, which is an abnormal fluid coming from the nipple.

If you have these or other breast changes, talk with your health care provider to get these changes checked as soon as possible.

Breast and Lymphatic System Basics

To better understand breast changes, it helps to know what the breasts and lymphatic system are made of.

Excerpted from "Understanding Breast Changes: A Health Guide for Women," by the National Cancer Institute (NCI, www.cancer.gov), part of the National Institutes of Health, January 1, 2011.

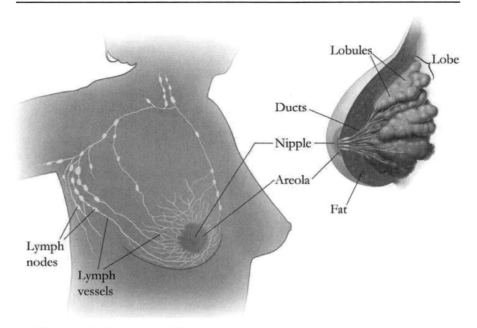

Figure 1.1. Anatomy of the breast.

The Breasts

Breasts are made of connective tissue, glandular tissue, and fatty tissue. Connective tissue and glandular tissue look dense, or white on a mammogram. Fatty tissue is non-dense, or black on a mammogram. Dense breasts can make mammograms harder to interpret.

Breasts have lobes, lobules, ducts, an areola, and a nipple.

- Lobes are sections of the glandular tissue. Lobes have smaller sections called lobules that end in tiny bulbs that can make milk.

- Ducts are thin tubes that connect the lobes and lobules. Milk flows from the lobules through the ducts to the nipple.

- The nipple is the small raised area at the tip of the breast. Milk flows through the nipple. The areola is the area of darker-colored skin around the nipple. Each breast also has lymph vessels.

The Lymphatic System

The lymphatic system, which is a part of your body's defense system, contains lymph vessels and lymph nodes.

- Lymph vessels are thin tubes that carry a fluid called lymph and white blood cells.

- Lymph vessels lead to small, bean-shaped organs called lymph nodes. Lymph nodes are found near your breast, under your arm, above your collarbone, in your chest, and in other parts of your body.

- Lymph nodes filter substances in lymph to help fight infection and disease. They also store disease-fighting white blood cells called lymphocytes.

Check with Your Health Care Provider about Breast Changes

Check with your health care provider if you notice that your breast looks or feels different. No change is too small to ask about. In fact, the best time to call is when you first notice a breast change.

Breast changes to see your health care provider about include the following:

- A lump (mass) or a firm feeling

- A lump in or near your breast or under your arm

- Thick or firm tissue in or near your breast or under your arm

- A change in the size or shape of your breast

Lumps come in different shapes and sizes. Most lumps are not cancer.

If you notice a lump in one breast, check your other breast. If both breasts feel the same, it may be normal. Normal breast tissue can sometimes feel lumpy.

Some women do regular breast self-exams (BSE). Doing a BSE regularly can help you learn how your breast normally feels and make it easier to notice and find any changes.

Doing a BSE regularly is not a substitute for regular mammograms. Always get a lump checked. Don't wait until your next mammogram. You may need to have tests to be sure that the lump is not cancer.

Nipple discharge or changes to see your health care provider about include the following:

- Nipple discharge (fluid that is not breast milk)

- Nipple changes, such as a nipple that points or faces inward (inverted) into the breast

Nipple discharge may be different colors or textures. Nipple discharge is not usually a sign of cancer. It can be caused by birth control pills, some medicines, and infections.

Get nipple discharge checked, especially fluid that comes out by itself or fluid that is bloody.

You should also see your health provider if you have skin changes, such as itching, redness, scaling, dimples, or puckers on your breast. If the skin on your breast changes, get it checked as soon as possible.

Finding Breast Changes

Here are some ways your health care provider can find breast changes.

Clinical Breast Exam

During a clinical breast exam, your health care provider checks your breasts and nipples and under your arms for any abnormal changes. This exam is part of a routine check-up.

Mammogram

A mammogram is an x-ray picture of your breast tissue. This test may find tumors that are too small to feel. During a mammogram, each breast is pressed between two plastic plates. Some discomfort is normal, but if it's painful, tell the mammography technician.

The best time to get a mammogram is at the end of your menstrual period. This is when your breasts are less tender. Some women have less breast tenderness if they don't have any caffeine for a couple of days before the mammogram.

After the x-ray pictures are taken, they are sent to a radiologist, who studies them and sends a report to your health care provider.

Both film and digital mammography use x-rays to make a picture of the breast tissue. The actual procedure for getting the mammogram is the same. The difference is in how the images are recorded and stored. It's like the difference between a film camera and a digital camera.

- Film mammography stores the image directly on x-ray film.

- Digital mammography takes an electronic image of the breast and stores it directly in a computer. Digital images can be made lighter, darker, or larger. Images can also be stored and shared electronically.

A research study sponsored by the National Cancer Institute (NCI) showed that digital mammography and film mammography are about the same in terms of detecting breast cancer. However, digital mammography may be better at detecting breast cancer in woman who are under age 50, have very dense breasts, or are premenopausal or perimenopausal (the times before and at the beginning of menopause).

Talk with your health care provider to learn more about what is best for you.

When you make your appointment, be sure to tell the staff if you have breast implants. Ask if they have specialists who are trained in taking and reading mammograms of women with breast implants. This is important because breast implants can make it harder to see cancer or other abnormal changes on the mammogram. A special technique called implant displacement views is used.

- If you have breast implants for cosmetic reasons, you may have either a screening mammogram or a diagnostic mammogram. This will depend on the facility that does the mammogram.

- If you have breast implant(s) after having a mastectomy for breast cancer, talk with your breast surgeon or oncologist to learn about the best screening test for you.

Magnetic Resonance Imaging (MRI)

Magnetic resonance imaging, also called MRI, uses a powerful magnet, radio waves, and a computer to take detailed pictures of areas inside the breast. MRI is another tool that can be used to find breast cancer. However, MRIs don't replace mammograms. They are used in addition to mammograms in women who are at increased risk of breast cancer.

MRIs have some limits. For example, they cannot find breast changes such as microcalcifications. MRIs are also less specific than other tests. This means that they may give false-positive test results—the test shows that there is cancer when there really is not.

Talk with your health care provider about having other screening tests, such as an MRI, in addition to mammograms. Ask your health care provider if you are at increased risk of breast cancer due to the following:

- Harmful changes (mutations) in the BRCA1 or BRCA2 [breast cancer 1 and breast cancer 2] gene

- A family history of breast cancer

- Your personal medical history

Getting Your Mammogram Results

You should get a written report of your mammogram results within 30 days of your mammogram, since this is the law. Be sure the mammography facility has your address and phone number. It's helpful to get your mammogram at the same place each year. This way, your current mammogram can be compared with past mammograms.

If your results were normal:

- Your breast tissue shows no signs of a mass or calcification.

- Visit your health care provider if you notice a breast change before your next appointment.

If your results were abnormal, here is what it means:

- A breast change was found. It may be benign (not cancer), premalignant (may become cancer), or cancer.

- It's important to get all the follow-up tests your health care provider asks you to.

If you don't get your results, call your health care provider.

Keep in mind that most breast changes are not cancer. But all changes need to be checked, and more tests may be needed.

Mammograms can show lumps, calcifications, and other changes in your breast. The radiologist will study the mammogram for breast changes that do not look normal and for differences between your breasts. When possible, he or she will compare your most recent mammogram with past mammograms to check for changes.

Lump (or Mass)

The size, shape, and edges of a lump give the radiologist important information. A lump that is not cancer often looks smooth and round and has a clear, defined edge. Lumps that look like this are often cysts. However, if the lump on the mammogram has a jagged outline and an irregular shape, more tests are needed.

Depending on the size and shape of the lump, your health care provider may ask you to have the following:

- Another clinical breast exam

- Another mammogram to have a closer look at the area

- An ultrasound exam to find out if the lump is solid or is filled with fluid

- A test called a biopsy to remove cells, or the entire lump, to look at under a microscope to check for signs of disease

Calcifications

Calcifications are deposits of calcium in the breast tissue. They are too small to be felt, but can be seen on a mammogram. There are two types:

- Macrocalcifications look like small white dots on a mammogram. They are common in women over 50 years old. Macrocalcifications are not related to cancer and usually don't need more testing.

- Microcalcifications look like tiny white specks on a mammogram. They are usually not a sign of cancer. However, if they are found in an area of rapidly dividing cells, or grouped together in a certain way, you may need more tests.

Depending on how many calcifications you have, their size, and where they are found, your health care provider may ask you to have the following:

- Another mammogram to have a closer look at the area

- A test called a biopsy to check for signs of disease

Mammography is an excellent tool to find breast changes in most women who have no signs of breast cancer. However, it may not detect all breast cancers. See your health care provider if you have a lump that was not seen on a mammogram or notice any other breast changes.

Follow-Up Tests to Diagnose Breast Changes

An ultrasound exam, an MRI, a biopsy, or other follow-up tests may be needed to learn more about a breast change.

Ultrasound

An ultrasound exam uses sound waves to make a picture of breast tissue. This picture is called a sonogram. It helps radiologists to see if a lump or mass is solid or filled with fluid. A fluid-filled lump is called a cyst.

MRI

Magnetic resonance imaging, also called MRI, uses a powerful magnet, radio waves, and a computer to take detailed pictures of areas inside the breast. Sometimes breast lumps or large lymph nodes are found during a clinical breast exam or breast self-exam that were not seen on a mammogram or ultrasound. In these cases, an MRI can be used to learn more about these changes.

Breast Biopsy

A breast biopsy is a procedure to remove a sample of breast cells or tissue, or an entire lump. A pathologist then looks at the sample under a microscope to check for signs of disease. A biopsy is the only way to find out if cells are cancer.

Biopsies are usually done in an office or a clinic on an outpatient basis. This means you will go home the same day as the procedure. Local anesthesia is used for some biopsies. This means you will be awake, but you won't feel pain in your breast during the procedure. General anesthesia is often used for a surgical biopsy. This means that you will be asleep and won't wake up during the procedure.

Common types of breast biopsies include the following:

- Fine-needle aspiration biopsy: A fine-needle aspiration biopsy is a simple procedure that takes only a few minutes. Your health care provider inserts a thin needle into the breast to take out fluid and cells.

- Core biopsy: A core biopsy, also called a core needle biopsy, uses a needle to remove small pieces or cores of breast tissue. The samples are about the size of a grain of rice. You may have a bruise, but usually not a scar.

- Vacuum-assisted biopsy: A vacuum-assisted biopsy uses a probe, connected to a vacuum device, to remove a small sample of breast tissue. The small cut made in the breast is much smaller than with surgical biopsy. This procedure causes very little scarring, and no stitches are needed.

- Surgical biopsy: A surgical biopsy is an operation to remove part, or all, of a lump so it can be looked at under a microscope to check for signs of disease. Sometimes a doctor will do a surgical biopsy as the first step. Other times, a doctor may do a surgical biopsy if the results of a needle biopsy do not give enough information.

When only a sample of breast tissue is removed, it's called an incisional biopsy. When the entire lump or suspicious area is removed, it's called an excisional biopsy.

If the breast change cannot be felt, wire localization, also called needle localization, may be used to find the breast change. During wire localization, a thin, hollow needle is inserted into the breast. A mammogram is taken to make sure that the needle is in the right place. Then a fine wire is inserted through the hollow needle, to mark the area of tissue to be removed. Next, the needle is removed, and another mammogram is taken. You then go to the operating room where the surgeon removes the wire and surrounding breast tissue. The tissue is sent to the lab to be checked for signs of disease.

Chapter 2

Benign Breast Changes

Most women have changes in their breasts during their lifetime. Many of these changes are caused by hormones. For example, your breasts may feel more lumpy or tender at different times in your menstrual cycle.

Other breast changes can be caused by the normal aging process. As you near menopause, your breasts may lose tissue and fat. They may become smaller and feel lumpy. Most of these changes are not cancer; they are called benign changes. However, if you notice a breast change, don't wait until your next mammogram. Make an appointment to get it checked.

Young women who have not gone through menopause often have more dense tissue in their breasts. Dense tissue has more glandular and connective tissue and less fat tissue. This kind of tissue makes mammograms harder to interpret—because both dense tissue and tumors show up as solid white areas on x-ray images. Breast tissue gets less dense as women get older.

Before or during your menstrual periods, your breasts may feel swollen, tender, or painful. You may also feel one or more lumps during this time because of extra fluid in your breasts. These changes usually go away by the end of your menstrual cycle. Because some lumps are caused by normal hormone changes, your health care provider may have you come back for a return visit, at a different time in your menstrual cycle.

Excerpted from "Understanding Breast Changes: A Health Guide for Women," by the National Cancer Institute (NCI, www.cancer.gov), part of the National Institutes of Health, January 1, 2011.

During pregnancy, your breasts may feel lumpy. This is usually because the glands that produce milk are increasing in number and getting larger.

While breastfeeding, you may get a condition called mastitis. This happens when a milk duct becomes blocked. Mastitis causes the breast to look red and feel lumpy, warm, and tender. It may be caused by an infection and it is often treated with antibiotics. Sometimes the duct may need to be drained. If the redness or mastitis does not go away with treatment, call your health care provider.

As you approach menopause, your menstrual periods may come less often. Your hormone levels also change. This can make your breasts feel tender, even when you are not having your menstrual period. Your breasts may also feel more lumpy than they did before.

If you are taking hormones (such as menopausal hormone therapy, birth control pills, or injections) your breasts may become more dense. This can make a mammogram harder to interpret. Be sure to let your health care provider know if you are taking hormones.

When you stop having menstrual periods (menopause), your hormone levels drop, and your breast tissue becomes less dense and more fatty. You may stop having any lumps, pain, or nipple discharge that you used to have. And because your breast tissue is less dense, mammograms may be easier to interpret.

Breast Changes That Are Not Cancer

These changes are not cancer and do not increase your risk of breast cancer. They are called benign changes.

- Adenosis: Small, round lumps, or a lumpy feeling that are caused by enlarged breast lobules. Sometimes the lumps are too small to be felt. If there is scar-like tissue, the condition may be painful and is called sclerosing adenosis.

- Cysts: Lumps filled with fluid. Breast cysts often get bigger and may be painful just before your menstrual period begins. Cysts are most common in premenopausal women and in women who are taking menopausal hormone therapy.

- Fat necrosis: Round, firm lumps that usually don't hurt. The lumps most often appear after an injury to the breast, surgery, or radiation therapy.

- Fibroadenomas: Hard, round lumps that may feel like a small marble and move around easily. They are usually painless and are most common in young women under 30 years old.

14

- Intraductal papilloma: A wart-like growth in a milk duct of the breast. It's usually found close to the nipple and may cause clear, sticky, or bloody discharge from the nipple. It may also cause pain and a lump. It is most common in women 35–55 years old.

Breast Changes That Are Not Cancer, But Increase Your Risk of Cancer

These conditions are not cancer, but having them increases your risk of breast cancer. They are considered risk factors for breast cancer. Other risk factors include, for example, your age and a family history of breast cancer.

- Atypical hyperplasia: Atypical lobular hyperplasia (ALH) is a condition in which abnormal cells are found in the breast lobules. Atypical ductal hyperplasia (ADH) is a condition in which abnormal cells are found in the breast ducts.

- Lobular carcinoma in situ (LCIS): This is a condition in which abnormal cells are found in the breast lobules. There are more abnormal cells in the lobule with LCIS than with ALH. Since these cells have not spread outside the breast lobules, it's called "*in situ*," which is a Latin term that means "in place."

The abnormal cells found in these conditions are not cancer cells. If you have ALH, ADH, or LCIS, talk with a doctor who specializes in breast health to make a plan that works best for you. Depending on your personal and family medical history, it may include the following:

- Mammograms every year
- Clinical breast exams every 6 to 12 months
- Tamoxifen (for all women) or raloxifene (for postmenopausal women). These drugs have been shown to lower some women's risk of breast cancer.
- Surgery
- Clinical trials

Breast Changes That May Become Cancer

Ductal carcinoma in situ (DCIS) is a condition in which abnormal cells are found in the lining of a breast duct. These cells have not spread outside the duct to the breast tissue. This is why it is called "in situ," which is a Latin term that means "in place." You may also hear DCIS called Stage 0 breast carcinoma in situ or noninvasive cancer.

Since it's not possible to determine which cases of DCIS will become invasive breast cancer, it's important to get treatment for DCIS. Talk with a doctor who specializes in breast health to learn more. Treatment for DCIS is based on how much of the breast is affected, where DCIS is in the breast, and its grade. Most women with DCIS are cured with proper treatment.

Treatment choices for DCIS include the following:

- Lumpectomy: This is a type of breast-conserving surgery or breast-sparing surgery. It is usually followed by radiation therapy.

- Mastectomy: This type of surgery is used to remove the breast or as much of the breast tissue as possible.

- Tamoxifen: This drug may also be taken to lower the chance that DCIS will come back, or to prevent invasive breast cancer.

- Clinical trials: Talk with your health care provider about whether a clinical trial is a good choice for you.

Breast Cancer

Breast cancer is a disease in which cancer cells form in the tissues of the breast. Breast cancer cells do the following:

- Grow and divide without control

- Invade nearby breast tissue

- May form a mass called a tumor

- May metastasize, or spread, to the lymph nodes or other parts of the body

After breast cancer has been diagnosed, tests are done to find out the extent, or stage, of the cancer. The stage is based on the size of the tumor and whether the cancer has spread. Treatment depends on the stage of the cancer.

Chapter 3

What You Need to Know about Breast Cancer

Breast cancer is the most common type of cancer among women in the United States (other than skin cancer). In 2012, about 227,000 women in the United States will be diagnosed with breast cancer.

The Breasts

Inside a woman's breast are 15 to 20 sections called lobes. Each lobe is made of many smaller sections called lobules. Lobules have groups of tiny glands that can make milk. After a baby is born, a woman's breast milk flows from the lobules through thin tubes called ducts to the nipple. Fat and fibrous tissue fill the spaces between the lobules and ducts.

The breasts also contain lymph vessels. These vessels are connected to small, round masses of tissue called lymph nodes. Groups of lymph nodes are near the breast in the underarm (axilla), above the collarbone, and in the chest behind the breastbone.

Cancer Cells

Cancer begins in cells, the building blocks that make up tissues. Tissues make up the breasts and other parts of the body.

Excerpted from "What You Need to Know about Breast Cancer," by the National Cancer Institute (NCI, www.cancer.gov), part of the National Institutes of Health, October 15, 2009.

Normal cells grow and divide to form new cells as the body needs them. When normal cells grow old or get damaged, they die, and new cells take their place.

Sometimes, this process goes wrong. New cells form when the body doesn't need them, and old or damaged cells don't die as they should. The buildup of extra cells often forms a mass of tissue called a lump, growth, or tumor.

Tumors in the breast can be benign (not cancer) or malignant (cancer). Benign tumors are not as harmful as malignant tumors.

Benign tumors:

- are rarely a threat to life;
- can be removed and usually don't grow back;
- don't invade the tissues around them;
- don't spread to other parts of the body.

Malignant tumors:

- may be a threat to life;
- often can be removed but sometimes grow back;
- can invade and damage nearby organs and tissues (such as the chest wall);
- can spread to other parts of the body.

Breast cancer cells can spread by breaking away from the original tumor. They enter blood vessels or lymph vessels, which branch into all the tissues of the body. The cancer cells may be found in lymph nodes near the breast. The cancer cells may attach to other tissues and grow to form new tumors that may damage those tissues.

The spread of cancer is called metastasis.

Detection and Diagnosis

Your doctor can check for breast cancer before you have any symptoms. During an office visit, your doctor will ask about your personal and family medical history. You'll have a physical exam. Your doctor may order one or more imaging tests, such as a mammogram.

Doctors recommend that women have regular clinical breast exams and mammograms to find breast cancer early. Treatment is more likely to work well when breast cancer is detected early.

Clinical Breast Exam

During a clinical breast exam, your health care provider checks your breasts. You may be asked to raise your arms over your head, let them hang by your sides, or press your hands against your hips.

Your health care provider looks for differences in size or shape between your breasts. The skin of your breasts is checked for a rash, dimpling, or other abnormal signs. Your nipples may be squeezed to check for fluid.

Using the pads of the fingers to feel for lumps, your health care provider checks your entire breast, underarm, and collarbone area. A lump is generally the size of a pea before anyone can feel it. The exam is done on one side and then the other. Your health care provider checks the lymph nodes near the breast to see if they are enlarged.

If you have a lump, your health care provider will feel its size, shape, and texture. Your health care provider will also check to see if the lump moves easily. Benign lumps often feel different from cancerous ones. Lumps that are soft, smooth, round, and movable are likely to be benign. A hard, oddly shaped lump that feels firmly attached within the breast is more likely to be cancer, but further tests are needed to diagnose the problem.

Mammogram

A mammogram is an x-ray picture of tissues inside the breast. Mammograms can often show a breast lump before it can be felt. They also can show a cluster of tiny specks of calcium. These specks are called microcalcifications. Lumps or specks can be from cancer, precancerous cells, or other conditions. Further tests are needed to find out if abnormal cells are present.

Before they have symptoms, women should get regular screening mammograms to detect breast cancer early:

- Women in their 40s and older should have mammograms every one or two years.

- Women who are younger than 40 and have risk factors for breast cancer should ask their health care provider whether to have mammograms and how often to have them.

If the mammogram shows an abnormal area of the breast, your doctor may order clearer, more detailed images of that area. Doctors use diagnostic mammograms to learn more about unusual breast changes, such as a lump, pain, thickening, nipple discharge, or change in breast size or shape. Diagnostic mammograms may focus on a specific area of the breast. They may involve special techniques and more views than screening mammograms.

Other Imaging Tests

If an abnormal area is found during a clinical breast exam or with a mammogram, the doctor may order other imaging tests:

- Ultrasound: A woman with a lump or other breast change may have an ultrasound test. An ultrasound device sends out sound waves that people can't hear. The sound waves bounce off breast tissues. A computer uses the echoes to create a picture. The picture may show whether a lump is solid, filled with fluid (a cyst), or a mixture of both. Cysts usually are not cancer. But a solid lump may be cancer.

- MRI (magnetic resonance imaging): MRI uses a powerful magnet linked to a computer. It makes detailed pictures of breast tissue. These pictures can show the difference between normal and diseased tissue.

Biopsy

A biopsy is the removal of tissue to look for cancer cells. A biopsy is the only way to tell for sure if cancer is present.

You may need to have a biopsy if an abnormal area is found. An abnormal area may be felt during a clinical breast exam but not seen on a mammogram. Or an abnormal area could be seen on a mammogram but not be felt during a clinical breast exam. In this case, doctors can use imaging procedures (such as a mammogram, an ultrasound, or MRI) to help see the area and remove tissue.

Your doctor may refer you to a surgeon or breast disease specialist for a biopsy. The surgeon or doctor will remove fluid or tissue from your breast in one of several ways:

- Fine-needle aspiration biopsy: Your doctor uses a thin needle to remove cells or fluid from a breast lump.

- Core biopsy: Your doctor uses a wide needle to remove a sample of breast tissue.

- Skin biopsy: If there are skin changes on your breast, your doctor may take a small sample of skin.

- Surgical biopsy: Your surgeon removes a sample of tissue.

- Incisional biopsy: An incisional biopsy takes a part of the lump or abnormal area.

- Excisional biopsy: An excisional biopsy takes the entire lump or abnormal area.

A pathologist will check the tissue or fluid removed from your breast for cancer cells. If cancer cells are found, the pathologist can tell what kind of cancer it is. The most common type of breast cancer is ductal carcinoma. It begins in the cells that line the breast ducts. Lobular carcinoma is another type. It begins in the lobules of the breast.

Lab Tests with Breast Tissue

If you are diagnosed with breast cancer, your doctor may order special lab tests on the breast tissue that was removed:

- Hormone receptor tests: Some breast tumors need hormones to grow. These tumors have receptors for the hormones estrogen, progesterone, or both. If the hormone receptor tests show that the breast tumor has these receptors, then hormone therapy is most often recommended as a treatment option.

- HER2 [human epidermal growth factor receptor 2]/neu test: HER2/neu protein is found on some types of cancer cells. This test shows whether the tissue either has too much HER2/neu protein or too many copies of its gene. If the breast tumor has too much HER2/neu, then targeted therapy may be a treatment option.

It may take several weeks to get the results of these tests. The test results help your doctor decide which cancer treatments may be options for you.

You may want to ask your doctor these questions before having a biopsy:

- What kind of biopsy will I have? Why?

- How long will it take? Will I be awake? Will it hurt? Will I have anesthesia? What kind?

- Are there any risks? What are the chances of infection or bleeding after the biopsy?

- Will I have a scar?

- How soon will I know the results?

- If I do have cancer, who will talk with me about the next steps? When?

Treatment

Women with breast cancer have many treatment options. The treatment that's best for one woman may not be best for another.

The options are surgery, radiation therapy, hormone therapy, chemotherapy, and targeted therapy. You may receive more than one type of treatment.

Surgery and radiation therapy are types of local therapy. They remove or destroy cancer in the breast.

Hormone therapy, chemotherapy, and targeted therapy are types of systemic therapy. The drug enters the bloodstream and destroys or controls cancer throughout the body.

The treatment that's right for you depends mainly on the stage of the cancer, the results of the hormone receptor tests, the result of the HER2/neu test, and your general health.

You may want to talk with your doctor about taking part in a clinical trial, a research study of new treatment methods. Clinical trials are an important option for women at any stage of breast cancer.

Your doctor can describe your treatment choices, the expected results, and the possible side effects. Because cancer therapy often damages healthy cells and tissues, side effects are common. Before treatment starts, ask your health care team about possible side effects, how to prevent or reduce these effects, and how treatment may change your normal activities.

You may want to know how you will look during and after treatment. You and your health care team can work together to develop a treatment plan that meets your medical and personal needs.

Your doctor may refer you to a specialist, or you may ask for a referral. Specialists who treat breast cancer include surgeons, medical oncologists, and radiation oncologists. You also may be referred to a plastic surgeon or reconstructive surgeon. Your health care team may also include an oncology nurse and a registered dietitian.

You may want to ask your doctor these questions before you begin treatment:

- What did the hormone receptor tests show? What did other lab tests show? Would genetic testing be helpful to me or my family?

- Do any lymph nodes show signs of cancer?

- What is the stage of the disease? Has the cancer spread?

- What are my treatment choices? Which do you recommend for me? Why?

- What are the expected benefits of each kind of treatment?
- What can I do to prepare for treatment?
- Will I need to stay in the hospital? If so, for how long?
- What are the risks and possible side effects of each treatment? How can side effects be managed?
- What is the treatment likely to cost? Will my insurance cover it?
- How will treatment affect my normal activities?
- Would a research study (clinical trial) be appropriate for me?
- Can you recommend other doctors who could give me a second opinion about my treatment options?
- How often should I have checkups?

Surgery

Surgery is the most common treatment for breast cancer. Your doctor can explain each type, discuss and compare the benefits and risks, and describe how each will change the way you look:

- Breast-sparing surgery: This is an operation to remove the cancer but not the breast. It's also called breast-conserving surgery. It can be a lumpectomy or a segmental mastectomy (also called a partial mastectomy). Sometimes an excisional biopsy is the only surgery a woman needs because the surgeon removed the whole lump.
- Mastectomy: This is an operation to remove the entire breast (or as much of the breast tissue as possible). In some cases, a skin-sparing mastectomy may be an option. For this approach, the surgeon removes as little skin as possible.

The surgeon usually removes one or more lymph nodes from under the arm to check for cancer cells. If cancer cells are found in the lymph nodes, other cancer treatments will be needed.

You may choose to have breast reconstruction. This is plastic surgery to rebuild the shape of the breast. It may be done at the same time as the cancer surgery or later. If you're considering breast reconstruction, you may wish to talk with a plastic surgeon before having cancer surgery.

In breast-sparing surgery, the surgeon removes the cancer in the breast and some normal tissue around it. The surgeon may also remove lymph nodes under the arm. The surgeon sometimes removes some of the lining over the chest muscles below the tumor.

In total (simple) mastectomy, the surgeon removes the whole breast. Some lymph nodes under the arm may also be removed.

In modified radical mastectomy, the surgeon removes the whole breast and most or all of the lymph nodes under the arm. Often, the lining over the chest muscles is removed. A small chest muscle also may be taken out to make it easier to remove the lymph nodes.

The time it takes to heal after surgery is different for each woman. Surgery causes pain and tenderness. Medicine can help control the pain. Before surgery, you should discuss the plan for pain relief with your doctor or nurse. After surgery, your doctor can adjust the plan if you need more relief.

Any kind of surgery also carries a risk of infection, bleeding, or other problems. You should tell your health care team right away if you develop any problems.

You may feel off balance if you've had one or both breasts removed. You may feel more off balance if you have large breasts. This imbalance can cause discomfort in your neck and back.

Also, the skin where your breast was removed may feel tight. Your arm and shoulder muscles may feel stiff and weak. These problems usually go away. The doctor, nurse, or physical therapist can suggest exercises to help you regain movement and strength in your arm and shoulder. Exercise can also reduce stiffness and pain. You may be able to begin gentle exercise within days of surgery.

Because nerves may be injured or cut during surgery, you may have numbness and tingling in your chest, underarm, shoulder, and upper arm. These feelings usually go away within a few weeks or months. But for some women, numbness does not go away.

Removing the lymph nodes under the arm slows the flow of lymph fluid. The fluid may build up in your arm and hand and cause swelling. This swelling is called lymphedema. It can develop soon after surgery or months or even years later. You'll always need to protect the arm and hand on the treated side of your body from cuts, burns, or other injuries.

You may want to ask your doctor these questions before having surgery:

- What kinds of surgery can I consider? Is breast-sparing surgery an option for me? Is a skin-sparing mastectomy an option? Which operation do you recommend for me? Why?

- Will any lymph nodes be removed? How many? Why?

- How will I feel after the operation? Will I have to stay in the hospital?

- Will I need to learn how to take care of myself or my incision when I get home?

- Where will the scars be? What will they look like?

- If I decide to have plastic surgery to rebuild my breast, how and when can that be done? Can you suggest a plastic surgeon for me to contact?

- Will I have to do special exercises to help regain motion and strength in my arm and shoulder? Will a physical therapist or nurse show me how to do the exercises?

- Is there someone I can talk with who has had the same surgery I'll be having?

- How often will I need checkups?

Radiation Therapy

Radiation therapy (also called radiotherapy) uses high-energy rays to kill cancer cells. It affects cells only in the part of the body that is treated. Radiation therapy may be used after surgery to destroy breast cancer cells that remain in the area.

Doctors use two types of radiation therapy to treat breast cancer. Some women receive both types:

- External radiation therapy: The radiation comes from a large machine outside the body. You will go to a hospital or clinic for treatment. Treatments are usually five days a week for four to six weeks. External radiation is the most common type used for breast cancer.

- Internal radiation therapy (implant radiation therapy or brachytherapy): The doctor places one or more thin tubes inside the breast through a tiny incision. A radioactive substance is loaded into the tube. The treatment session may last for a few minutes, and the substance is removed. When it's removed, no radioactivity remains in your body. Internal radiation therapy may be repeated every day for a week.

Side effects depend mainly on the dose and type of radiation. It's common for the skin in the treated area to become red, dry, tender, and itchy. Your breast may feel heavy and tight. Internal radiation therapy may make your breast look red or bruised. These problems usually go away over time.

25

Bras and tight clothes may rub your skin and cause soreness. You may want to wear loose-fitting cotton clothes during this time.

Gentle skin care also is important. You should check with your doctor before using any deodorants, lotions, or creams on the treated area. Toward the end of treatment, your skin may become moist and "weepy." Exposing this area to air as much as possible can help the skin heal. After treatment is over, the skin will slowly heal. However, there may be a lasting change in the color of your skin.

You're likely to become very tired during radiation therapy, especially in the later weeks of treatment. Resting is important, but doctors usually advise patients to try to stay active, unless it leads to pain or other problems.

You may wish to discuss with your doctor the possible long-term effects of radiation therapy. For example, radiation therapy to the chest may harm the lung or heart. Also, it can change the size of your breast and the way it looks. If any of these problems occur, your health care team can tell you how to manage them.

You may want to ask your doctor these questions before having radiation therapy:

- Which type of radiation therapy can I consider? Are both types an option for me?

- When will treatment start? When will it end? How often will I have treatments?

- How will I feel during treatment? Will I need to stay in the hospital? Will I be able to drive myself to and from treatment?

- What can I do to take care of myself before, during, and after treatment?

- How will we know the treatment is working?

- Will treatment harm my skin?

- How will my chest look afterward?

- Are there any lasting effects?

- What is the chance that the cancer will come back in my breast?

- How often will I need checkups?

Hormone Therapy

Hormone therapy may also be called anti-hormone treatment. If lab tests show that the tumor in your breast has hormone receptors, then hormone therapy may be an option. Hormone therapy keeps cancer cells from getting or using the natural hormones (estrogen and progesterone) they need to grow.

If you have not gone through menopause, the options include the following:

- Tamoxifen: This drug can prevent the original breast cancer from returning and also helps prevent the development of new cancers in the other breast. As treatment for metastatic breast cancer, tamoxifen slows or stops the growth of cancer cells that are in the body. It's a pill that you take every day for five years. In general, the side effects of tamoxifen are similar to some of the symptoms of menopause. The most common are hot flashes and vaginal discharge. Others are irregular menstrual periods, thinning bones, headaches, fatigue, nausea, vomiting, vaginal dryness or itching, irritation of the skin around the vagina, and skin rash. Serious side effects are rare, but they include blood clots, strokes, uterine cancer, and cataracts.

- LH-RH [luteinizing hormone releasing hormone] agonist: This type of drug can prevent the ovaries from making estrogen. The estrogen level falls slowly. Examples are leuprolide and goserelin. This type of drug may be given by injection under the skin in the stomach area. Side effects include hot flashes, headaches, weight gain, thinning bones, and bone pain.

- Surgery to remove your ovaries: Until you go through menopause, your ovaries are your body's main source of estrogen. When the surgeon removes your ovaries, this source of estrogen is also removed. (A woman who has gone through menopause wouldn't benefit from this kind of surgery because her ovaries produce much less estrogen.) When the ovaries are removed, menopause occurs right away. The side effects are often more severe than those caused by natural menopause. Your health care team can suggest ways to cope with these side effects.

If you have gone through menopause, the options include:

- Aromatase inhibitor: This type of drug prevents the body from making a form of estrogen (estradiol). Examples are anastrazole, exemestane, and letrozole. Common side effects include hot flashes, nausea, vomiting, and painful bones or joints. Serious side effects include thinning bones and an increase in cholesterol.

- Tamoxifen: Hormone therapy is given for at least five years. Women who have gone through menopause receive tamoxifen for two to five years. If tamoxifen is given for less than five years, then an aromatase inhibitor often is given to complete the five years. Some women have hormone therapy for more than five years.

Chemotherapy

Chemotherapy uses drugs to kill cancer cells. The drugs that treat breast cancer are usually given through a vein (intravenous) or as a pill. You'll probably receive a combination of drugs.

You may receive chemotherapy in an outpatient part of the hospital, at the doctor's office, or at home. Some women need to stay in the hospital during treatment.

The side effects depend mainly on which drugs are given and how much. Chemotherapy kills fast-growing cancer cells, but the drugs can also harm normal cells that divide rapidly:

- Blood cells: When drugs lower the levels of healthy blood cells, you're more likely to get infections, bruise or bleed easily, and feel very weak and tired. Your health care team will check for low levels of blood cells. If your levels are low, your health care team may stop the chemotherapy for a while or reduce the dose of the drug. There are also medicines that can help your body make new blood cells.

- Cells in hair roots: Chemotherapy may cause hair loss. If you lose your hair, it will grow back after treatment, but the color and texture may be changed.

- Cells that line the digestive tract: Chemotherapy can cause a poor appetite, nausea and vomiting, diarrhea, or mouth and lip sores. Your health care team can give you medicines and suggest other ways to help with these problems.

Some drugs used for breast cancer can cause tingling or numbness in the hands or feet. This problem often goes away after treatment is over.

Other problems may not go away. For example, some of the drugs used for breast cancer may weaken the heart. Your doctor may check your heart before, during, and after treatment. A rare side effect of chemotherapy is that years after treatment, a few women have developed leukemia (cancer of the blood cells).

Some anticancer drugs can damage the ovaries. If you have not gone through menopause yet, you may have hot flashes and vaginal dryness.

Your menstrual periods may no longer be regular or may stop. You may become infertile (unable to become pregnant). For women over the age of 35, this damage to the ovaries is likely to be permanent.

On the other hand, you may remain able to become pregnant during chemotherapy. Before treatment begins, you should talk with your doctor about birth control because many drugs given during the first trimester are known to cause birth defects.

Targeted Therapy

Some women with breast cancer may receive drugs called targeted therapy. Targeted therapy uses drugs that block the growth of breast cancer cells. For example, targeted therapy may block the action of an abnormal protein (such as HER2) that stimulates the growth of breast cancer cells.

Trastuzumab (Herceptin) or lapatinib (TYKERB) may be given to a woman whose lab tests show that her breast tumor has too much HER2:

- Trastuzumab: This drug is given through a vein. It may be given alone or with chemotherapy. Side effects that most commonly occur during the first treatment include fever and chills. Other possible side effects include weakness, nausea, vomiting, diarrhea, headaches, difficulty breathing, and rashes. These side effects generally become less severe after the first treatment. Trastuzumab also may cause heart damage, heart failure, and serious breathing problems. Before and during treatment, your doctor will check your heart and lungs.

- Lapatinib: The tablet is taken by mouth. Lapatinib is given with chemotherapy. Side effects include nausea, vomiting, diarrhea, tiredness, mouth sores, and rashes. It can also cause red, painful hands and feet. Before treatment, your doctor will check your heart and liver. During treatment, your doctor will watch for signs of heart, lung, or liver problems.

You may want to ask your doctor these questions before having hormone therapy, chemotherapy, or targeted therapy:

- What drugs will I be taking? What will they do?

- When will treatment start? When will it end? How often will I have treatments?

- Where will I have treatment?

- What can I do to take care of myself during treatment?
- How will we know the treatment is working?
- Which side effects should I tell you about?
- Will there be long-term effects?
- How often will I need checkups?

Second Opinion

Before starting treatment, you might want a second opinion from another doctor about your diagnosis and treatment plan. Some women worry that their doctor will be offended if they ask for a second opinion. Usually the opposite is true. Most doctors welcome a second opinion. And many health insurance companies will pay for a second opinion if you or your doctor requests it. Some companies require a second opinion.

If you get a second opinion, the doctor may agree with your first doctor's diagnosis and treatment plan. Or the second doctor may suggest another approach. Either way, you'll have more information and perhaps a greater sense of control. You may also feel more confident about the decisions you make, knowing that you've looked carefully at your options.

It may take some time and effort to gather your medical records and see another doctor. Usually it's not a problem if it takes you several weeks to get a second opinion. In most cases, the delay in starting treatment will not make treatment less effective. To make sure, you should discuss this possible delay with your doctor. Some women with breast cancer need treatment right away.

There are many ways to find a doctor for a second opinion. You can ask your doctor, a local or state medical society, a nearby hospital, or a medical school for names of specialists.

Breast Reconstruction

Some women who plan to have a mastectomy decide to have breast reconstruction. Other women prefer to wear a breast form (prosthesis) inside their bra. Others decide to do nothing after surgery. All of these options have pros and cons. What is right for one woman may not be right for another. What is important is that nearly every woman treated for breast cancer has choices.

Breast reconstruction may be done at the same time as the mastectomy, or later on. If radiation therapy is part of the treatment plan, some doctors suggest waiting until after radiation therapy is complete.

If you are thinking about breast reconstruction, you should talk to a plastic surgeon before the mastectomy, even if you plan to have your reconstruction later on.

There are many ways for a surgeon to reconstruct the breast. Some women choose to have breast implants, which are filled with saline or silicone gel.

You also may have breast reconstruction with tissue that the plastic surgeon removes from another part of your body. Skin, muscle, and fat can come from your lower abdomen, back, or buttocks. The surgeon uses this tissue to create a breast shape.

The type of reconstruction that is best for you depends on your age, body type, and the type of cancer surgery that you had. The plastic surgeon can explain the risks and benefits of each type of reconstruction.

Nutrition and Physical Activity

It's important for you to take very good care of yourself before, during, and after cancer treatment. Taking care of yourself includes eating well and staying as active as you can.

You need the right amount of calories to maintain a good weight. You also need enough protein to keep up your strength. Eating well may help you feel better and have more energy.

Sometimes, especially during or soon after treatment, you may not feel like eating. You may be uncomfortable or tired. You may find that foods don't taste as good as they used to. In addition, the side effects of treatment (such as poor appetite, nausea, vomiting, or mouth blisters) can make it hard to eat well. On the other hand, some women treated for breast cancer may have a problem with weight gain.

Your doctor, a registered dietitian, or another health care provider can suggest ways to help you meet your nutrition needs.

Many women find that they feel better when they stay active. Walking, yoga, swimming, and other activities can keep you strong and increase your energy. Exercise may reduce nausea and pain and make treatment easier to handle. It also can help relieve stress. Whatever physical activity you choose, be sure to talk to your doctor before you start. Also, if your activity causes you pain or other problems, be sure to let your doctor or nurse know.

Follow-up Care

You'll need regular checkups after treatment for breast cancer. Checkups help ensure that any changes in your health are noted and

31

treated if needed. If you have any health problems between checkups, you should contact your doctor.

Your doctor will check for return of the cancer. Also, checkups help detect health problems that can result from cancer treatment.

You should report any changes in the treated area or in your other breast to the doctor right away. Tell your doctor about any health problems, such as pain, loss of appetite or weight, changes in menstrual cycles, unusual vaginal bleeding, or blurred vision. Also talk to your doctor about headaches, dizziness, shortness of breath, coughing or hoarseness, backaches, or digestive problems that seem unusual or that don't go away. Such problems may arise months or years after treatment. They may suggest that the cancer has returned, but they can also be symptoms of other health problems. It's important to share your concerns with your doctor so that problems can be diagnosed and treated as soon as possible.

Checkups usually include an exam of the neck, underarm, chest, and breast areas. Since a new breast cancer may develop, you should have regular mammograms. You probably won't need a mammogram of a reconstructed breast or if you had a mastectomy without reconstruction. Your doctor may order other imaging procedures or lab tests.

Sources of Support

Learning that you have breast cancer can change your life and the lives of those close to you. These changes can be hard to handle. It's normal for you, your family, and your friends to need help coping with the feelings that such a diagnosis can bring.

Concerns about treatments and managing side effects, hospital stays, and medical bills are common. You may also worry about caring for your family, keeping your job, or continuing daily activities.

Several organizations offer special programs for women with breast cancer. Women who have had the disease serve as trained volunteers. They may talk with or visit women who have breast cancer, provide information, and lend emotional support. They often share their experiences with breast cancer treatment, breast reconstruction, and recovery.

You may be afraid that changes to your body will affect not only how you look but also how other people feel about you. You may worry that breast cancer and its treatment will affect your sexual relationships. Many couples find it helps to talk about their concerns. Some find that counseling or a couples' support group can be helpful.

Here's where you can go for support:

- Doctors, nurses, and other members of your health care team can answer questions about treatment, working, or other activities.

- Social workers, counselors, or members of the clergy can be helpful if you want to talk about your feelings or concerns. Often, social workers can suggest resources for financial aid, transportation, home care, or emotional support.

- Support groups also can help. In these groups, women with breast cancer or their family members meet with other patients or their families to share what they have learned about coping with the disease and the effects of treatment. Groups may offer support in person, over the telephone, or on the internet. You may want to talk with a member of your health care team about finding a support group.

- Women with breast cancer often get together in support groups, but please keep in mind that each woman is different. Ways that one woman deals with cancer may not be right for another. You may want to ask your health care provider about advice you receive from other women with breast cancer.

- Information specialists at 800-4-CANCER (800-422-6237) and at LiveHelp (www.cancer.gov/livehelp) can help you locate programs, services, and publications. They can send you a list of organizations that offer services to women with cancer.

Taking Part in Cancer Research

Cancer research has led to real progress in the prevention, detection, and treatment of breast cancer. Continuing research offers hope that in the future even more women with breast cancer will be treated successfully.

Doctors all over the country are conducting many types of clinical trials (research studies in which people volunteer to take part). Clinical trials are designed to find out whether new approaches are safe and effective.

Even if the people in a trial do not benefit directly, they may still make an important contribution by helping doctors learn more about breast cancer and how to control it. Although clinical trials may pose some risks, doctors do all they can to protect their patients.

Doctors are trying to find better ways to care for women with breast cancer. They are studying many types of treatment and their combinations:

- Radiation therapy: In women with early breast cancer who have had a lumpectomy, doctors are comparing the effectiveness of standard radiation therapy aimed at the whole breast to that of radiation therapy aimed at a smaller part of the breast.

- Chemotherapy and targeted therapy: Researchers are testing new anticancer drugs and doses. They are looking at new drug combinations before surgery. They are also looking at new ways of combining chemotherapy with targeted therapy, hormone therapy, or radiation therapy. In addition, they are studying lab tests that may predict whether a woman might be helped by chemotherapy.

- Hormone therapy: Doctors are testing several types of hormone therapy, including aromatase inhibitors. They are looking at whether hormone therapy before surgery may help shrink the tumor.

- Supportive care: Doctors are looking at ways to lessen the side effects of treatment, such as lymphedema after surgery. They are looking at ways to reduce pain and improve quality of life.

If you're interested in being part of a clinical trial, talk with your doctor. The NCI website includes a section on clinical trials at www.cancer .gov/clinicaltrials.

Chapter 4

The Role of Estrogen in Breast Cancer Development

What Are Estrogens?

Estrogens are a family of related molecules that stimulate the development and maintenance of female characteristics and sexual reproduction.

The natural estrogens produced by women are steroid molecules, which means that they are derived from a particular type of molecular skeleton containing four rings of carbon atoms. The most prevalent forms of human estrogen are estradiol and estrone. Both are produced and secreted by the ovaries, although estrone is also made in the adrenal glands and other organs.

Estrogen Targets Tissue

Estrogens are hormones, which means that they function as signaling molecules. A signaling molecule exerts its effects by traveling through the bloodstream and interacting with cells in a variety of target tissues.

The breast and the uterus, which play central roles in sexual reproduction, are two of the main targets of estrogen. In addition, estrogen molecules act on the brain, bone, liver, and heart.

"Estrogen Receptors/SERMs," by the National Cancer Institute (NCI, www.cancer.gov), part of the National Institutes of Health, October 15, 2010.

Estrogen Receptors

Estrogens act on target tissues by binding to parts of cells called estrogen receptors.

An estrogen receptor is a protein molecule found inside those cells that are targets for estrogen action. Estrogen receptors contain a specific site to which only estrogens (or closely related molecules) can bind.

The target tissues affected by estrogen molecules all contain estrogen receptors; other organs and tissues in the body do not. Therefore, when estrogen molecules circulate in the bloodstream and move throughout the body, they exert effects only on cells that contain estrogen receptors.

Estrogen Receptors Trigger Gene Activation

Estrogen receptors normally reside in the cell's nucleus, along with DNA [deoxyribonucleic acid] molecules.

In the absence of estrogen molecules, these estrogen receptors are inactive and have no influence on DNA (which contains the cell's genes). But when an estrogen molecule enters a cell and passes into the nucleus, the estrogen binds to its receptor, thereby causing the shape of the receptor to change. This estrogen-receptor complex then binds to specific DNA sites, called estrogen response elements, which are located near genes that are controlled by estrogen.

After it has become attached to estrogen response elements in DNA, this estrogen-receptor complex binds to coactivator proteins and more nearby genes become active. The active genes produce molecules of messenger RNA [ribonucleic acid], which guide the synthesis of specific proteins. These proteins can then influence cell behavior in different ways, depending on the cell type involved.

Estrogen-Induced Changes in Cell Behavior

In liver cells, for example, estrogen alters the production of proteins that influence cholesterol levels in the blood.

Cholesterol does not readily dissolve in blood, so before it can be transported through the body, it first becomes bound to special cholesterol-carrying proteins called lipoproteins. The liver produces two such lipoproteins, called low-density lipoprotein (LDL) and high-density lipoprotein (HDL).

LDL cholesterol is considered to be the bad form of cholesterol because it tends to release cholesterol directly onto the inner wall of arteries, creating the plaque that can lead to heart disease. In contrast, HDL is considered to be the good form of cholesterol because it inhibits the formation of plaque and carries cholesterol away from the arteries and back to the liver.

The net effect of estrogen's action on liver cells is to increase the amount of HDL cholesterol and to decrease the amount of LDL cholesterol. By increasing HDL and decreasing LDL, estrogen helps to lower the risk of heart disease.

Estrogen-Induced Stimulation of Cell Proliferation

In some target tissues, the main effect of estrogen is to cause cells to grow and divide, a process called cell proliferation.

In breast tissue, for example, estrogen triggers the proliferation of cells lining the milk glands, thereby preparing the breast to produce milk if the woman should become pregnant.

Estrogen also promotes proliferation of the cells that form the inner lining, or endometrium, of the uterus, thereby preparing the uterus for possible implantation of an embryo. During a normal menstrual cycle, estrogen levels fall dramatically at the end of each cycle if pregnancy does not occur. As a result, the endometrium disintegrates and is shed from the uterus and vagina in a bleeding process called menstruation.

Estrogen and Cancer

Paradoxically, estrogen can be both a beneficial and a harmful molecule. The main beneficial effects of estrogen include its roles in the following:

- Programming the breast and uterus for sexual reproduction

- Controlling cholesterol production in ways that limit the buildup of plaque in the coronary arteries

- Preserving bone strength by helping to maintain the proper balance between bone buildup and breakdown

Unfortunately, in addition to these important beneficial effects, estrogen can also be harmful. The most serious problem arises from the ability of estrogen to promote the proliferation of cells in the breast and uterus. Although this ability to stimulate cell proliferation is one of estrogen's normal roles, it can also increase a woman's chance of developing breast or uterine cancer.

Estrogen and Breast Cancer

During each menstrual cycle, estrogen normally triggers the proliferation of cells that form the inner lining of the milk glands in the breast.

If pregnancy does not occur, estrogen levels fall dramatically at the end of each monthly menstrual cycle. In the absence of high estrogen levels, those milk gland cells that have proliferated in any given month will deteriorate and die, followed by a similar cycle of cell proliferation and cell death the following month. For the average woman, this means hundreds of cycles of breast cell division and cell death repeated over a span of roughly 40 years, from puberty to menopause.

But how do these estrogen-induced cycles of breast cell proliferation increase the risk of developing cancer?

Cancer Arises from DNA Mutations in Cells

Cancer is caused by DNA damage (i.e., mutations) in genes that regulate cell growth and division.

Some mutations are inherited, while others are caused by exposure to radiation or to mutation-inducing chemicals such as those found in cigarette smoke.

Mutations also can occur spontaneously as a result of mistakes that are made when a cell duplicates its DNA molecules prior to cell division.

When cells acquire mutations in specific genes that control proliferation, such as proto-oncogenes or tumor suppressor genes, these changes are copied with each new generation of cells. Later, more mutations in these altered cells can lead to uncontrolled proliferation and the onset of cancer.

Estrogen-Induced Proliferation of Existing Mutant Cells

Although estrogen does not appear to directly cause the DNA mutations that trigger the development of human cancer, estrogen does stimulate cell proliferation.

Therefore, if breast cells already possess a DNA mutation that increases the risk of developing cancer, these cells will proliferate (along with normal breast cells) in response to estrogen stimulation. The result will be an increase in the total number of mutant cells, any of which might thereafter acquire the additional mutations that lead to uncontrolled proliferation and the onset of cancer.

In other words, estrogen-induced cell production leads to an increase in the total number of mutant cells that exist. These cells are at increased risk of becoming cancerous, so the chances that cancer may actually develop are increased.

Estrogen-Induced Proliferation and Spontaneous New Mutations

Even in women who do not have any mutant breast cells, estrogen-induced proliferation of normal breast cells may still increase the risk of developing cancer.

The reason involves DNA. A cell must duplicate its DNA molecules prior to each cell division, thereby ensuring that the two new cells resulting from the process of cell division each receive one complete set of DNA molecules. But the process of DNA duplication occasionally makes mistakes, so the resulting DNA copies may contain a small number of errors (i.e., mutations). If one of these spontaneous mutations occurs in a gene that controls cell growth and division, it could lead to the development of cancer.

Proliferation of normal cells from exposure to estrogen creates a vulnerability to spontaneous mutations, some of which might represent a first step on the pathway to cancer.

Estrogen and Uterine Cancer

In the uterus, estrogen triggers the proliferation of endometrial-lining cells during each month of the menstrual cycle, followed by death of these cells during menstruation. Over a span of 40 years, from puberty to menopause, hundreds of cycles of cell division and cell death will occur.

These repeated cycles of estrogen-induced cell division tend to increase the risk of developing cancer in the same two ways as in the breast: Estrogen can stimulate the division of uterine cells that already have DNA mutations, and it also increases the chances of developing new, spontaneous mutations when estrogen stimulates cell proliferation. Whether the mutations are inherited or spontaneous, estrogen-driven proliferation will increase the number of these altered cells that can ultimately lead to the development of uterine cancer.

Antiestrogens

Since estrogen can promote the development of cancer in the breast and uterus, it seems logical to postulate that substances that block the action of estrogen might be helpful in preventing or treating these two types of cancer.

This rationale has led scientists to work on the development of antiestrogen drugs that can block the action of estrogens and thereby interfere with, or even prevent, the proliferation of breast and uterine cancer cells. Antiestrogens work by binding to estrogen receptors so that the estrogen molecules themselves cannot bind to those receptors. This also blocks estrogen from activating genes for specific growth-promoting proteins.

SERMS

In working on the development of antiestrogens, scientists have made a somewhat surprising discovery. Some drugs that block the action of estrogen in certain tissues actually can mimic the action of estrogen in other tissues.

Such selectivity is made possible by the fact that the estrogen receptors of different target tissues vary in chemical structure. These differences allow estrogen-like drugs to interact in different ways with the estrogen receptors of different tissues. Such drugs are called selective estrogen receptor modulators, or SERMs, because they selectively stimulate or inhibit the estrogen receptors of different target tissues. For example, a SERM might inhibit the estrogen receptor found in breast cells but activate the estrogen receptor present in uterine endometrial cells. A SERM of this type would inhibit cell proliferation in breast cells, but stimulate the proliferation of uterine endometrial cells.

Tamoxifen and Cancer

The first SERM to be investigated extensively for its anticancer properties is a drug called tamoxifen (Nolvadex).

Tamoxifen blocks the action of estrogen in breast tissue by binding to the estrogen receptors of breast cells, thereby preventing estrogen molecules from binding to these receptors. But unlike what occurs when estrogen binds to its receptor, tamoxifen binds but does not change the receptor's shape, so coactivators are unable to bind. As a result, the genes that stimulate cell proliferation cannot be activated.

By interfering with estrogen receptors in this way, tamoxifen blocks the ability of estrogen to stimulate the proliferation of breast cells.

Tamoxifen and Breast Cancer Treatment

In women who have breast cancer, proliferation of the breast cancer cells is often driven by estrogen, just as in the case of normal breast cells.

Since tamoxifen (Nolvadex) can block the effects of estrogen on breast cells, scientists predicted that breast cancer could be treated by using tamoxifen to interfere with estrogen-induced cell proliferation. Based on encouraging results obtained in experimental trials, tamoxifen was first approved for such use in breast cancer treatment in the 1970s.

The first step in treating women with breast cancer is to surgically remove the cancer from the breast. It is difficult to be certain that every cancer cell has been removed at the time of surgery because some breast cancer cells could have spread to surrounding tissues or other organs prior to the operation. Therefore, women often receive some type of treatment after surgery (adjuvant therapy) to prevent the growth of any cancer cells that might remain in the body. Studies show that when tamoxifen is used for this purpose, the risk of cancer recurrence is reduced.

Aromatase Inhibitors

Many breast tumors are estrogen sensitive, meaning the hormone estrogen helps them to grow. Aromatase inhibitors (AIs) can help block the growth of these tumors by lowering the amount of estrogen in the body.

Using a substance called aromatase, the ovaries and other tissues of the body produce estrogen. AIs do not block estrogen production by the ovaries, but they can block other tissues from making this hormone. That's why AIs are used mostly in women who have reached menopause, when the ovaries are no longer producing estrogen.

Tamoxifen (Nolvadex) also helps to prevent the growth of estrogen-sensitive breast tumors, but it works differently from AIs. Whereas AIs reduce the amount of estrogen in the body, tamoxifen blocks a tumor's ability to use estrogen.

Currently, three AIs are approved by the U.S. Food and Drug Administration (FDA): Anastrazole (Arimidex), exemestane (Aromasin), and letrozole (Femara).

Estrogen Receptor-Negative Breast Cancer

Unlike normal breast cells, cancer cells arising in the breast do not always have receptors for estrogen.

Breast cancers that do have estrogen receptors are said to be estrogen receptor-positive, while those breast cancers that do not possess estrogen receptors are estrogen receptor-negative. In women with estrogen receptor-positive cancers, cancer cell growth is under the control of estrogen.

41

Therefore, such cancers are often susceptible to treatment with tamoxifen (Nolvadex), because tamoxifen works by blocking the interaction between estrogen and the estrogen receptor.

In contrast, the growth of estrogen receptor-negative cancer cells is not governed by estrogen and is not treated with tamoxifen.

Tamoxifen and Breast Cancer Prevention

Once tamoxifen (Nolvadex) had been shown to reduce the risk of cancer reappearing after breast cancer surgery (in women with estrogen receptor-positive cancers), the question arose whether tamoxifen might also be helpful in preventing breast cancer in women at high risk of developing the disease.

The rationale for using tamoxifen to try to prevent breast cancer is similar to the rationale for using tamoxifen in breast cancer treatment. Estrogen-induced cycles of breast cell proliferation increase a woman's risk of developing breast cancer. Therefore, using tamoxifen to block the action of estrogen in the breast in healthy women might be expected to decrease a woman's chances of developing cancer in the future.

In 1992, the National Cancer Institute opened a study involving more than 13,000 healthy women considered to be at high risk for breast cancer based on their family or medical history. Half the women were given tamoxifen, while the other half were given a placebo. After five years, the group receiving tamoxifen had a lower rate of breast cancer.

Tamoxifen as a Cause of Uterine Cancer

Although tamoxifen (Nolvadex) has been useful both in treating breast cancer patients and in decreasing the risk of getting breast cancer in women at high risk, it also has some serious side effects.

These side effects arise from the fact that while tamoxifen acts as an antiestrogen that blocks the effects of estrogen on breast cells, it mimics the actions of estrogen in other tissues such as the uterus. Its estrogen-like effects on the uterus stimulate proliferation of the uterine endometrium and increase the risk of uterine cancer.

The Need for Better SERMs

The fact that tamoxifen (Nolvadex) blocks the action of estrogen in breast tissue while mimicking the action of estrogen in the uterus means that it functions as a SERM, selectively blocking or stimulating the estrogen receptors of different target tissues.

In addition to acting like estrogen in the uterus, tamoxifen resembles estrogen in its ability to lower LDL cholesterol levels. And in postmenopausal women, tamoxifen also resembles estrogen in its ability to preserve or increase bone density. Thus, aside from its tendency to increase the risk of uterine cancer, tamoxifen has a number of potentially beneficial properties.

As a result, scientists have been actively working on the development of other SERMs that might exhibit some of the beneficial properties of tamoxifen without sharing its potentially harmful effects.

Estrogen Replacement in Menopause

In addition to their relevance for cancer treatment and prevention, SERMs may also be potentially important for women who have passed through menopause and therefore produce little estrogen.

The lack of estrogen in postmenopausal women is linked to several health problems. For example, estrogen has positive effects on blood vessels and on bones. After menopause, though, women are at increased risk for heart disease and for osteoporosis, a weakening of the bones that causes them to become more vulnerable to fractures.

To counteract these potential problems, some postmenopausal women take hormone pills containing estrogen to strengthen bones and help control other menopausal symptoms. But, as a consequence, such women are subjecting themselves to the harmful effects of estrogen—namely, an increased risk for invasive breast cancer and uterine cancer.

Estrogen Plus Progestin Replacement

Studies carried out in the 1980s suggested that adding the hormone progesterone to estrogen could offset the increased risk of uterine cancer linked to the use of estrogen by itself. For this reason, hormone replacement therapy using estrogen plus progestin (a synthetic form of progesterone) became a common way of treating women with menopausal symptoms.

However, a study of 16,000 menopausal women carried out by the Women's Health Initiative was prematurely halted in 2002 when preliminary results indicated that the harm associated with this type of treatment outweighs the potential benefits. The major risks detected were an increased chance of developing invasive breast cancer, as well as an increased risk of strokes, heart attacks, and blood clots. While the data also revealed that hormone replacement with estrogen plus progestin lowered the risk of osteoporosis and colon cancer, these benefits were not considered to be sufficient to outweigh the other risks.

Searches for the Perfect SERM

Because of the potential cancer and cardiovascular risks inherent in hormone pills containing estrogen and progestin, scientists are working on the development of SERMs for postmenopausal women that can mimic the beneficial effects of estrogen without exerting any of its harmful effects.

The ideal drug, of course, would be a SERM exhibiting the positive effects of estrogen on bones, heart, and blood vessels without exhibiting the potentially harmful effects of estrogen on the breast and uterus.

Raloxifene and the Prevention of Osteoporosis

One SERM that may exhibit some of these properties is raloxifene (Evista), a drug approved by the FDA in 1997 for preventing osteoporosis in postmenopausal women.

Raloxifene appears to function like estrogen in bone, acting to maintain bone strength and increase bone density. In addition, raloxifene also resembles estrogen in its ability to lower LDL cholesterol levels, thereby decreasing the risk of heart disease.

Although information on the long-term risks and benefits of raloxifene is limited compared to tamoxifen, preliminary evidence suggests that raloxifene may exert these beneficial effects on bones, heart, and blood vessels without increasing a woman's risk of developing cancer.

Raloxifene and Risk of Invasive Breast Cancer

In animal studies, raloxifene (Evista) reduced the incidence of both breast and uterine cancer. And in preliminary human trials, raloxifene reduced the risk of breast cancer without the unwanted stimulation of uterine cell division that is exhibited by tamoxifen (Nolvadex). As a result of these findings, the National Cancer Institute sponsored a human clinical study to directly compare the effects of tamoxifen and raloxifene in postmenopausal women at higher than average risk for this disease. The trial, named STAR (Study of Tamoxifen and Raloxifene), was begun in 1999 and is following more than 19,000 women for a period of 5 to 10 years.

Early STAR trial results show that raloxifene works as well as tamoxifen in reducing risk by about 50 percent for invasive breast cancer in postmenopausal women. And raloxifene has fewer side effects. Participants in STAR who were assigned to take raloxifene had 36 percent fewer uterine cancers and 29 percent fewer blood clots from that drug than did the women assigned to take tamoxifen.

On the other hand, tamoxifen reduces the incidence of lobular carcinoma in situ (LCIS) and ductal carcinoma in situ (DCIS) by half, while raloxifene did not have an effect on these diagnoses. (LCIS and DCIS are sometimes called noninvasive or stage 0 breast cancers.)

A woman can go to www.cancer.gov/bcrisktool to determine if her individual risk for invasive breast cancer is above average.

Chapter 5

The Link between Breast and Ovarian Cancer

Among women, breast cancer is the most commonly diagnosed cancer after nonmelanoma skin cancer, and it is the second leading cause of cancer deaths after lung cancer. In 2012, an estimated 229,060 new cases will be diagnosed, and 39,920 deaths from breast cancer will occur. The incidence of breast cancer, particularly for estrogen receptor-positive cancers occurring after age 50 years, is declining and has declined at a faster rate since 2003; this may be temporally related to a decrease in hormone replacement therapy (HRT) following early reports from the Women's Health Initiative. Ovarian cancer is the ninth most common cancer, with an estimated 22,280 new cases in 2012, but is the fifth most deadly, with an estimated 15,500 deaths in 2012.

A possible genetic contribution to both breast and ovarian cancer risk is indicated by the increased incidence of these cancers among women with a family history, and by the observation of some families in which multiple family members are affected with breast and/or ovarian cancer, in a pattern compatible with an inheritance of autosomal dominant cancer susceptibility. Formal studies of families (linkage analysis) have subsequently proven the existence of autosomal dominant predispositions to breast and ovarian cancer and have led to the identification of several highly penetrant genes as the cause of inherited cancer risk in many families. Mutations in these genes are

Excerpted from PDQ® Cancer Information Summary. National Cancer Institute; Bethesda, MD. Genetics of Breast and Ovarian Cancer (PDQ)—Health Professional version. Updated 01/2012. Available at: www.cancer.gov. Accessed February 1, 2012.

rare in the general population and are estimated to account for no more than 5% to 10% of breast and ovarian cancer cases overall. It is likely that other genetic factors contribute to the etiology of some of these cancers.

Family History as a Risk Factor for Breast Cancer

In cross-sectional studies of adult populations, 5% to 10% of women have a mother or sister with breast cancer, and about twice as many have either a first-degree relative (FDR) or a second-degree relative with breast cancer. The risk conferred by a family history of breast cancer has been assessed in both case-control and cohort studies, using volunteer and population-based samples, with generally consistent results. In a pooled analysis of 38 studies, the relative risk (RR) of breast cancer conferred by an FDR with breast cancer was 2.1. Risk increases with the number of affected relatives and age at diagnosis.

Family History as a Risk Factor for Ovarian Cancer

Although reproductive, demographic, and lifestyle factors affect risk of ovarian cancer, the single greatest ovarian cancer risk factor is a family history of the disease. A large meta-analysis of 15 published studies estimated an odds ratio (OR) of 3.1 for the risk of ovarian cancer associated with at least one FDR with ovarian cancer.

Autosomal Dominant Inheritance of Breast/Ovarian Cancer Predisposition

Autosomal dominant inheritance of breast/ovarian cancer is characterized by transmission of cancer predisposition from generation to generation, through either the mother's or the father's side of the family, with the following characteristics:

- Inheritance risk of 50%: When a parent carries an autosomal dominant genetic predisposition, each child has a 50:50 chance of inheriting the predisposition. Although the risk of inheriting the predisposition is 50%, not everyone with the predisposition will develop cancer because of incomplete penetrance and/or gender-restricted or gender-related expression.

- Both males and females can inherit and transmit an autosomal dominant cancer predisposition. A male who inherits a cancer predisposition can still pass the altered gene on to his sons and daughters.

Breast and ovarian cancer are components of several autosomal dominant cancer syndromes. The syndromes most strongly associated with both cancers are the BRCA1 or BRCA2 [breast cancer gene 1 or breast cancer gene 2] mutation syndromes. Breast cancer is also a common feature of Li-Fraumeni syndrome due to TP53 mutations and of Cowden syndrome due to PTEN mutations. Other genetic syndromes that may include breast cancer as an associated feature include heterozygous carriers of the ataxia telangiectasia (AT) gene and Peutz-Jeghers syndrome. Ovarian cancer has also been associated with Lynch syndrome, basal cell nevus (Gorlin) syndrome (OMIM), and multiple endocrine neoplasia type 1 (MEN1) (OMIM). Germline mutations in the genes responsible for those syndromes produce different clinical phenotypes of characteristic malignancies and, in some instances, associated nonmalignant abnormalities.

The family characteristics that suggest hereditary breast and ovarian cancer predisposition include the following:

- Multiple cancers within a family suggest a predisposition.

- Cancers typically occur at an earlier age than in sporadic cases (defined as cases not associated with genetic risk).

- Two or more primary cancers in a single individual suggest predisposition. These could be multiple primary cancers of the same type (e.g., bilateral breast cancer) or primary cancer of different types (e.g., breast and ovarian cancer in the same individual).

- Cases of male breast cancer suggest predisposition.

There are no pathognomonic features distinguishing breast and ovarian cancers occurring in BRCA1 or BRCA2 mutation carriers from those occurring in noncarriers. Breast cancers occurring in BRCA1 mutation carriers are more likely to be estrogen receptor (ER)-negative, progesterone receptor (PR)-negative, and HER2/neu receptor-negative and have a basal phenotype. BRCA1-associated ovarian cancers are more likely to be high grade and of serous histopathology.

Difficulties in Identifying a Family History of Breast and Ovarian Cancer Risk

When using family history to assess risk, the accuracy and completeness of family history data must be taken into account. A reported family history may be erroneous, or a person may be unaware of relatives affected with cancer. In addition, small family sizes and premature deaths may limit the information obtained from a family history. Breast or ovarian cancer on the paternal side of the family usually involves more distant relatives than on the maternal side and thus may be more difficult to obtain. When comparing self-reported information with independently verified cases, the sensitivity of a history of breast cancer is relatively high, at 83% to 97%, but lower for ovarian cancer, at 60%.

Other Risk Factors for Breast Cancer

Other risk factors for breast cancer include age, reproductive and menstrual history, hormone therapy, radiation exposure, mammographic breast density, alcohol intake, physical activity, anthropometric variables, and a history of benign breast disease.

Age

Cumulative risk of breast cancer increases with age, with most breast cancers occurring after age 50 years. In women with a genetic susceptibility, breast cancer, and to a lesser degree, ovarian cancer, tends to occur at an earlier age than in sporadic cases.

Reproductive and Menstrual History

In general, breast cancer risk increases with early menarche and late menopause and is reduced by early first full-term pregnancy. Although results have been complex and may be gene dependent, several studies have suggested that the influence of these factors on risk in BRCA1/BRCA2 mutation carriers appear to be similar to noncarriers. Evidence suggests that reproductive history may be differentially associated with breast cancer subtype (i.e., triple-negative vs. ER-positive breast cancers). In contrast to ER-positive breast cancers, parity has been positively associated with triple-negative disease, with no association with ages at menarche and menopause.

Oral Contraceptives

Oral contraceptives (OCs) may produce a slight increase in breast cancer risk among long-term users, but this appears to be a short-term effect. In a meta-analysis of data from 54 studies, the risk of breast cancer associated with OC use did not vary in relationship to a family history of breast cancer.

OCs are sometimes recommended for ovarian cancer prevention in BRCA1 and BRCA2 mutation carriers. Although the data are not entirely consistent, a meta-analysis concluded that there was no significant increased risk of breast cancer with OC use in BRCA1/BRCA2 mutation carriers. However, use of OCs formulated before 1975 was associated with an increased risk of breast cancer.

Hormone Replacement Therapy

Data exist from both observational and randomized clinical trials regarding the association between postmenopausal HRT and breast cancer. A meta-analysis of data from 51 observational studies indicated a RR of breast cancer of 1.35 for women who had used HRT for five or more years after menopause. The Women's Health Initiative (WHI), a randomized controlled of about 160,000 postmenopausal women, investigated the risks and benefits of HRT. The estrogen-plus-progestin arm of the study, which randomized more than 16,000 women to receive combined HRT or placebo, was halted early because health risks exceeded benefits. Adverse outcomes prompting closure included significant increase in both total (245 vs. 185 cases) and invasive (199 vs. 150 cases) breast cancers and increased risks of coronary heart disease, stroke, and pulmonary embolism. Similar findings were seen in the estrogen-progestin arm of the prospective observational Million Women's Study in the United Kingdom. The risk of breast cancer was not elevated, however, in women randomly assigned to estrogen-only versus placebo in the WHI study. Eligibility for the estrogen-only arm of this study required hysterectomy, and 40% of these patients also had undergone oophorectomy, which potentially could have impacted breast cancer risk.

The association between HRT and breast cancer risk among women with a family history of breast cancer has not been consistent; some studies suggest risk is particularly elevated among women with a family history, while others have not found evidence for an interaction between these factors. The increased risk of breast cancer associated with HRT use in the large meta-analysis did not differ significantly between subjects with and without a family history. The WHI study has not reported analyses stratified on breast cancer family history, and subjects have not been systematically tested for BRCA1/BRCA2 mutations. Short-term use of hormones for treatment of menopausal symptoms appears to confer little or no breast cancer risk. The effect of HRT on breast cancer risk among carriers of BRCA1 or BRCA2 mutations has been studied only in the context of bilateral risk-reducing oophorectomy, in which short-term replacement does not appear to reduce the protective effect of oophorectomy on breast cancer risk.

Radiation Exposure

Observations in survivors of the atomic bombings of Hiroshima and Nagasaki and in women who have received therapeutic radiation treatments to the chest and upper body document increased breast cancer risk as a result of radiation exposure. The significance of this risk factor in women with a genetic susceptibility to breast cancer is unclear.

Preliminary data suggest that increased sensitivity to radiation could be a cause of cancer susceptibility in carriers of BRCA1 or BRCA2 mutations, and in association with germline ATM and TP53 mutations.

The possibility that genetic susceptibility to breast cancer occurs via a mechanism of radiation sensitivity raises questions about radiation exposure. It is possible that diagnostic radiation exposure, including mammography, poses more risk in genetically susceptible women than in women of average risk. Therapeutic radiation could also pose carcinogenic risk. A cohort study of BRCA1 and BRCA2 mutation carriers treated with breast-conserving therapy, however, showed no evidence of increased radiation sensitivity or sequelae in the breast, lung, or bone marrow of mutation carriers. Conversely, radiation sensitivity could make tumors in women with genetic susceptibility to breast cancer more responsive to radiation treatment. Studies examining the impact of mammography and chest x-ray exposure in BRCA1 and BRCA2 mutation carriers have had conflicting results.

Alcohol Intake

The risk of breast cancer increases by approximately 10% for each 10 g of daily alcohol intake (approximately one drink or less) in the general population. Prior studies of BRCA1/BRCA2 mutation carriers have found no increased risk associated with alcohol consumption.

Physical Activity and Anthropometry

Weight gain and being overweight are commonly recognized risk factors for breast cancer. In general, overweight women are most commonly observed to be at increased risk of postmenopausal breast cancer and at reduced risk of premenopausal breast cancer. Sedentary lifestyle may also be a risk factor. These factors have not been systematically evaluated in women with a positive family history of breast cancer or in carriers of cancer-predisposing mutations, but one study suggested a reduced risk of cancer associated with exercise among BRCA1 and BRCA2 mutation carriers.

Benign Breast Disease and Mammographic Density

Benign breast disease (BBD) is a risk factor for breast cancer, independent of the effects of other major risk factors for breast cancer (age, age at menarche, age at first live birth, and family history of breast cancer). There may also be an association between BBD and family history of breast cancer.

An increased risk of breast cancer has also been demonstrated for women who have increased density of breast tissue as assessed by mammogram, and breast density is likely to have a genetic component in its etiology.

Other Factors

Other risk factors, including those that are only weakly associated with breast cancer and those that have been inconsistently associated with the disease in epidemiologic studies (e.g., cigarette smoking), may be important in women who are in specific genotypically defined subgroups. For example, some studies have suggested that certain N-acetyl transferase alleles may influence female smokers' risk of developing breast cancer. One study found a reduced risk of breast cancer among BRCA1/BRCA2 mutation carriers who smoked, but an expanded follow-up study failed to find an association.

Other Risk Factors for Ovarian Cancer

Factors that increase risk for ovarian cancer include increasing age and nulliparity, while those that decrease risk include surgical history and use of OCs. Relatively few studies have addressed the effect of these risk factors in women who are genetically susceptible to ovarian cancer.

Age

Ovarian cancer incidence rises in a linear fashion from age 30 years to age 50 years and continues to increase, though at a slower rate, thereafter. Before age 30 years, the risk of developing epithelial ovarian cancer is remote; even in hereditary cancer families.

Reproductive History

Nulliparity is consistently associated with an increased risk of ovarian cancer, including among BRCA1/BRCA2 mutation carriers. Risk may also be increased among women who have used fertility drugs, especially those who remain nulligravid. Evidence is growing that the use of menopausal HRT is associated with an increased risk of ovarian cancer, particularly in long-time users and users of sequential estrogen-progesterone schedules.

Surgical History

Bilateral tubal ligation and hysterectomy are associated with reduced ovarian cancer risk, including in BRCA1/BRCA2 mutation carriers. Ovarian cancer risk is reduced more than 90% in women with documented BRCA1 or BRCA2 mutations who chose risk-reducing salpingo-oophorectomy (RRSO). In this same population, prophylactic removal of the ovaries also resulted in a nearly 50% reduction in the risk of subsequent breast cancer.

Oral Contraceptives

Use of OCs for four or more years is associated with an approximately 50% reduction in ovarian cancer risk in the general population. A majority of, but not all, studies also support OCs being protective among BRCA1/BRCA2 mutation carriers. A meta-analysis of 18 studies including 13,627 BRCA mutation carriers reported a significantly reduced risk of ovarian cancer associated with OC use.

Major Genes

Epidemiologic studies have clearly established the role of family history as an important risk factor for both breast and ovarian cancer. After gender and age, a positive family history is the strongest known predictive risk factor for breast cancer. In most cases an extensive family history (more than four affected relatives in the same biologic line) is not present. However, it has long been recognized that in some families, there is hereditary breast cancer, which is characterized by an early age of onset, bilaterality, and the presence of breast cancer in multiple generations in an apparent autosomal dominant pattern of transmission (through either the maternal or paternal lineage), sometimes including tumors of other organs, particularly the ovary and prostate gland. It is now known that some of these "cancer families" can be explained by specific mutations in single cancer susceptibility genes. The isolation of several of these genes, which when mutated are associated with a significantly increased risk of breast/ovarian cancer, makes it possible to identify individuals at risk. Although such cancer susceptibility genes are very important, highly penetrant germline mutations are estimated to account for only 5% to 10% of breast cancers overall.

A 1988 study reported the first quantitative evidence that breast cancer segregated as an autosomal dominant trait in some families. The search for genes associated with hereditary susceptibility to breast cancer has been facilitated by studies of large kindreds with multiple affected individuals, and has led to the identification of several susceptibility genes, including BRCA1, BRCA2, TP53, PTEN/MMAC1, and STK11. Other genes, such as the mismatch repair genes MLH1, MSH2, MSH6, and PMS2, have been associated with an increased risk of ovarian cancer, but have not been consistently associated with breast cancer.

BRCA1

In 1990, a susceptibility gene for breast cancer was mapped by genetic linkage to the long arm of chromosome 17, in the interval 17q12-21. The linkage between breast cancer and genetic markers on chromosome 17q was soon confirmed by others, and evidence for the coincident transmission of both breast and ovarian cancer susceptibility in linked families was observed. The BRCA1 gene (OMIM) was subsequently identified by positional cloning methods and has been found to contain 24 exons that encode a protein of 1,863 amino acids. Germline mutations in BRCA1 are associated with early-onset breast cancer, ovarian cancer, and fallopian tube cancer. Male breast cancer, pancreatic cancer, testicular cancer, and early-onset prostate cancer may also be associated with mutations in BRCA1; however, male breast cancer, pancreatic cancer, and prostate cancer are more strongly associated with mutations in BRCA2.

BRCA2

A second breast cancer susceptibility gene, BRCA2, was localized to the long arm of chromosome 13 through linkage studies of 15 families with multiple cases of breast cancer that were not linked to BRCA1. Mutations in BRCA2 (OMIM) are associated with multiple cases of breast cancer in families, and are also associated with male breast cancer, ovarian cancer, prostate cancer, melanoma, and pancreatic cancer. BRCA2 is a large gene with 27 exons that encode a protein of 3,418 amino acids. While not homologous genes, both BRCA1 and BRCA2 have an unusually large exon 11 and translational start sites in exon 2. Like BRCA1, BRCA2 appears to behave like a tumor suppressor gene. In tumors associated with both BRCA1 and BRCA2 mutations, there is often loss of the wild-type (nonmutated) allele.

Mutations in BRCA1 and BRCA2 appear to be responsible for disease in 45% of families with multiple cases of breast cancer only and in up to 90% of families with both breast and ovarian cancer.

BRCA1 and BRCA2 Function

Most BRCA1 and BRCA2 mutations are predicted to produce a truncated protein product, and thus loss of protein function, although some missense mutations cause loss of function without truncation. Because inherited breast/ovarian cancer is an autosomal dominant condition, persons with a BRCA1 or BRCA2 mutation on one copy of chromosome 17 or 13 also carry a normal allele on the other paired chromosome. In most breast and ovarian cancers that have been studied from mutation carriers, deletion of the normal allele results in loss of all function, leading to the classification of BRCA1 and BRCA2 as tumor suppressor genes. In addition to, and as part of, their roles as tumor suppressor genes, BRCA1 and BRCA2 are involved in myriad functions within cells, including homologous DNA repair, genomic stability, transcriptional regulation, protein ubiquitination, chromatin remodeling, and cell cycle control.

Population Estimates of the Likelihood of Having a BRCA1 or BRCA2 Mutation

Statistics regarding the percentage of individuals found to be BRCA mutation carriers among samples of women and men with a variety of personal cancer histories regardless of family history are provided in the following text. These data can help determine who might best benefit from a referral for cancer genetic counseling and consideration of genetic testing, but cannot replace a personalized risk assessment, which might indicate a higher or lower mutation likelihood based on additional personal and family history characteristics.

In some cases, the same mutation has been found in multiple apparently unrelated families. This observation is consistent with a founder effect, wherein a mutation identified in a contemporary population can be traced back to a small group of founders isolated by geographic, cultural, or other factors. Most notably, two specific BRCA1 mutations (185delAG and 5382insC) and a BRCA2 mutation (6174delT) have been reported to be common in Ashkenazi Jews. However, other founder mutations have been identified in African Americans and Hispanics. The presence of these founder mutations has practical implications for genetic testing. Many laboratories offer directed testing specifically for ethnic-specific alleles. This greatly simplifies the technical aspects of the test but is not without limitations. For example, it is estimated that up to 15% of BRCA1 and BRCA2 mutations that occur among Ashkenazim are nonfounder mutations.

Among the general population, the likelihood of having any BRCA mutation is as follows:

- General population (excluding Ashkenazim): About 1 in 400 (~0.25%)
- Women with breast cancer (any age): 1 in 50 (2%)
- Women with breast cancer (younger than 40 years): 1 in 10 (10%)
- Men with breast cancer (any age): 1 in 20 (5%)
- Women with ovarian cancer (any age): 1 in 8 to 1 in 10 (10%–15%)

Among Ashkenazi Jewish individuals, the likelihood of having any BRCA mutation is as follows:

- General Ashkenazi Jewish population: 1 in 40 (2.5%)
- Women with breast cancer (any age): 1 in 10 (10%)
- Women with breast cancer (younger than 40 years): 1 in 3 (30%–35%)
- Men with breast cancer (any age): 1 in 5 (19%)
- Women with ovarian cancer or primary peritoneal cancer (all ages): 1 in 3 (36%–41%)

Two large U.S. population-based studies of breast cancer patients younger than age 65 years examined the prevalence of BRCA1 and BRCA2 mutations in various ethnic groups. The prevalence of BRCA1 mutations in breast cancer patients by ethnic group was 3.5% in Hispanics, 1.3% to 1.4% in African Americans, 0.5% in Asian Americans, 2.2% to 2.9% in non-Ashkenazi Caucasians, and 8.3% to 10.2% in Ashkenazi Jewish individuals. The prevalence of BRCA2 mutations by ethnic group was 2.6% in African Americans and 2.1% in Caucasians.

A retrospective review of 29 Ashkenazi Jewish patients with primary fallopian tube tumors identified germline BRCA mutations in 17%. Another study of 108 women with fallopian tube cancer identified mutations in 55.6% of the Jewish women and 26.4% of non-Jewish women (30.6% overall).

Chapter 6

Statistics on Breast Cancer in the United States

Probability of Breast Cancer in American Women

Risk of Developing Breast Cancer

The National Cancer Institute's (NCI) Surveillance, Epidemiology, and End Results (SEER) Program report estimates that, based on current rates, 12.2 percent of women born in the United States today will develop breast cancer at some time in their lives. This estimate is based on breast cancer statistics for the years 2005 through 2007.

This estimate means that, if the current rate stays the same, women born now have an average risk of 12.2 percent (often expressed as "one in eight") of being diagnosed with breast cancer at some time in their lives. On the other hand, the chance that they will never have breast cancer is 87.8 percent (expressed as "seven in eight").

In the 1970s, the lifetime risk of being diagnosed with breast cancer in the United States was just under 10 percent (often expressed as "one in 10").

The last five annual SEER reports show these estimates of lifetime risk:

This chapter contains text from "Probability of Breast Cancer in American Women," by the National Cancer Institute (NCI, www.cancer.gov), part of the National Institutes of Health, September 17, 2010, and, under the heading, "Facts about Breast Cancer Mortality and Lifetime Risk," text excerpted from "SEER Stat Fact Sheets: Breast," by Surveillance Epidemiology and End Results (SEER), of the NCI, November 10, 2011.

- 13.2 percent for 2000 through 2002 ("1 in 7.58," often expressed as "one in eight")

- 12.7 percent for 2001 through 2003 ("1 in 7.87," often expressed as "one in eight")

- 12.3 percent for 2002 through 2004 ("1 in 8.13," often expressed as "one in eight")

- 12.0 percent for 2003 through 2005 ("1 in 8.33," often expressed as "one in eight")

- 12.1 percent for 2004 through 2006 ("1 in 8.26," often expressed as "one in eight")

SEER statisticians expect some variability from year to year. Slight changes, such as the one reported this year, may be explained by a variety of factors, including minor changes in risk factor levels in the population, slight changes in screening rates, or just random variability inherent in the data.

Risk of Being Diagnosed with Breast Cancer at Different Ages

The estimated probability of being diagnosed with breast cancer for specific age groups and for specific time periods is generally more informative than lifetime probabilities. Estimates by decade of life are less influenced by changes in life expectancy and incidence rates. The SEER report estimates the risk of developing breast cancer in 10-year age intervals. These calculations factor in the proportion of women who live to each age. In other words, they take into account that not all women live to older ages, when breast cancer risk becomes the greatest.

A woman's chance of being diagnosed with breast cancer is the following:

- From age 30 through age 39 is 0.43 percent (often expressed as "1 in 233")

- From age 40 through age 49 is 1.45 percent (often expressed as "1 in 69")

- From age 50 through age 59 is 2.38 percent (often expressed as "1 in 42")

- From age 60 through age 69 is 3.45 percent (often expressed as "1 in 29")

These probabilities are averages for the whole population. An individual woman's breast cancer risk may be higher or lower, depending on a number of factors, including her family history, reproductive history, race/ethnicity, and other factors that are not yet fully understood.

Facts about Breast Cancer Mortality and Lifetime Risk

It is estimated that 230,480 women will be diagnosed with and 39,520 women will die of cancer of the breast in 2011.

Incidence and Mortality

SEER incidence: From 2004–2008, the median age at diagnosis for cancer of the breast was 61 years of age. Approximately 0.0% were diagnosed under age 20; 1.9% between 20 and 34; 10.2% between 35 and 44; 22.6% between 45 and 54; 24.4% between 55 and 64; 19.7% between 65 and 74; 15.5% between 75 and 84; and 5.6% 85+ years of age.

The age-adjusted incidence rate was 124.0 per 100,000 women per year. These rates are based on cases diagnosed in 2004–2008 from 17 Surveillance Epidemiology and End Results (SEER) geographic areas. See Table 6.1.

Table 6.1. Incidence Rates by Race

Race/Ethnicity	Female
All Races	124.0 per 100,000 women
White	127.3 per 100,000 women
Black	119.9 per 100,000 women
Asian/Pacific Islander	93.7 per 100,000 women
American Indian/Alaska Native	77.9 per 100,000 women
Hispanic	92.1 per 100,000 women

U.S. mortality: From 2004–2008, the median age at death for cancer of the breast was 68 years of age. Approximately 0.0% died under age 20; 0.9% between 20 and 34; 5.7% between 35 and 44; 14.9% between 45 and 54; 21.1% between 55 and 64; 19.8% between 65 and 74; 22.3% between 75 and 84; and 15.3% 85+ years of age.

The age-adjusted death rate was 23.5 per 100,000 women per year. These rates are based on patients who died in 2004–2008 in the United States. See Table 6.2.

61

Table 6.2. Death Rates by Race

Race/Ethnicity	Female
All Races	23.5 per 100,000 women
White	22.8 per 100,000 women
Black	32.0 per 100,000 women
Asian/Pacific Islander	12.2 per 100,000 women
American Indian/Alaska Native	17.2 per 100,000 women
Hispanic	15.1 per 100,000 women

Survival and Stage

Survival examines how long after diagnosis people live. Cancer survival is measured in a number of different ways depending on the intended purpose. The survival statistics presented here are based on relative survival.

The overall five-year relative survival for 2001–2007 from 17 SEER geographic areas was 89.1%. Five-year relative survival by race was: 90.4% for white women; 77.0% for black women. See Table 6.3.

Table 6.3. Stage Distribution and Five-Year Relative Survival by Stage at Diagnosis for 2001–2007, All Races, Females

Stage at Diagnosis	Stage Distribution (%)	Five-year Relative Survival (%)
Localized (confined to primary site)	60	98.6
Regional (spread to regional lymph nodes)	33	83.8
Distant (cancer has metastasized)	5	23.3
Unknown (unstaged)	2	52.4

Lifetime Risk

Based on rates from 2006–2008, 12.29% of women born today will be diagnosed with cancer of the breast at some time during their lifetime. This number can also be expressed as one in eight women will be diagnosed with cancer of the breast during their lifetime. These statistics are called the lifetime risk.

Lifetime risk may also be discussed in terms of the probability of developing or of dying from cancer. Based on cancer rates from 2006 to 2008, it was estimated that men had about a 45 percent chance of developing cancer in their lifetimes, while women had about a 38 percent chance of developing cancer. Sometimes it is more useful to look at the probability of developing cancer of the breast between two age groups. For example, 5.68% of women will develop cancer of the breast between their 50th and 70th birthdays.

Prevalence

On January 1, 2008, in the United States there were approximately 2,632,005 women alive who had a history of cancer of the breast. This includes any person alive on January 1, 2008 who had been diagnosed with cancer of the breast at any point prior to January 1, 2008 and includes persons with active disease and those who are cured of their disease.

Chapter 7

Recent Research Advances in Breast Cancer

Yesterday

- In 1975, the incidence rate for female breast cancer in the United States was 105 new cases diagnosed for every 100,000 women in the population; the mortality rate was 31 deaths for every 100,000 women.

- Among women diagnosed with breast cancer during the period from 1975 through 1977, about 75% survived their disease at least five years. Among white women, the five-year relative survival rate was 76%; among African-American women, it was 62%.

- Mastectomy was the only accepted surgical option for breast cancer treatment.

- Only one randomized trial of mammography for breast cancer screening had been completed. Several other trials and the joint National Institutes of Health (NIH) and American Cancer Society (ACS) Breast Cancer Detection Demonstration Projects were just beginning.

- Clinical investigation of combination chemotherapy, using multiple drugs with different mechanisms of action, and of hormonal therapy as postsurgical (adjuvant) treatment for breast cancer was in its earliest stages.

From "Cancer Advances in Focus: Breast Cancer," by the National Cancer Institute (NCI, www.cancer.gov), part of the National Institutes of Health, September 23, 2010.

65

- In the mid-1970s, clinical evaluation of the drug tamoxifen, a selective estrogen receptor modulator (SERM), as a hormonal treatment for breast cancer was just beginning.

- No gene associated with an increased risk of breast cancer had yet been identified.

Today

- In 2007, the latest year for which we have updated statistics, the U.S. incidence rate for female breast cancer was approximately 125 new cases diagnosed for every 100,000 women in the population; the mortality rate was approximately 23 deaths for every 100,000 women. Although the incidence rate in 2007 was higher than that in 1975, this rate has been declining since 1998–1999, when it peaked at a rate of 141 new cases for every 100,000 women in the population. The breast cancer death rate in the United States has been declining steadily since 1989–1990, when it peaked at a rate of 33 deaths for every 100,000 women.

- Among women diagnosed with breast cancer during the period from 1999 through 2006, 90% were expected to survive their disease at least five years. Among white women, the five-year relative survival rate was 91%; among African-American women, it was 78%. The increase in breast cancer survival seen since the mid-1970s has been attributed to both screening and improved treatment.

- Breast-conserving surgery (lumpectomy) followed by local radiation therapy has replaced mastectomy as the preferred surgical approach for treating early-stage breast cancer.

- Routine mammographic screening is an accepted standard for the early detection of breast cancer. The results of eight randomized trials, the NIH-ACS Breast Cancer Detection Demonstration Projects, and other research studies showed that mammographic screening can reduce the mortality from breast cancer.

- Combination chemotherapy is a standard of care in the adjuvant treatment of operable breast cancer. The goal of this systemic therapy is to eradicate cancer cells that may have spread beyond the breast. Neoadjuvant chemotherapy, or chemotherapy given before surgery to reduce the size of the tumor and to increase the chance of breast-conserving surgery, is also an option.

- Hormonal therapy with SERMs (such as tamoxifen) and aromatase inhibitors is now standard in the treatment of women with estrogen receptor-positive breast cancer, both as adjuvant therapy and in the treatment of advanced disease. Estrogen receptor-positive breast cancer cells can be stimulated to grow by the hormone estrogen. SERMs interfere with this growth stimulation by preventing estrogen from binding to the estrogen receptor. In contrast, aromatase inhibitors block estrogen production by the body. Food and Drug Administration (FDA)-approved aromatase inhibitors include anastrozole, exemestane, and letrozole.

- Tamoxifen and another SERM, raloxifene, have been approved by the FDA as treatments to reduce the risk of breast cancer in women who have an increased risk of developing the disease.

- The monoclonal antibody trastuzumab is an accepted treatment for breast cancers that overproduce a protein called human epidermal growth factor receptor 2, or HER2. This protein is produced in abnormally high amounts by about 20% of breast tumors. Breast cancers that overproduce HER2 tend to be more aggressive and are more likely to recur. Trastuzumab targets the HER2 protein specifically, and this antibody, in conjunction with adjuvant chemotherapy, can lower the risk of recurrence of HER2-overproducing breast cancers by about 50% in comparison with chemotherapy alone.

- Several breast cancer susceptibility genes have now been identified, including BRCA1, BRCA2, TP53, and PTEN/MMAC1. Approximately 60% of women with an inherited mutation in BRCA1 or BRCA2 will develop breast cancer sometime during their lives, compared with about 12% of women in the general population. Women with inherited BRCA1 or BRCA2 gene mutations also have an increased risk of ovarian cancer.

Tomorrow

We will use our rapidly increasing knowledge in the fields of cancer genomics and cell biology to develop more effective and less toxic treatments for breast cancer and to improve our ability to identify cancers that are more likely to recur. Moreover, we will use this knowledge to tailor breast cancer therapy to the individual patient. For example, gene expression analysis has led to the identification of five subtypes of breast cancer that have distinct biological features, clinical outcomes, and responses to chemotherapy. This knowledge can be exploited in the development of treatment strategies based on the specific characteristics of a woman's tumor. Furthermore, a patient's response to chemotherapy is influenced not only by the genetic characteristics of their tumor but also by inherited variations in genes that affect the body's ability to absorb, metabolize, and eliminate drugs. Our growing knowledge should enable prediction of tumor responses to individual chemotherapy drugs or classes of drugs, as well as the likelihood of severe adverse effects from them. This knowledge should also aid in the development of more individualized treatments and permit the design of more effective and less toxic chemotherapy agents.

We will use our increasing knowledge of the immune system to enhance the body's ability to recognize and destroy cancer cells. The knowledge we have acquired thus far has facilitated the development of several promising breast cancer treatment vaccines that are currently under clinical evaluation.

We will use advanced technologies, including genomic technologies, to improve our ability to detect breast cancer at its earliest stages, when it is most treatable, and to better define individual risk for this disease.

We will strive to understand, address, and eliminate factors that contribute to the higher mortality from breast cancer experienced by African-American women compared with women of other racial and ethnic groups.

Part Two

Types of Breast Cancer

Chapter 8

Ductal Carcinoma in Situ (DCIS)

What is ductal carcinoma in situ (DCIS)?

Ductal carcinoma in situ is the earliest possible and most treatable diagnosis of breast cancer. Some experts consider it to be premalignant. The most common form of non-invasive breast cancer, DCIS accounts for about 20 percent of all newly diagnosed breast cancers, according to the National Cancer Institute. Sometimes, DCIS is seen in association with an invasive form of breast cancer.

The diagnosis of DCIS is increasing because more women are receiving regular mammograms—and because of advancements in mammography technology, which can now find small areas of calcification in the breast. Experts estimate that about one-third of women with DCIS will develop invasive breast cancer within 10 years if the disease is left untreated.

Who is most likely to have DCIS?

Because of how DCIS is detected, it can be found in women earlier than age 45, which is the age breast cancer becomes more common. However, as a woman ages, breast cancer risk does not decline; therefore, DCIS can be found at any age. Less than 10 percent of women with breast cancer have a family history of the disease.

71

Other factors increasing the risk of having breast cancer include having no children or the first child after age 30, early menstruation, and consuming three or more alcoholic drinks a day.

What characterizes DCIS?

DCIS is characterized by pre-cancerous or early stage cell abnormalities in the breast ducts. On a mammogram, DCIS appears as areas of calcification.

How does the pathologist make a diagnosis?

The pathologist examines biopsy specimens, along with other tests if necessary. If mammography shows suspicious findings, a biopsy may be recommended. A biopsy is the most widely used method for making a firm diagnosis of breast cancer. During a biopsy procedure, a primary care physician removes cells or tissues from the suspicious area for the pathologist to examine more closely in the laboratory. In some cases a biopsy may be performed with surgery.

To make a firm diagnosis of DCIS, the pathologist will investigate whether the malignancy has invaded tissue surrounding the ducts. A diagnosis of DCIS means the tumor remains only in its original place—in situ.

What else does the pathologist look for?

The biopsy sample is tested for the presence of estrogen receptors. Women with DCIS containing this receptor are more likely to respond positively to hormone therapy. Due to continual advances in research, other tests may be used as well.

With all necessary tests completed, pathologists determine the cancer's stage. All DCIS tumors are Stage Tis, which means the tumor is in situ and has not spread. The cure rate for stage Tis tumors is close to 100 percent if standard forms of treatment are followed.

How do doctors determine what surgery or treatment will be necessary?

The pathologist consults with your primary care physician after reviewing the test results. Together, using their combined experience and knowledge, they determine treatment options most appropriate for your condition.

What kinds of treatments are available for DCIS?

DCIS is treated through surgery, which is sometimes supplemented by radiation therapy. It's important to learn as much as you can about your treatment options and to make the decision that's right for you. Because having DCIS is not an emergency situation, you can take your time making your choices.

Advancements in surgical techniques have enabled about 70 percent of women to choose breast-conserving surgical treatments like lumpectomy rather than mastectomy, where the entire breast is removed. If you have DCIS, which is confined to one area of one breast, you are likely to be a good candidate for lumpectomy. If your breast cannot be conserved, breast reconstruction surgery may be a possibility after you recover from your initial operation to remove the cancer.

Radiation therapy is often used after lumpectomy and sometimes after mastectomy to rid the body of any microscopic remnants of the cancer in the area where the original tumor was found and removed.

For more information, visit the American Cancer Society, Y-ME National Breast Cancer Organization, or Cancer.Net websites.

What kinds of questions should I ask my doctors?

Ask any question you want. There are no questions you should be reluctant to ask. Here are a few to consider:

- Please describe the type of cancer I have and what treatment options are available.

- What are the chances for full remission?

- What treatment options do you recommend? Why do you believe these are the best treatments?

- What are the pros and cons of these treatment options?

- What are the side effects?

- Should I receive a second opinion?

- Is your medical team experienced in treating the type of cancer I have?

- Can you provide me with information about the physicians and others on the medical team?

Chapter 9

Lobular Carcinoma in Situ (LCIS)

What is lobular carcinoma in situ (LCIS)?

Lobular carcinoma in situ, also known as lobular neoplasia, is not technically a cancer or a carcinoma. The alternate name for this condition—lobular neoplasia—is more technically accurate, since LCIS is only a marker of cancer in most women. In women who develop invasive lobular carcinoma, LCIS is a direct precursor. An LCIS diagnosis means there is abnormal cell growth that increases your chances for developing breast cancer later in life. While having LCIS increases the chances of someday having breast cancer, most women with LCIS do not develop breast cancer. Due to improvements in breast cancer screening, the diagnosis of LCIS is increasing.

Who is most likely to have LCIS?

LCIS is more common in pre-menopausal women; however, LCIS can be found at any age. Less than 10 percent of women with breast cancer have a family history of the disease. Other factors increasing the risk of having breast cancer include having no children or the first child after age 30, early menstruation, and consuming three or more alcoholic drinks a day.

What characterizes LCIS?

LCIS is characterized by the appearance of abnormal cells in the milk-producing lobules of the breast. LCIS rarely shows on a mammogram; instead, it is usually discovered by chance as part of a biopsy sample for a breast lump, which a pathologist examines.

How does the pathologist make a diagnosis?

The pathologist examines biopsy specimens along with other tests if necessary. A biopsy is the most widely used method for detecting breast cancer. During a biopsy procedure, the primary care doctor removes cells or tissues from the suspicious area for the pathologist to examine more closely in the laboratory. In some cases, a biopsy may be performed with surgery.

The pathologist also will note the size and location of the cell abnormalities. To make a firm diagnosis of LCIS, the pathologist will investigate whether the abnormal cells have invaded outside lobules into the surrounding tissue. A diagnosis of LCIS means the cell abnormalities remain only in their original place—in situ.

What else does the pathologist look for?

The biopsy sample is at this time not tested any further. All LCIS tumors are stage 0, which means the tumor is not cancerous. The cure rate for stage 0 tumors is close to 100 percent if standard forms of treatment are followed.

How do doctors determine what surgery or treatment will be necessary?

The pathologist consults with your primary care physician after reviewing the test results. Together, using their combined experience and knowledge, they determine treatment options most appropriate for your condition.

What kinds of treatments are available for LCIS?

Most women with LCIS do not receive immediate treatment; instead, they are closely monitored through regular clinical breast exams and mammography. In addition, they are encouraged to do self-exams each month and to report unusual lumps or changes to a physician.

Some women with LCIS, usually those with a strong family history of breast cancer, choose the preventive removal of both breasts, a procedure known as prophylactic mastectomy, often followed with breast reconstruction. This treatment significantly reduces the risk of breast cancer.

Another option is to consider taking the drug tamoxifen, which was proved to reduce the risk of breast cancer in a recent clinical trial conducted by the National Surgical Adjuvant Breast and Bowel Project (NSABP). A second NSABP clinical trial, known as the STAR (Study of Tamoxifen and Raloxifene) trial, is now under way to compare the effectiveness of tamoxifen with raloxifene, a promising new anti-cancer drug. If you are interested, ask your physician about these drug therapy options.

For more information, visit the American Cancer Society, Y-ME National Breast Cancer Organization, or Cancer.Net websites.

What kinds of questions should I ask my doctors?

Ask any question you want. There are no questions you should be reluctant to ask. Here are a few to consider:

- Please describe the type of condition I have and what kind of preventive measures I can take.

- Is any type of treatment recommended at this stage?

- What are the pros and cons of these treatment options?

- What are the side effects?

- Should I receive a second opinion?

- Is your medical team experienced in treating the condition I have?

- Can you provide me with information about the physicians and others on the medical team?

Chapter 10

Invasive Carcinoma of the Breast

Chapter Contents

Section 10.1

Understanding Invasive Breast Cancer

This section contains text, under the heading "What Is Invasive Breast Cancer?" excerpted from Curtis RE, Freedman DM, Ron E, Ries LAG, Hacker DG, Edwards BK, Tucker MA, Fraumeni JF Jr. (eds). New Malignancies Among Cancer Survivors: SEER Cancer Registries, 1973–2000. National Cancer Institute. NIH Publ. No. 05-5302. Bethesda, MD, 2006. Reviewed by David A. Cooke, MD, FACP, April 2, 2012. This section also contains text from "More Accurate Method of Estimating Invasive Breast Cancer Risk in African American Women Developed," National Cancer Institute (NCI, www.cancer.gov), part of the National Institutes of Health, November 27, 2007, and "Single-Dose Partial Breast Irradiation Safe for Some Women with Invasive Breast Cancer," by the NCI, August 4, 2010.

What Is Invasive Breast Cancer?

Invasive breast cancer is the most frequently diagnosed new malignancy and the second most common cause of cancer death, after lung cancer, among women in the United States.

This malignancy currently accounts for 32% of all new cancer cases and 15% of cancer deaths among American women. Incidence rates in the SEER [Surveillance Epidemiology and End Results] database vary greatly by race and ethnic group, with lower rates seen for black, Asian, and Hispanic women than for white women. Although breast cancer incidence rates have been increasing since the 1980s, death rates have declined by about 2.3% per year since 1990, with some of the downturn related to increases in early detection by mammography and to effective treatment with adjuvant chemotherapy. About 72% of the invasive breast cancers reported to SEER are ductal carcinomas, not otherwise specified (NOS); 9% are lobular carcinomas; and the remaining 19% are other histologic types. The current relative survival rates for all breast cancers combined are 88.8% at five years (79.5% at 10 years) for white females, but only 75.3% at five years (63.9% at 10 years) for black females. Treatment for early-stage invasive breast cancer shifted in the 1980s and 1990s from radical mastectomy with or without regional radiotherapy to the chest wall and lymph nodes (postmastectomy radiation) to increasing use of breast-conserving surgery followed by breast radiation (postlumpectomy radiation). Adjuvant chemotherapy (including alkylating agents) and hormones (tamoxifen) are also widely used.

A large body of epidemiologic evidence links reproductive risk factors to breast cancer risk. There is strong evidence that exogenous estrogens increase breast cancer risk close in time to the diagnosis, and that specific endogenous hormones play an important role in explaining risk. Factors consistently associated with an increased risk of breast cancer include late age at first birth, low parity (less than two births), early onset of menarche, late age at menopause, and hormone replacement therapy, while early menopause from ovarian ablation and longer lactation periods are associated with a reduction in risk. In addition, physical inactivity, regular alcohol use (more than one drink/day), greater height, and postmenopausal obesity have been shown to heighten risk. Breast cancer incidence is positively associated with higher socioeconomic status, which has been explained largely by known lifestyle and reproductive risk factors. Although relatively uncommon, exposure to ionizing radiation before the age of 40 years increases the risk of breast cancer, with elevated risks detected even from low-dose exposures.

A family history of breast cancer is an important risk factor for this disease. The increased risk of breast cancer among women with at least one affected first-degree relative is about two-fold, and the risk rises with increasing numbers and younger ages of affected relatives. Approximately 2% to 5% of breast cancers are probably attributable to the inheritance of rare, highly penetrant susceptibility genes, such as BRCA1/2 [breast cancer genes 1 and 2]. Women with BRCA1/2 mutations have a high cumulative risk of developing cancers of the breast (35%–84% by age 70 years) and ovary (10%–50%), with tumors tending to arise at an earlier age compared with sporadic cases. Germline mutations of p53 (Li-Fraumeni syndrome) and the PTEN [phosphatase and tensin homolog] gene are rare and account for less than 1% of inherited breast cancer.

More Accurate Method of Estimating Invasive Breast Cancer Risk in African American Women Developed

A model for calculating invasive breast cancer risk, called the CARE model, has been found to give better estimates of the number of breast cancers that would develop in African-American women 50 to 79 years of age than an earlier model which was based primarily on data from white women. Both models were designed to be used by health care professionals and should either be used by them or in consultation with them. Researchers at the National Cancer Institute (NCI), part of the National Institutes of Health, and their collaborators report on the study methodology and results online in *JNCI* [*Journal of the National Cancer Institute*] on November 27, 2007.

"NCI's Breast Cancer Risk Assessment Tool has been widely used for counseling women and determining eligibility for breast cancer prevention trials," said NCI Director John E. Niederhuber, MD. "The development of the CARE model highlights the need to develop targeted tools to assess an individual woman's risk, and those tools must be based on many factors that also assure that the tool can be used in a non-discriminatory manner."

The NCI investigators worked with colleagues from the Women's Contraceptive and Reproductive Experiences (CARE) Study, the Women's Health Initiative, and the Study of Tamoxifen and Raloxifene trial (a breast cancer prevention trial) to produce and test the new model. Some members of the team had worked on both the CARE and earlier model, called BCRAT (Breast Cancer Risk Assessment Tool). Because of the higher accuracy of the CARE model for African-American women, the NCI authors are now recommending its use for counseling these women regarding their risk of breast cancer.

While the BCRAT allows for projections for African-American women and for women from other racial and ethnic groups, these projections are based on certain assumptions. In particular, it is assumed that the relative risk of breast cancer associated with having a specific profile of risk factors for white women applies to African American women and to women from other racial and ethnic groups as well. Because of the need to rely on these various assumptions, rather than on sufficient data from African-American women and women in other racial and ethnic groups, BCRAT, which can be found on the NCI website at www.cancer.gov/bcrisktool, includes a disclaimer for African-American women and for women in other groups that their projections might be inaccurate.

To develop a new model that would more accurately assess an African-American woman's chance of developing breast cancer, researchers in the CARE study examined data from 1,607 African-American women with invasive breast cancer and 1,637 African-American women of similar ages who did not have breast cancer. The factors used in the model were age at first menstrual period, number of first-degree relatives (mother or sisters) who had breast cancer, and number of previous benign breast biopsy examinations. A woman's age at the birth of her first child, a risk factor for white women, did not improve prediction in African-American women and so was not included in the model. Risk was calculated by combining information on these factors with African-American rates of new invasive breast cancer from NCI's Surveillance, Epidemiology and End Results Program and with national mortality data.

To test the accuracy of the model, researchers compared data in the CARE model with data from the 14,059 African-American women aged 50 to 79 in the Women's Health Initiative (WHI) study who had no prior history of breast cancer. From the risk factor profiles for breast cancer that were collected at entry into the WHI, the researchers used the CARE model to estimate the number of women who would be expected to develop invasive breast cancer and found that the model predicted that 323 would be affected, close to the 350 breast cancers in African-American women that actually occurred during the WHI follow up. According to Mitchell H. Gail, MD, NCI, the lead author of this study, "The CARE model predicted the numbers of breast cancer diagnoses well overall, and in most categories."

One of the key uses of the BCRAT has been to determine eligibility criteria for a number of breast cancer prevention trials. For African-American women 45 and older, the CARE model risk projections were usually higher than those from the BCRAT. To assess what the impact of using the CARE model might have been on a recently completed prevention trial, the researchers used eligibility screening data from 20,278 African-American women who were examined in the Study of Tamoxifen and Raloxifene (STAR) trial between 1999 and 2004. The investigators estimated that 30.3 percent of African-American women would have had significant five-year invasive breast cancer risks based on the CARE model, compared to only 14.5 percent based on BCRAT.

"African-American women were both more interested in and more likely to enroll in the STAR trial compared to the earlier Breast Cancer Prevention Trial, but the recruitment process and our enrollment task would have been easier if the CARE model had been available," said Worta McCaskill-Stevens, MD, NCI, one of the leaders of the STAR trial.

Additionally, inaccurate projections using the BCRAT could result in African-American women receiving an underestimate of their breast cancer risk. As a result of this underestimate, African American women might not get counseling about actions they could take to reduce their risk. "There has been great interest in developing race- or ethnicity-specific adaptations of the BCRAT model that are based on sufficient race- or ethnicity-specific data, and the CARE data enabled us to develop the new model," said Gail.

It should be noted that the CARE model, like the BCRAT, needs to be approached with caution or avoided for certain special populations. These models should not be used for women with a previous history of breast cancer. The models tend to underestimate risk in women who have received radiation to the chest and in women who are known to carry mutations associated with increased risk of breast cancer, such as mutations in the BRCA1 and BRCA2 [breast cancer gene 1 and 2] genes.

Reference: Gail MH, Costantino JP, Pee D, Bondy M, Newman L, Selvan M, Anderson GL, Malone KE, Marchbanks PA, McCaskill-Stevens W, Norman SA, Simon MS, Spirtas R, Ursin G, and Bernstein L. Projecting Individualized Absolute Invasive Breast Cancer Risk in African American Women. *JNCI*. Vol. 99, No. 23.

Single-Dose Partial Breast Irradiation Safe for Some Women with Invasive Breast Cancer

In a randomized phase III trial, women who received single-dose partial-breast irradiation during breast-conserving surgery had the same likelihood of having their cancer recur in the same breast after four years of follow-up as women who received standard whole-breast external beam radiation therapy after surgery.

Background

Women with early-stage breast cancer often undergo breast-conserving surgery (BCS) instead of mastectomy (removal of the entire breast). During BCS, only the portion of the breast containing the tumor and a few nearby lymph nodes are removed. To reduce the likelihood of cancer recurrence, standard treatment includes a course of external-beam radiation therapy (EBRT) to the whole breast after BCS. This type of radiation therapy is given in small doses given five times a week for about six weeks.

Because EBRT requires a large amount of time, as well as travel to and from a treatment center, researchers are developing ways to deliver radiation therapy in fewer treatment sessions to women receiving BCS. One such method is accelerated partial-breast irradiation, in which radiation is delivered specifically to the area of the breast that contained the tumor instead of to the whole breast. Partial-breast irradiation is given in fewer, higher doses than EBRT.

Many types of technology to deliver partial-breast irradiation are under development. In a randomized phase III clinical trial called TARGIT-A, researchers compared partial-breast irradiation given during surgery (i.e., intraoperatively) with standard whole-breast EBRT for women receiving BCS for invasive breast cancer.

The Study

Researchers from nine countries randomly assigned 1,113 women to receive a single dose of approximately 20 Gy of intraoperative partial breast irradiation using a device called the Intrabeam and 1,119 to receive whole-breast EBRT at a dose of 40 Gy to 56 Gy (gray) given in a total of 15 to 25 fractions (with an optional booster dose at the end of treatment). All participating doctors received special training in the use of the Intrabeam device.

All of the women were 45 years of age or older and eligible for BCS for a single invasive tumor. The trial was restricted to patients with ductal carcinoma; patients with lobular carcinoma, which has a higher risk of recurrence, were excluded. However, some patients in the intraoperative treatment group (about 15 percent) were found to have lobular carcinoma or other high-risk disease during surgery, and these patients later received additional EBRT. Women in both groups received hormone therapy and chemotherapy as needed.

The women returned for initial follow-up visits three and six months after treatment, after which they were scheduled for assessment every six months for up to five years and then annually for up to 10 years. The primary outcome was local cancer recurrence in the same breast. The trial was a non-inferiority trial, which means that it aimed to show that intraoperative partial breast irradiation did not result in worse outcomes than standard EBRT. The researchers also recorded side effects from both treatments.

The study was led by Dr. Jayant S. Vaidya from the Research Department of Surgery, University College London, in the United Kingdom and was published online in *Lancet*, June 4, 2010.

Results

Most women participating in TARGIT-A had small tumors: 36 percent had tumors smaller than 1 cm in diameter (about the size of a pencil eraser) and 50 percent had tumors of between 1 cm and 2 cm in diameter. Only 14 percent of the women had tumors that were larger than 2 cm in diameter. The majority of tumors were of low grade, and in more than 80 percent of the women cancer had not spread to any lymph nodes.

After four years of follow-up, only five women in the EBRT group and six in the intraoperative partial-breast irradiation group had experienced a local recurrence of their cancer—a nearly identical rate. This result indicates that intraoperative partial breast irradiation was not inferior to standard EBRT in this trial.

The occurrence of side effects was also similar between the two groups. Women who underwent intraoperative partial-breast irradiation had more instances of wound seroma (development of fluid pockets at the site of surgery) requiring frequent drainage, but major complications related to radiation therapy were more common in the EBRT group.

Limitations

Dr. Bhadrasain Vikram, Chief of NCI's Clinical Radiation Oncology Branch, noted that these results cannot be generalized to other types of partial-breast irradiation. "If you want these results, you have to use this device and this treatment schedule," he said. Other clinical trials, including one by the National Surgical Adjuvant Breast and Bowel Project, are currently comparing different methods of partial-breast irradiation with standard EBRT.

In addition, explained Dr. Vikram, partial-breast irradiation is not appropriate for every patient with invasive ductal breast carcinoma. The overwhelming majority of patients in this trial had small tumors that were estrogen-receptor positive and no cancer spread to the lymph nodes. Therefore, that's the group of patients that this technique would be most applicable to. Giving this regimen to patients who don't meet that profile would be somewhat risky, because we don't know if partial-breast irradiation would be adequate for preventing recurrence.

Comments

The risk of local recurrence in patients receiving BCS followed by EBRT is highest in the second and third years after treatment. Because the local recurrence rate was similar in the two groups in this trial and no local recurrences were seen in either group during the fourth year of follow-up, the authors conclude that their trial "provides robust and mature evidence that substantiates previous findings showing that targeted intraoperative radiotherapy is safe," stated the authors. "These results challenge . . . that whole-breast radiotherapy is necessary in this group of patients," they concluded.

This trial may be particularly relevant to women over the age of 70 with early-stage breast cancer, said Dr. Vikram. Another recent clinical trial suggested that the inconvenience of EBRT may outweigh its benefits for these women. However, "for those patients, intraoperative partial-breast irradiation would be almost ideal, because treatment would be over by the time they woke up from anesthesia, and they wouldn't have to come back for weeks and weeks of radiation treatment," he explained.

But younger patients would also benefit, he concluded. "This technique takes out the hassle factor from radiation therapy and allows a patient to preserve her breast and not have to worry about recurrence. Appropriate patients would definitely benefit from using this technique versus skipping radiation altogether."

Section 10.2

Invasive Lobular Carcinoma

What is invasive lobular carcinoma (ILC)?

Invasive lobular carcinoma, also known as infiltrating lobular carcinoma, is a type of breast cancer that starts in a lobule and spreads to surrounding breast tissue. If not treated at an early stage, ILC also can move into other parts of the body, such as the uterus or ovaries. ILC is the second most common type of invasive breast cancer, accounting for 10 to 15 percent of all breast cancer cases.

Who is most likely to have ILC?

Women between the ages of 45 and 56 are most likely to have ILC. Less than 10 percent of women with breast cancer have a family history of the disease. Other factors increasing the risk of having breast cancer include having no children or the first child after age 30, early menstruation, and consuming three or more alcoholic drinks a day.

What characterizes ILC?

ILC is characterized by a general thickening of an area of the breast, usually the section above the nipple and toward the arm. You may not be able to feel a breast lump or hard mass. Instead, an area of breast tissue may only feel differently than the rest of your breast. ILC also is less likely to appear on a mammogram. When it does appear, it may show as a mass with fine spikes radiating from the edges or appear as an asymmetry compared to the other breast.

How does the pathologist make a diagnosis?

The pathologist examines a biopsy specimen, along with other tests if necessary. A biopsy is the most widely used method for detecting ILC breast cancer. During a biopsy procedure, the surgeon removes cells or tissues from the suspicious area for the pathologist to examine more closely in the laboratory. In some cases, a biopsy may be performed with surgery. The surgeon removes all or part of the tumor for the pathologist to examine.

Laboratory testing enables the pathologist to determine the type of cancer and whether it is invasive. The pathologist examines the tissue sample under a microscope and assigns a histologic type and histologic tumor grade to it. Grade 1 cancers tend to grow the slowest, while Grade 3 tumors spread more aggressively. The pathologist also notes the size of the tumor, how close the cancer is to the edge of the tissue removed by the surgeon, and whether the tumor invaded blood or lymphatic vessels. These factors help pathologists determine the likelihood of the cancer remaining in or returning to the affected area.

What else does the pathologist look for?

The biopsy sample is tested for the presence of estrogen (ER) and progesterone receptors (PgR) using a method called immunohistochemistry, or IHC. Women with cancers containing these receptors are more likely to respond positively to hormonal therapy such as tamoxifen. If breast cancer cells have estrogen receptors, the cancer is called ER-positive breast cancer. If breast cancer cells have progesterone receptors, the cancer is called PgR-positive breast cancer. About 75 percent to 80 percent of breast cancers are ER- and/or PgR-positive. Low-grade cancers are even more likely to be ER- and/The College of American Pathology (CAP) and the American Society of Clinical Oncology (ASCO) have issued a joint guideline aimed at improving the accuracy of IHC testing for the presence of ER and PgR in breast cancer.

Pathologists also may check for a protein called HER2 [human epidermal growth factor receptor 2]. There is also a guideline developed by the CAP and ASCO in 2007 that details how this test should be done so that it will be accurate and reproducible. Laboratories doing testing for HER2 should be following these guidelines. The recommendations are very similar to the new ER and PgR recommendations. Cancers with too much HER2 are very likely to respond to targeted therapy with trastuzumab or lapatinib. Due to continual advances in research, other tests may be used as well.

After reviewing the results of the laboratory tests, your clinician may recommend additional tests to determine to what extent malignant cells may have spread to other parts of the body.

Depending on your situation, these tests may include a chest x-ray; a bone scan; and imaging tests including computed tomography (CT), magnetic resonance imaging (MRI), or PET (positron emission tomography). All these tests can detect signs that the cancer may have spread to other parts of the body.

By completing necessary tests, pathologists determine the cancer's stage. Stage 1 ILC tumors are confined to the breast, and Stage 4 tumors spread beyond areas near the breast. Stages 2 and 3 describe conditions between these two extremes.

How do doctors determine what surgery or treatment will be necessary?

The pathologist consults with your primary physician after reviewing the test results and determining the cancer's stage. Together, using their combined experience and knowledge, they determine treatment options most appropriate for your condition.

What kinds of treatments are available for ILC?

ILC is treated through one or more of the following: Surgery, chemotherapy, hormonal therapy, and radiation therapy. It's important to learn as much as you can about your treatment options and to make the right decision.

Most women choose surgery. Advancements in surgical techniques have enabled about 70 percent of women to choose breast-conserving surgical treatments like lumpectomy rather than mastectomy, where the entire breast and often some or all lymph nodes near the breast are removed. Mastectomy reduces the chances the cancer will return. Lumpectomy is an option when the cancer is in a relatively small part of one breast. How far your tumor has grown and advanced will determine if breast-conserving treatments are possible. If your breast cannot be conserved, breast reconstruction surgery may be a possibility after you recover from your initial operation to remove the cancer.

Most women with invasive breast cancer will be offered chemotherapy and/or hormonal therapy. Chemotherapy drugs kill rapidly dividing tumor cells that may be spreading through the body, reducing the risk of the cancer coming back in another body site. Drugs affecting hormone responsiveness also kill tumor cells, which require hormones to grow, and prevent these cells from spreading or coming back. Drugs targeting HER2 receptor specifically kill cells having large amounts of this protein and prevent these cells from spreading or coming back. Radiation therapy is used to rid the body of any microscopic remnants of the cancer in the area where the original tumor was found and removed.

Clinical trials of new treatments for ILC may be found at www.cancer.gov/clinicaltrials. These treatments are highly experimental in nature but may be an option for advanced cancers.

For more information, go to www.cancer.org (American Cancer Society), www.y-me.org (Y-ME National Breast Cancer Organization), or www.cancer.net (American Society of Clinical Oncology).

What kinds of questions should I ask my doctors?

Ask any question you want. There are no questions you should be reluctant to ask. Here are a few to consider:

- Please describe the type of cancer I have and what treatment options are available.
- What stage is the cancer?
- What are the chances for full remission?
- What treatment options do you recommend? Why do you believe these are the best treatments?
- What are the pros and cons of these treatment options?
- What are the side effects?
- Is your medical team experienced in treating the type of cancer I have?
- Can you provide me with information about the physicians and others on the medical team?
- Is the laboratory doing the testing for my cancer following the new guidelines for the ER, PgR, and HER2 tests?

Chapter 11

Medullary Breast Carcinoma

What Is Medullary Breast Cancer?

Medullary breast cancer is a rare type of breast cancer that accounts for around 3–5% of all breast cancers. It can occur at any age and is more common in women who inherit a faulty copy of the BRCA1 gene [breast cancer gene 1].

Medullary breast cancer can also occur in men but this is very rare.

It is an invasive type of cancer, which means it has spread from the ducts into the surrounding breast tissue and has the potential to spread to other parts of the body, although this is not common with this type of breast cancer.

Medullary breast cancer will usually have a clear, well-defined border between the cancer and the breast tissue that surrounds it when looked at under a microscope. This is one feature which pathologists (doctors who examine tissue removed during a biopsy or surgery) use to distinguish it from the much more common invasive ductal cancer (also known as no special type).

Other features of medullary breast cancer are that the individual cancer cells are often large and variable in size and shape. Pathologists will often also find lymphocytes (white blood cells) within and surrounding a medullary cancer.

Excerpted from "Medullary breast cancer fact sheet," © Breast Cancer Care, 2012. All rights reserved. Reprinted with permission. To view the complete text of this fact sheet and additional information, visit www.breastcancercare.org.uk.

Although each case is different, the outlook for medullary breast cancer is often thought to be better than for other more common types of invasive breast cancer.

How Is Medullary Breast Cancer Diagnosed?

Medullary breast cancer is diagnosed in the same way as other breast cancers. Investigations include a mammogram (breast x-ray) and/or an ultrasound scan, followed by a fine needle aspiration (FNA) and/or core biopsy.

How Is Medullary Breast Cancer Treated?

Medullary cancer is treated in a similar way to other types of breast cancer. As with all types of breast cancer, certain features of medullary breast cancer will affect what treatments might be offered. Breast surgery is often the first treatment for breast cancer. This may be breast-conserving surgery (usually referred to as wide local excision or lumpectomy), and is the removal of the cancer with a margin (border) of normal breast tissue around it, or a mastectomy (removal of all the breast tissue including the nipple area). The amount of tissue removed depends on the size of the cancer and the size of your breast. Your breast surgeon will discuss this with you.

If you are going to have a mastectomy, you will usually be able to consider breast reconstruction. This can be done at the same time as your mastectomy (known as immediate reconstruction) or at a later date some time in the future (known as delayed reconstruction).

Your doctors will also want to check whether breast cancer cells have spread from the breast to the lymph nodes (glands) under the arm (the axilla), although this is less common with medullary breast cancer than with other, more common, types of breast cancer. This helps them decide whether you will benefit from additional treatment after surgery.

To see whether or not any of the lymph nodes under the arm are affected, your breast surgeon may wish to remove some (lymph node sample) or all of them (lymph node clearance) during breast surgery. Another way of checking the lymph nodes under the arm is called sentinel node biopsy. This identifies whether or not the first lymph node (or nodes) is clear of cancer cells. If it is, this usually means the other nodes are clear too, so no more will need to be removed. However, sentinel node biopsy is not appropriate for everyone and your surgeon will discuss whether or not this procedure is an option for you.

What Are the Adjuvant (Additional) Treatments?

After surgery you are likely to need further medical treatment. This is called adjuvant (additional) therapy and includes chemotherapy, radiotherapy, hormone therapy, and targeted therapy.

The aim of these treatments is to reduce the risk of breast cancer cells returning in the same breast or the opposite breast or spreading somewhere else in the body.

Radiotherapy

If you have breast-conserving surgery, you will usually be given radiotherapy to reduce the risk of the breast cancer returning in the same breast. Radiotherapy may also be given to the chest wall following a mastectomy in some circumstances, for example, if a number of lymph nodes in the armpit are affected.

Chemotherapy

For some people, chemotherapy (anti-cancer drugs which aim to destroy cancer cells) is recommended. Whether you are offered chemotherapy will depend on various features of the cancer such as its size and grade (how different the cells look under the microscope compared to normal cells and how quickly they are growing) and whether or not the lymph nodes are affected.

Hormone (Endocrine) Therapy

As the female hormone estrogen can play a part in stimulating some breast cancers to grow, there are a number of hormone therapies that work in different ways to block the effect of estrogen on cancer cells.

Hormone therapy will only be prescribed if your breast cancer has receptors within the cell that bind to the female hormone estrogen and stimulate the cancer to grow (known as estrogen receptor positive or ER+ breast cancer). All breast cancers are tested for estrogen receptors using tissue from a biopsy or after surgery.

If your cancer is estrogen receptor positive, your doctors will discuss with you which hormone therapy they think is most appropriate.

When estrogen receptors are not found (estrogen receptor negative or ER- breast cancer) tests may be done for progesterone (another female hormone) receptors. As estrogen receptors play a more important role than progesterone receptors, the benefits of hormone therapy are less clear for people whose breast cancer is only progesterone receptor positive (PR+ and ER-). If this is the case, your specialist will discuss with you whether hormone therapy is appropriate.

Medullary breast cancer is more likely to be ER-. If this is the case, then hormone therapy will not be of any benefit to you.

Targeted Therapies

This group of drugs works by blocking specific ways that breast cancer cells divide and grow. The most well-known targeted therapy is trastuzumab (Herceptin) but the benefits of others are being looked at in clinical trials so it is likely more targeted therapies will become available in the future. Only people whose cancer has high levels of HER2 [human epidermal growth factor receptor 2], a protein that makes cancer cells grow, will benefit from having trastuzumab.

Various tests to measure HER2 levels can be done on breast tissue removed by biopsy or during surgery. If your cancer is found to be HER2 negative, then trastuzumab will not be of benefit to you. Medullary breast cancer tends to be HER2 negative, meaning that trastuzumab will not have any benefit.

Some breast cancers are HER2 and estrogen receptor negative (known as triple negative breast cancer when progesterone receptors are also negative). This is quite common in medullary breast cancer. If you have triple negative breast cancer, you may feel concerned that you are not able to have treatments such as trastuzumab or hormone therapy. However, people diagnosed with medullary breast cancer often have a better prognosis (outlook) than people with other types of breast cancer.

Further Support

Being told you have breast cancer can be a very anxious, frightening, and sometimes isolating time. It can be particularly difficult to be diagnosed with a rare type of breast cancer such as medullary breast cancer, as you may not meet any other people with exactly the same diagnosis as you.

There are people who can support you so don't be afraid to ask for help if you need it. You can let other people know how you are feeling, particularly your family and friends, so that they can be more supportive. Some people find it helpful to discuss their feelings and concerns with their breast care nurse or specialist. If you feel you'd like to talk through your feelings and concerns in more depth over time, a counselor or psychologist may be appropriate. Your breast care nurse, specialist, or health care provider can arrange this.

You may also find it helpful to talk to someone who has had a similar experience to you. You can do this one-to-one or in a support group.

Chapter 12

Inflammatory Breast Cancer

What is inflammatory breast cancer (IBC)?

Inflammatory breast cancer is a rare but very aggressive type of breast cancer in which the cancer cells block the lymph vessels in the skin of the breast. This type of breast cancer is called "inflammatory" because the breast often looks swollen and red, or "inflamed." IBC accounts for 1 to 5 percent of all breast cancer cases in the United States. It tends to be diagnosed in younger women compared to non-IBC breast cancer. It occurs more frequently and at a younger age in African Americans than in Whites. Like other types of breast cancer, IBC can occur in men, but usually at an older age than in women. Some studies have shown an association between family history of breast cancer and IBC, but more studies are needed to draw firm conclusions.

What are the symptoms of IBC?

Symptoms of IBC may include redness, swelling, and warmth in the breast, often without a distinct lump in the breast. The redness and warmth are caused by cancer cells blocking the lymph vessels in the skin. The skin of the breast may also appear pink, reddish purple, or bruised. The skin may also have ridges or appear pitted, like the skin of

Excerpted from "Inflammatory Breast Cancer: Questions and Answers," by the National Cancer Institute (NCI, www.cancer.gov), part of the National Institutes of Health, August 29, 2006. Reviewed by David A. Cooke, MD, FACP, February 12, 2012.

an orange (called peau d'orange), which is caused by a buildup of fluid and edema (swelling) in the breast. Other symptoms include heaviness, burning, aching, increase in breast size, tenderness, or a nipple that is inverted (facing inward). These symptoms usually develop quickly—over a period of weeks or months. Swollen lymph nodes may also be present under the arm, above the collarbone, or in both places. However, it is important to note that these symptoms may also be signs of other conditions such as infection, injury, or other types of cancer.

How is IBC diagnosed?

Diagnosis of IBC is based primarily on the results of a doctor's clinical examination. Biopsy, mammogram, and breast ultrasound are used to confirm the diagnosis. IBC is classified as either stage IIIB or stage IV breast cancer. Stage IIIB breast cancers are locally advanced; stage IV breast cancer is cancer that has spread to other organs. IBC tends to grow rapidly, and the physical appearance of the breast of patients with IBC is different from that of patients with other stage III breast cancers. IBC is an especially aggressive, locally advanced breast cancer.

Cancer staging describes the extent or severity of an individual's cancer. Knowing a cancer's stage helps the doctor develop a treatment plan and estimate prognosis (the likely outcome or course of the disease; the chance of recovery or recurrence).

How is IBC treated?

Treatment consisting of chemotherapy, targeted therapy, surgery, radiation therapy, and hormonal therapy is used to treat IBC. Patients may also receive supportive care to help manage the side effects of the cancer and its treatment. Chemotherapy (anticancer drugs) is generally the first treatment for patients with IBC, and is called neoadjuvant therapy. Chemotherapy is systemic treatment, which means that it affects cells throughout the body. The purpose of chemotherapy is to control or kill cancer cells, including those that may have spread to other parts of the body.

After chemotherapy, patients with IBC may undergo surgery and radiation therapy to the chest wall. Both radiation and surgery are local treatments that affect only cells in the tumor and the immediately surrounding area. The purpose of surgery is to remove the tumor from the body, while the purpose of radiation therapy is to destroy remaining cancer cells. Surgery to remove the breast (or as much of the breast tissue as possible) is called a mastectomy. Lymph node dissection (removal of the lymph nodes in the underarm area for examination under a microscope) is also done during this surgery.

After initial systemic and local treatment, patients with IBC may receive additional systemic treatments to reduce the risk of recurrence (cancer coming back). Such treatments may include additional chemotherapy, hormonal therapy (treatment that interferes with the effects of the female hormone estrogen, which can promote the growth of breast cancer cells), targeted therapy (such as trastuzumab, also known as Herceptin), or all three. Trastuzumab is administered to patients whose tumors overexpress the HER2 (human epidermal growth factor receptor 2) tumor protein.

Supportive care is treatment given to improve the quality of life of patients who have a serious or life-threatening disease, such as cancer. It prevents or treats as early as possible the symptoms of the disease, side effects caused by treatment of the disease, and psychological, social, and spiritual problems related to the disease or its treatment. For example, compression garments may be used to treat lymphedema (swelling caused by excess fluid buildup) resulting from radiation therapy or the removal of lymph nodes. Additionally, meeting with a social worker, counselor, or member of the clergy can be helpful to those who want to talk about their feelings or discuss their concerns. A social worker can often suggest resources for help with recovery, emotional support, financial aid, transportation, or home care.

Are clinical trials (research studies with people) available? Where can people get more information about clinical trials?

Yes. The NCI is sponsoring clinical trials that are designed to find new treatments and better ways to use current treatments. Before any new treatment can be recommended for general use, doctors conduct clinical trials to find out whether the treatment is safe for patients and effective against the disease. Participation in clinical trials is a treatment option for many patients with IBC, and all patients with IBC are encouraged to consider treatment in a clinical trial.

People interested in taking part in a clinical trial should talk with their doctor. Information about clinical trials is available at www.cancer.gov/clinicaltrials.

What is the prognosis for patients with IBC?

Prognosis describes the likely course and outcome of a disease— that is, the chance that a patient will recover or have a recurrence.

IBC is more likely to have metastasized (spread to other areas of the body) at the time of diagnosis than non-IBC cases. As a result, the five-year survival rate for patients with IBC is between 25 and 50 percent, which is significantly lower than the survival rate for patients with non-IBC breast cancer. It is important to keep in mind, however, that these statistics are averages based on large numbers of patients. Statistics cannot be used to predict what will happen to a particular patient because each person's situation is unique. Patients are encouraged to talk to their doctors about their prognosis given their particular situation.

Chapter 13

Paget Disease of the Nipple

What is Paget disease of the nipple?

Paget disease of the nipple, also called Paget disease of the breast, is an uncommon type of cancer that forms in or around the nipple. More than 95 percent of people with Paget disease of the nipple also have underlying breast cancer; however, Paget disease of the nipple accounts for less than 5 percent of all breast cancers. For instance, of the 211,240 new cases of breast cancer projected to be diagnosed in 2005, fewer than 11,000 will also involve Paget disease of the nipple.

Most patients diagnosed with Paget disease of the nipple are over age 50, but rare cases have been diagnosed in patients in their 20s. The average age at diagnosis is 62 for women and 69 for men. The disease is rare among both women and men.

Paget disease of the nipple was named after Sir James Paget, a scientist who noted an association between changes in the appearance of the nipple and underlying breast cancer. There are several other unrelated diseases named after Paget, including Paget disease of the bone and Paget disease of the vulva; this text discusses only Paget disease of the nipple.

What are the possible causes of Paget disease of the nipple?

Scientists do not know exactly what causes Paget disease of the nipple, but two major theories have been suggested for how it develops.

Excerpted from "Paget Disease of the Nipple," by the National Cancer Institute (NCI, www.cancer.gov), part of the National Institutes of Health, June 27, 2005. Reviewed by David A. Cooke, MD, FACP, February 12, 2012.

One theory proposes that cancer cells, called Paget cells, break off from a tumor inside the breast and move through the milk ducts to the surface of the nipple, resulting in Paget disease of the nipple. This theory is supported by the fact that more than 97 percent of patients with Paget disease also have underlying invasive breast cancer or ductal carcinoma in situ (DCIS). DCIS, also called intraductal carcinoma, is a condition in which abnormal cells are present only in the lining of the milk ducts in the breast, and have not invaded surrounding tissue or spread to the lymph nodes. DCIS sometimes becomes invasive breast cancer. Invasive breast cancer is cancer that has spread outside the duct into the breast tissue, and possibly into the lymph nodes under the arm or into other parts of the body.

The other theory suggests that skin cells of the nipple spontaneously become Paget cells. This theory is supported by the rare cases of Paget disease in which there is no underlying breast cancer, and the cases in which the underlying breast cancer is found to be a separate tumor from the Paget disease.

What are the symptoms of Paget disease of the nipple?

Symptoms of early Paget disease of the nipple include redness and mild scaling and flaking of the nipple skin. Early symptoms may cause only mild irritation and may not be enough to prompt a visit to the doctor. Improvement in the skin can occur spontaneously, but this should not be taken as a sign that the disease has disappeared. More advanced disease may show more serious destruction of the skin. At this stage, the symptoms may include tingling, itching, increased sensitivity, burning, and pain. There may also be discharge from the nipple, and the nipple can appear flattened against the breast.

In approximately half of patients with Paget disease of the nipple, a lump or mass in the breast can be felt during physical examination. In most cases, Paget disease of the nipple is initially confined to the nipple, later spreading to the areola or other regions of the breast. The areola is the circular area of darker skin that surrounds the nipple. Paget disease of the nipple can also be found only on the areola, where it may resemble eczema, a noncancerous itchy red rash. Although rare, Paget disease of the nipple can occur in both breasts.

How is Paget disease of the nipple diagnosed?

If a health care provider suspects Paget disease of the nipple, a biopsy of the nipple skin is performed. In a biopsy, the doctor removes a small sample of tissue. A pathologist examines the tissue under a microscope to see if Paget cells are present. The pathologist may use a technique called immunohistochemistry (staining tissues to identify specific cells) to differentiate Paget cells from other cell types. A sample of nipple discharge may also be examined under a microscope for the presence of Paget cells.

Because most people with Paget disease of the nipple also have underlying breast cancer, physical examination and mammography (x-ray of the breast) are used to make a complete diagnosis.

How is Paget disease of the nipple treated?

Surgery is the most common treatment for Paget disease of the nipple. The specific treatment often depends on the characteristics of the underlying breast cancer.

A modified radical mastectomy may be recommended when invasive cancer or extensive DCIS has been diagnosed. In this operation, the surgeon removes the breast, the lining over the chest muscles, and some of the lymph nodes under the arm. In cases where underlying breast cancer is not invasive, the surgeon may perform a simple mastectomy to remove only the breast and the lining over the chest muscles.

Alternatively, patients whose disease is confined to the nipple and the surrounding area may undergo breast-conserving surgery or lumpectomy followed by radiation therapy. During breast-conserving surgery, the surgeon removes the nipple, areola, and the entire portion of the breast believed to contain the cancer. In most cases, radiation therapy is also used to help prevent recurrence (return of the cancer).

During surgery, particularly modified radical mastectomy, the doctor may perform an axillary node dissection to remove the lymph nodes under the arm. The lymph nodes are then examined to see if the cancer has spread to them. In some cases, a sentinel lymph node biopsy may be performed to remove only one or a few lymph nodes.

Adjuvant treatment (treatment that is given in addition to surgery to prevent the cancer from coming back) may be part of the treatment plan, depending on the type of cancer and whether cancer cells have spread to the lymph nodes. Radiation treatment is a common adjuvant therapy for Paget disease of the nipple following breast-conserving surgery. Adjuvant treatment with anticancer drugs or hormone therapies may also be recommended, depending on the extent of the disease and prognostic factors (estimated chance of recovery from the disease or chance that the disease will recur).

Chapter 14

Triple-Negative Breast Cancer

What is triple-negative breast cancer? About 10 to 20 percent of breast cancers are triple-negative, but you may never have heard of triple-negative breast cancer before you received your test results.

Hearing new words and not understanding what they mean may make you feel scared and overwhelmed.

Knowing breast cancer basics can help you understand how triple-negative breast cancer is different from other types of breast cancer.

To find out what type of breast cancer you have, your doctors search for the presence or absence of three receptors, proteins that live inside or on the surface of a cell and bind to something in the body to cause the cell to react. You may have heard of the estrogen receptor (ER), progesterone receptor (PR), and human epidermal growth factor receptor 2 (HER2).

In estrogen receptor-positive breast cancer, progesterone receptor-positive breast cancer and HER2 positive breast cancer, treatments prevent, slow, or stop cancer growth with medicines that target those receptors. But triple-negative breast cancers need different types of treatments because they are estrogen receptor-negative, progesterone receptor negative, and HER2 negative. Medicines like tamoxifen, which targets the estrogen receptor, and trastuzumab (Herceptin), which targets HER2, are not helpful in treating triple-negative breast cancer. Instead, chemotherapy has been shown to be the most effective treatment for triple-negative breast cancer.

Researchers are working to improve their understanding of the biology of triple-negative breast cancers, how these types of cancers behave, and what puts people at risk for them. Their goals are to find out the best ways to use treatments that already exist and to develop new ones.

Understanding the Basal-Like Subtype

Most triple-negative breast cancers have a basal-like cell pattern. This term means the cells look like the basal cells that line the breast ducts, the tubes in the breast where milk travels.

You might have heard your doctor call triple-negative breast cancer a basal tumor, basal breast cancer, or basal-like disease.

Basal-like breast cancers tend to overexpress, or make too much of, certain genes that encourage cancer growth. Not all triple-negative breast cancers are basal-like, and not all basal-like breast cancers are triple-negative. About 70 to 90 percent of triple-negative breast cancers are basal-like.

Doctors choose treatments because the cancer is triple-negative, not because it is basal-like. The basal status of the cancer does not factor into treatment decisions, but your doctor may tell you if the cancer is basal-like because the term appears in breast cancer resources and information.

Three Myths about Triple-Negative Breast Cancer

Myth: Women with triple-negative breast cancer can have the same treatments as all other women with breast cancer.

Fact: Many people do not understand that there are different kinds of breast cancer. Even some women who have had breast cancer do not understand the differences between triple-negative breast cancers and breast cancers that are hormone receptor-positive or HER2 positive.

Women you meet may have taken a hormonal treatment pill for five years to protect them from recurrence (a return of the cancer), or they may know someone who has. These women may not understand that this option does not exist for you. Having to explain the differences between triple-negative and other breast cancers can be frustrating, especially if you are just learning about this diagnosis yourself. On the other hand, you may take some of the same chemotherapy medicines as women with other types of breast cancer.

Myth: Triple-negative breast cancers are always hard to treat.

Fact: Your doctor may tell you triple-negative breast cancer is harder to treat than other types of breast cancer. While many triple-negative cancers are aggressive, your doctor's prediction of how well your treatment will work depends on the tumor size and whether the cancer has traveled to the lymph nodes in your armpit just as much as it does on its triple-negative status. There are some very effective treatments for triple-negative breast cancer. Your doctor will work with you to find the treatment that is right for you.

Myth: Only African-American women get triple-negative breast cancer.

Fact: Triple-negative breast cancers affect women of all races. Breast cancers in African-American women are more likely to be triple-negative than those in white women.

Triple-Negative Breast Cancer Risk Factors

Researchers are still learning why some women are more likely than others to develop triple-negative breast cancer. Research supports a relationship between risk and your genes, age, race, and ethnicity.

Breast Cancer Gene Mutations

Everyone has BRCA1 and BRCA2 genes [breast cancer gene 1 and breast cancer gene 2], which we get from our mother and father. When they work properly, these genes prevent the development of cancers. However, less than 10 percent of people with breast cancer are born with a mutation, or abnormality, in BRCA1 or BRCA2.

If you are born with a BRCA1 or BRCA2 gene mutation, you are at increased risk for developing breast, ovarian, and other cancers throughout your life. The BRCA1 mutation puts you at higher risk for developing a basal-like breast cancer. Scientists are still trying to find out why BRCA1 mutations increase the risk of developing triple-negative breast cancer. Keep in mind, not all breast cancers from BRCA mutations are triple-negative. In fact, BRCA2 mutations are more likely to be present in estrogen receptor-positive breast cancer.

If you have a family history of breast cancer, you and your relatives could carry a BRCA1 or BRCA2 mutation. You could also be the first person in your family known to develop breast cancer because of a BRCA mutation. Knowing your BRCA status can help you and your doctors discuss an effective treatment plan and learn ways to reduce your risk for recurrence. A genetic counselor can talk with you about genetic testing.

Age, Race, or Ethnicity

Several studies suggest that being premenopausal, African-American, Latina, or Caribbean increases your risk of developing basal-like or triple-negative breast cancer. Among African-American women who develop breast cancer, there is an estimated 20 to 40 percent chance of the breast cancer being triple-negative.

Researchers do not yet understand why premenopausal women and women in some ethnic groups have higher rates of triple-negative breast cancer than other groups of women.

Common Treatments for Triple-Negative Breast Cancer

Doctors use the same tests and surgeries to figure out treatments for triple-negative breast cancers as they do for other kinds of breast cancer. Your treatment will be based on whether the cancer has traveled to the lymph nodes near your breast, the size of the main tumor and details of pathology tests such as the tumor grade, which shows how quickly the cancer cells are dividing.

With early-stage disease, you are likely to have some type of surgery and chemotherapy; you also may have radiation.

Surgery

Your doctor will recommend some type of surgery, with the goal of removing the cancer from your breast. The two types of surgery for breast cancer are lumpectomy and mastectomy.

In lumpectomy, also called breast-conserving surgery, the surgeon removes the tumor plus a small rim of normal tissue around the tumor, called a margin.

Radiation therapy usually is given after lumpectomy. Sometimes radiation is needed after mastectomy.

Your doctor may recommend mastectomy, or removal of the entire breast, if:

- you have multiple tumors in the breast;
- the cancer is in your skin;
- the tumor is in the nipple area;
- you had cancer before in the same breast;

- you have a large tumor;
- you have calcifications (calcium deposits) or other abnormal cells over a large area of your breast.

You do not have to have a mastectomy just because you have triple-negative breast cancer.

Your surgeon should explain which surgery you need and the reasons why. In many cases, lumpectomy and mastectomy work equally well.

If you have a choice, know that studies show lumpectomy followed by radiation therapy works as well as mastectomy in treating breast cancers similar to yours.

As you consider your options, think about how this decision will impact your emotions, lifestyle, and practical needs. Ask yourself if you can accept losing your breast or if you can manage weeks of radiation after surgery if you keep your breast. Will keeping your breast impact your fear of recurrence? If you're interested, explore your breast reconstruction options. Consider talking it over with someone on the LBBC Survivors' Helpline (888-753-LBBC [753-5222]) who has made the same decision.

If you have a BRCA mutation, you may discuss with your doctors the option of removing both breasts. Depending on where you are in your life and whether you want to have biological children, you also may consider removing your ovaries to reduce your risk of ovarian cancer. Your doctor can help you understand how these decisions impact your treatment and quality of life.

Chemotherapy

You are likely to receive chemotherapy, medicine that kills cancer cells everywhere in your body.

This type of treatment is called systemic, or whole-body, therapy, and it may be given by vein or in some cases by pill. The goal of chemotherapy is to prevent metastasis, when breast cancer comes back and spreads to other parts of the body. A metastatic recurrence occurs when cancer cells travel away from the breast and start growing in other organs such as the bones, liver, lungs, or brain.

Chemotherapy may be given before or after surgery. If you have a tumor that is very large or you have a sizable tumor and want a lumpectomy, your doctor may recommend chemotherapy before surgery, also called neoadjuvant therapy. This therapy shrinks the tumor and helps your doctor learn how sensitive the tumor is to chemotherapy.

Chemotherapy is the most effective treatment for triple-negative breast cancer. The reason is that chemotherapy works better than other treatments at killing cancer cells that divide quickly, which is very common in triple-negative disease. When triple-negative breast cancers are found early, response rates to chemotherapy are high. Doctors try to lessen the chance of a metastatic recurrence by treating the whole body, including any areas where very tiny cancer cells may have traveled.

Often, the chemotherapy that you receive will be the same type given to women with hormone receptor-positive or HER2 positive breast cancer.

Studies show chemotherapy works better against triple-negative cancers than hormone receptor positive breast cancers. There are many types of chemotherapy, and you and your doctor will choose the best one for you.

In rare cases, you might not receive chemotherapy; for example, if you have a very low-grade tumor (the cancer cells are not dividing quickly), if the tumor is very small, or if the risks of chemotherapy outweigh the benefits. Because chemotherapy is a common treatment for triple-negative breast cancer, always ask your doctor to explain the reasons why you would not receive it.

Common Chemotherapies for Early-Stage, Triple-Negative Breast Cancer

AC: One common treatment for triple-negative breast cancer is doxorubicin (Adriamycin) with cyclophosphamide (Cytoxan), also known as AC chemotherapy. Adriamycin belongs to a family of medicines called anthracyclines, which work by stopping cancer cell growth and repair.

Cytoxan is in the family of alkylating agents that halt fast-growing cells.

FEC and FAC (or CAF): Some doctors give another medicine, fluorouracil (5FU), in addition to AC, and the regimen is called FAC or CAF. Sometimes a medicine called epirubicin (Ellence) is given in place of doxorubicin. Similar regimens with epirubicin are called FEC, CEF, or EC.

These combinations work by stopping the function of cancer cells and limiting cell division and growth.

Taxanes: Often, taxanes are given alongside or after AC or FEC. Taxanes work by blocking cell division and stopping the advance and growth of cancer cells, and they include paclitaxel (Taxol) and docetaxel

(Taxotere). When Taxol or Taxotere is added to AC, the regimen may be called AC-T, AC-D, or TAC. When Taxotere is added to FEC, the regimen is called FEC-T. Your doctor may also suggest other combinations of medicines to treat triple-negative cancer.

Radiation

Radiation is a local therapy that kills any cancer cells left after surgery in the area where the breast cancer was found. It helps protect you from a local recurrence, cancer coming back in the same place.

Radiation usually is given from outside your body by an external beam. It can be given inside the body in some circumstances.

If you have a lumpectomy, you will need radiation to kill any cancer cells left in the breast and sometimes in the underarm area.

Radiation also may be given after mastectomy if your surgeon found cancer close to your chest wall or in your lymph nodes. Ask a member of your healthcare team to explain the reasons why you need the treatment.

Finding a Doctor Who Understands Triple-Negative Breast Cancer

When selecting your healthcare team, choose providers with experience treating triple-negative breast cancer. Look online for oncologists and surgeons who say they specialize in breast cancer.

Search your region for clinical trials on triple-negative breast cancer, and find the names of doctors coordinating the studies. If you do not live near a health center with a doctor specializing in triple-negative breast cancer, consider traveling outside your area for a second opinion on your treatment plan.

For Young Women

No matter what type of breast cancer you have, a diagnosis can be overwhelming, especially when you are young. It can be upsetting and disruptive when you are looking for a job or starting your career; taking classes; single, dating, or newly married; struggling with finances or raising small children.

Balancing your daily responsibilities with your treatment can be very challenging. You may wonder, "How am I going to make it through financially?" Your friends might not be able to relate to what you are going through, and at times you could feel you lack support.

If you want children, you may worry about how treatments could affect your fertility. To learn about your options, talk with your doctor before treatment begins. Try to visit a fertility specialist with experience treating people with cancer.

For ways to cope, call the LBBC Survivors' Helpline at 888-753-LBBC (753-5222) or the Triple Negative Breast Cancer Foundation Helpline at 877-880-TNBC (880-8622). LBBC and TNBCF can match you with someone in a similar situation. The websites of Young Survival Coalition at www.youngsurvival.org or LIVESTRONG at www.livestrong.org/fertilehope have information to help you.

Ten Questions to Ask Your Doctor or Nurse

1. Have you treated other women with triple-negative breast cancer?

2. Is the cancer invasive or noninvasive? What is the cancer stage? What is the cancer grade? How will these features impact treatment decisions?

3. What treatments do I need?

4. What side effects might I have? Are there ways to prevent or lessen side effects?

5. Are there long-term effects of treatment? How do those risks compare to the benefits of therapy?

6. Am I able to get treatment through a clinical trial?

7. Should I take steps to preserve my fertility now if I want to have children after treatment? What are my options?

8. Could you connect me to someone else who has been treated for triple-negative breast cancer? Do you know of support groups?

9. What can I do to protect myself from recurrence?

10. Should I speak with a genetic counselor about genetic testing?

Find more detailed questions at www.tnbcfoundation.org.

Part Three

Risk Factors, Symptoms, and Prevention of Breast Cancer

Chapter 15

Breast Cancer Risk Factors and Symptoms

Overview

When you're told that you have breast cancer, it's natural to wonder what may have caused the disease. But no one knows the exact causes of breast cancer. Doctors seldom know why one woman develops breast cancer and another doesn't.

Doctors do know that bumping, bruising, or touching the breast does not cause cancer. And breast cancer is not contagious. You can't catch it from another person.

Doctors also know that women with certain risk factors are more likely than others to develop breast cancer. A risk factor is something that may increase the chance of getting a disease.

What Are Breast Cancer Risk Factors?

Some risk factors (such as drinking alcohol) can be avoided. But most risk factors (such as having a family history of breast cancer) can't be avoided.

The text in this chapter under the heading "Overview " is excerpted from "What You Need to Know about Breast Cancer," by the National Cancer Institute (NCI, www.cancer.gov), part of the National Institutes of Health, October 15, 2009. The text in this chapter under the heading "How Do Risk Factors Apply to You?" is from "Breast Cancer—Step 2: Which Risk Factors May Apply to You?" and the text under "What to Do about Your Risk Factors" is from "Breast Cancer—Step 3: Take Action," from "Cancer Risk: Understanding the Puzzle," by the National Cancer Institute, http://understandingrisk.cancer.gov. Both documents are undated and have been reviewed by David A. Cooke, MD, FACP, April 2, 2012.

Studies have found the following risk factors for breast cancer:

- **Age:** The chance of getting breast cancer increases as you get older. Most women are over 60 years old when they are diagnosed.

- **Personal health history:** Having breast cancer in one breast increases your risk of getting cancer in your other breast. Also, having certain types of abnormal breast cells (atypical hyperplasia, lobular carcinoma in situ [LCIS], or ductal carcinoma in situ [DCIS]) increases the risk of invasive breast cancer. These conditions are found with a breast biopsy.

- **Family health history:** Your risk of breast cancer is higher if your mother, father, sister, or daughter had breast cancer. The risk is even higher if your family member had breast cancer before age 50. Having other relatives (in either your mother's or father's family) with breast cancer or ovarian cancer may also increase your risk.

- **Certain genome changes:** Changes in certain genes, such as BRCA1 or BRCA2 [breast cancer gene 1 or breast cancer gene 2], substantially increase the risk of breast cancer. Tests can sometimes show the presence of these rare, specific gene changes in families with many women who have had breast cancer, and health care providers may suggest ways to try to reduce the risk of breast cancer or to improve the detection of this disease in women who have these genetic changes. Also, researchers have found specific regions on certain chromosomes that are linked to the risk of breast cancer. If a woman has a genetic change in one or more of these regions, the risk of breast cancer may be slightly increased. The risk increases with the number of genetic changes that are found. Although these genetic changes are more common among women than BRCA1 or BRCA2, the risk of breast cancer is far lower.

- **Radiation therapy to the chest:** Women who had radiation therapy to the chest (including the breasts) before age 30 are at an increased risk of breast cancer. This includes women treated with radiation for Hodgkin lymphoma. Studies show that the younger a woman was when she received radiation treatment, the higher her risk of breast cancer later in life.

- **Reproductive and menstrual history:**
  - The older a woman is when she has her first child, the greater her chance of breast cancer.

- Women who never had children are at an increased risk of breast cancer.

- Women who had their first menstrual period before age 12 are at an increased risk of breast cancer.

- Women who went through menopause after age 55 are at an increased risk of breast cancer.

- Women who take menopausal hormone therapy for many years have an increased risk of breast cancer.

- **Race:** In the United States, breast cancer is diagnosed more often in white women than in African American/black, Hispanic/Latina, Asian/Pacific Islander, or American Indian/Alaska Native women.

- **Breast density:** Breasts appear on a mammogram (breast x-ray) as having areas of dense and fatty (not dense) tissue. Women whose mammograms show a larger area of dense tissue than the mammograms of women of the same age are at increased risk of breast cancer.

- **History of taking DES (diethylstilbestrol):** DES was given to some pregnant women in the United States between about 1940 and 1971. (It is no longer given to pregnant women.) Women who took DES during pregnancy may have a slightly increased risk of breast cancer. The possible effects on their daughters are under study.

- **Being overweight or obese after menopause:** The chance of getting breast cancer after menopause is higher in women who are overweight or obese.

- **Lack of physical activity:** Women who are physically inactive throughout life may have an increased risk of breast cancer.

- **Drinking alcohol:** Studies suggest that the more alcohol a woman drinks, the greater her risk of breast cancer.

Having a risk factor does not mean that a woman will get breast cancer. Most women who have risk factors never develop breast cancer.

Many other possible risk factors have been studied. For example, researchers are studying whether women who have a diet high in fat or who are exposed to certain substances in the environment have an increased risk of breast cancer. Researchers continue to study these and other possible risk factors.

115

What Are Breast Cancer Symptoms?

Early breast cancer usually doesn't cause symptoms. But as the tumor grows, it can change how the breast looks or feels. The common changes include the following:

- A lump or thickening in or near the breast or in the underarm area
- A change in the size or shape of the breast
- Dimpling or puckering in the skin of the breast
- A nipple turned inward into the breast
- Discharge (fluid) from the nipple, especially if it's bloody
- Scaly, red, or swollen skin on the breast, nipple, or areola (the dark area of skin at the center of the breast
- Ridges or pitting on the skin so that it looks like the skin of an orange)

You should see your health care provider about any symptom that does not go away. Most often, these symptoms are not due to cancer. Another health problem could cause them. If you have any of these symptoms, you should tell your health care provider so that the problems can be diagnosed and treated.

How Risk Factors Apply to You

Age

The chance of getting breast cancer increases as you get older. If you are over age 60, you are at greatest risk. If you have not yet gone through menopause, your risk of breast cancer is lower than for women who have gone through menopause.

Personal History of Breast Cancer

If you have had breast cancer in one breast, you have an increased risk of getting it in the other breast.

Family History of Breast Cancer

If your mother, sister, or daughter has had breast cancer (especially before age 40), your risk is higher. Having other relatives with breast cancer (on either your mother's side or your father's side) may increase your risk.

Certain Breast Changes

Breast changes occur in almost all women. You might notice different kinds of breast changes at different times of your life. Most of these changes are not cancer. However, some changes may be signs of cancer.

Genetic Alterations

Approximately 5 to 10 percent of American women who get breast cancer each year have a hereditary form of the disease. You are at increased risk for this form of the disease if the following are true:

- If your family has a history of multiple cases of breast cancer
- If your family has a history of cases of both breast and ovarian cancer
- If you have one or more family members with two primary cancers at different sites
- If you are of Ashkenazi (Eastern European) Jewish background

Menstrual History

If you began to menstruate early (before age 12), you are at increased risk. If you went through menopause late (after age 55), you are at increased risk.

Radiation Therapy to the Chest

If you had radiation therapy to the chest (including your breasts) before age 30, you may be at increased risk. The younger you were when you received the radiation treatment, the higher your risk of breast cancer later in life.

Breast Density

If you are an older woman who has dense (not fatty) tissue on a mammogram, you are at increased risk. Research has shown that women age 45 or older who have at least 75 percent dense tissue on a mammogram are at increased risk of developing breast cancer. Scientists do not completely understand the reasons for this.

DES (Diethylstilbestrol)

DES is a synthetic form of estrogen that was given to some pregnant women in the United States between about 1940 and 1971. It is no longer given to pregnant women. If you took DES during pregnancy, you have a slightly increased risk of breast cancer. This does not appear to be the case for the daughters exposed to DES when their mothers were pregnant. However, as those daughters grow older, more studies of breast cancer risk are needed.

Reproductive History

The older you were when you had your first child, the greater your risk of developing breast cancer. If you have never had children, you also are at increased risk.

Hormone Use (Such as Estrogen and Progestin)

If you have used menopausal hormones (also called hormone replacement therapy or HRT)—either estrogen alone or estrogen plus progestin—for 5 or more years after menopause, you may have an increased risk of developing breast cancer.

Here are the basic facts about menopausal hormone use. They are based on the results of a large clinical trial, called the Women's Health Initiative:

- Estrogen plus progestin (combined therapy) increases the risk of breast cancer (as well as heart disease, stroke, and blood clots).

- Women over age 65 who took the combined therapy doubled their risk of developing dementia.

- There were fewer cases of hip fractures and colon cancer among women who used the combined therapy.

Obesity after Menopause

If you are obese after menopause, you have 1.5 times the risk of developing breast cancer compared to women of a healthy weight. This risk seems to apply only to postmenopausal women who do not use menopausal hormones. Among women who use these hormones, there is no significant difference in breast cancer risk between obese women and women of a healthy weight.

Physical Inactivity

There is a strong correlation between lack of physical activity and obesity. A recent study from the Women's Health Initiative found that physical activity among postmenopausal women who walked about 30 minutes per day was associated with a 20 percent reduction of breast cancer risk. However, this reduction in risk was greatest among women who were of normal weight. For these women, physical activity was associated with a 37 percent decrease in risk. The protective effect of physical activity was not found among overweight or obese women.

Alcoholic Beverages

Having two or more drinks each day increases your risk of getting breast cancer by about 25 percent. (A drink is defined as 12 ounces of regular beer, 5 ounces of wine, or 1.5 ounces of 80-proof liquor.)

What to Do about Your Risk Factors

Age

Follow your doctor's recommendations for screening.

Personal History of Breast Cancer

Follow your doctor's recommendations for follow-up visits.

Family History of Breast Cancer

Follow your doctor's recommendations for screening.

Certain Breast Changes

See your doctor about a breast change when you have any of the following:

- A lump in or near your breast or under your arm
- Thick or firm tissue in or near your breast or under your arm
- Nipple discharge or tenderness
- A nipple pulled back (inverted) into the breast
- Itching or skin changes such as redness, scales, dimples, or puckers
- A change in breast size or shape

Genetic Alterations

There are three things you can do.

- You can consider genetic testing. It's important to think about the advantages and disadvantages of testing.

119

- You may choose to be monitored more closely for any sign of cancer. This may include more frequent mammograms, breast exams by your doctor, breast self-exams, and an ultrasound exam of the ovaries.

- You may choose to join a research study that is looking at ways to reduce cancer risk. This may entail changing your diet, reducing the amount of alcohol you drink, or trying new drugs to reduce the risk of cancer.

Menstrual History

Follow your doctor's recommendations for screening.

Radiation Therapy to the Chest

Follow your doctor's recommendations for screening.

Breast Density

Follow your doctor's recommendations for screening if you are age 45 or older and have at least 75 percent dense tissue on a mammogram.

DES (Diethylstilbestrol)

Follow your doctor's recommendations for screening and follow-up. If your daughter was exposed to DES because you received it when you were pregnant, she also should follow the doctor's screening guidelines. More studies are needed to see if DES will affect the breast cancer risk for children of women who took it.

Reproductive History

Follow your doctor's recommendations for screening.

Hormone Use (Such as Estrogen and Progestin)

If you are using menopausal hormones (also called hormone replacement therapy), you should talk to your health care provider about whether the advantages to continuing to use them outweigh the disadvantages in your case. Every woman is different.

Obesity after Menopause

This one is complex. Before menopause, if you are obese you have a lower risk of developing breast cancer than do women of a healthy weight. After menopause, if you are obese your risk of developing breast cancer is 1.5 times the risk of women of a healthy weight. But this risk applies only if you do not use menopausal hormones. Among women who use menopausal hormones, there is no significant difference in breast cancer risk between obese women and women of a healthy weight.

To date, there have been no controlled clinical trials to determine whether avoiding weight gain decreases the risk of cancer. However, many observational studies have shown that avoiding weight gain lowers the risk of postmenopausal breast cancer. There is insufficient evidence that intentional weight loss will affect cancer risk for any cancer.

Physical Inactivity

If you are a postmenopausal woman of normal weight, the Women's Health Initiative clinical trial found that increased physical activity (walking about 30 minutes per day) was associated with a 37 percent decrease in risk. This protective effect of physical activity was not found among overweight or obese women. You may want to consider increasing your physical activity for its overall health benefits. Talk to your doctor.

Alcoholic Beverages

If you drink two or more drinks a day, your risk of getting breast cancer increases by about 25 percent. (A drink is defined as 12 ounces of regular beer, 5 ounces of wine, or 1.5 ounces of 80-proof liquor.) You may want to talk to your doctor about cutting down on alcoholic beverages.

Chapter 16

Alcohol Consumption and Breast Cancer Risk

While the potential health benefits of moderate alcohol consumption have garnered a lot of public attention, alcohol's impact on cancer risk has received much less. Epidemiological studies have consistently found that heavy drinking can increase the risk of liver, head and neck, and esophageal cancers, and even moderate drinking has been shown to increase the risk of breast cancer.

At the 2008 American Association for Cancer Research (AACR) annual meeting in San Diego, two new studies were presented that shed additional light on the alcohol-breast cancer connection, including one study that linked alcohol consumption with a significantly increased risk of the most common type of breast cancer.

Even though these studies grabbed headlines, researchers stress that important questions remain unanswered, such as which women who drink are at greatest risk, and what biological mechanism(s) alcohol might trigger to cause breast cancer. In short, researchers are still accumulating evidence that can form the basis for personalized clinical recommendations.

Nevertheless, some recommendations have already been made. As part of a far larger report on cancer prevention released last year, a consensus panel formed by the American Institute for Cancer Research (AICR) concluded: "The evidence on cancer justifies a recommendation not to drink alcoholic drinks."

"Alcohol and Breast Cancer Risk: New Findings," adapted from the *NCI Cancer Bulletin*, by the National Cancer Institute (NCI, www.cancer.gov), part of the National Institutes of Health, April 30, 2008.

The AICR report also acknowledged, however, the consistent findings that moderate alcohol consumption can protect against heart disease, and offered that, if individuals choose to drink, women should limit their consumption to one alcoholic beverage per day and men to two.

But even a highly consistent association between alcohol intake and breast cancer risk "is not the same as saying causality has been proven," says Dr. Arthur Schatzkin, chief of the Nutritional Epidemiology Branch in the National Cancer Institute's (NCI) Division of Cancer Epidemiology and Genetics. The same, he adds, holds true for the protection against heart disease.

"The breast cancer risks involved with alcohol are indeed modest; nothing like the magnitude of the risks between smoking and lung cancer or HPV [human papillomavirus] and cervical cancer," Dr. Schatzkin continues. "So it's difficult to be absolutely certain from the available studies that it's not some other biologic or behavioral factors associated with moderate drinking that are the real etiologic agents in breast cancer."

The important point, he stresses, is that "Drinking alcohol is an entirely avoidable risk factor," especially for women with established risks like a family history of breast cancer.

Studies dating back to the 1920s show that alcohol consumption and mortality risk are represented by a J-shaped curve: Risk of death is somewhat elevated in teetotalers, dips for moderate drinkers, and then climbs steadily as consumption increases.

According to long-term studies performed by Dr. Arthur Klatsky and colleagues at Kaiser Permanente in Oakland, CA, the vast bulk of the benefit of light-to-moderate alcohol consumption is due to an apparent protective effect against cardiovascular disease, primarily in middle-aged people.

Incidence data presented by NCI researchers at the AACR meeting were somewhat consistent with a J-curve, at least in terms of excessive alcohol consumption. Based on an analysis of more than 180,000 women in the NIH-AARP [National Institutes of Health-American Association of Retired Persons] Diet and Health Study, they found that women who consumed three or more alcoholic drinks a day had more than a 50-percent increased risk of ER+/PR+ [estrogen receptor positive/progesterone receptor positive] breast cancer, while women who drank smaller amounts also had an elevated risk, regardless of alcohol type.

The results, Dr. Klatsky notes, are mostly consistent with data from his studies and support the hypothesis that alcohol may increase breast cancer risk via an effect on estrogen. However, the results are not entirely consistent and highlight the difficulty in establishing a risk "threshold," Dr. Klatsky explains.

"Our data show that women who report having just several drinks a week don't have an increased [breast cancer] risk, and the risk begins somewhere between that and two drinks per day," he says.

In addition to the interplay between alcohol and estrogen, research has focused on several genes that code for the enzyme alcohol dehydrogenase (ADH), which is involved in alcohol metabolism. ADH initiates the breakdown of alcohol into acetaldehyde, ethanol's first metabolite, which is carcinogenic in animal models.

At the AACR meeting, researchers from Georgetown University's Lombardi Comprehensive Cancer Center and the State University of New York at Buffalo, using data from the Western New York Exposure and Breast Cancer Study, reported finding an increased breast cancer risk among postmenopausal women who drank and had variations in a gene that codes for ADH. The more the women reported drinking, the greater their risk.

"This is what we're really trying to get at now," says Lombardi's Deputy Director, Dr. Peter Shields, who co-led the study. "We're assuming that there are certain genetic susceptibilities. There's some evidence for it, but not enough studies to say that, for women who drink, certain genes put you at increased risk of breast cancer."

But other molecular players may be at work. Dr. Shields' lab has received funding from the Department of Defense to take a more systematic look at four potential causal mechanisms suggested by previous studies. These include the alcohol-estrogen link and the role of acetaldehyde, as well as alcohol-induced oxidative damage and disruption of folic acid pathways.

"We want to take this type of beverage that many women are going to drink," Dr. Shields says, "and figure out when they are really putting themselves at risk."

Chapter 17

Diethylstilbestrol (DES) and Breast Cancer Risk

What is DES?

Diethylstilbestrol (DES) is a synthetic form of the female hormone estrogen. It was prescribed to pregnant women between 1940 and 1971 to prevent miscarriage, premature labor, and related complications of pregnancy. The use of DES declined after studies in the 1950s showed that it was not effective in preventing these problems.

In 1971, researchers linked prenatal (before birth) DES exposure to a type of cancer of the cervix and vagina called clear cell adeno-carcinoma in a small group of women. Soon after, the Food and Drug Administration (FDA) notified physicians throughout the country that DES should not be prescribed to pregnant women. The drug continued to be prescribed to pregnant women in Europe until 1978.

DES is now known to be an endocrine-disrupting chemical, one of a number of substances that interfere with the endocrine system to cause cancer, birth defects, and other developmental abnormalities. The effects of endocrine-disrupting chemicals are most severe when exposure occurs during fetal development.

Excerpted from "Diethylstilbestrol (DES) and Cancer," by the National Cancer Institute (NCI, www.cancer.gov), part of the National Institutes of Health, October 5, 2011.

What is the cancer risk of women who were exposed to DES before birth?

The daughters of women who used DES while pregnant—commonly called DES daughters—have about 40 times the risk of developing clear cell adenocarcinoma of the lower genital tract than unexposed women. However, this type of cancer is still rare; approximately 1 in 1,000 DES daughters develops it.

The first DES daughters who were diagnosed with clear cell adenocarcinoma were very young at the time of their diagnoses. Subsequent research has shown that the risk of developing this disease remains elevated as women age into their 40s.

DES daughters have an increased risk of developing abnormal cells in the cervix and the vagina that are precursors of cancer (dysplasia, cervical intraepithelial neoplasia, and squamous intraepithelial lesions). These abnormal cells resemble cancer cells, but they do not invade nearby healthy tissue and are not cancer. They may develop into cancer, however, if left untreated. Scientists estimated that DES-exposed daughters were 2.2 times more likely to have these abnormal cell changes in the cervix than unexposed women. Approximately 4 percent of DES daughters developed these conditions because of their exposure. It has been recommended that DES daughters have a yearly Pap test and pelvic exam to check for abnormal cells.

DES daughters may also have a slightly increased risk of breast cancer after age 40. A 2006 study from the United States suggested that, overall, breast cancer risk is not increased in DES daughters, but that, after age 40, DES daughters have approximately twice the risk of breast cancer as unexposed women of the same age and with similar risk factors. However, a 2010 study from Europe found no difference in breast cancer risk between DES daughters and unexposed women and no difference in overall cancer risk. A 2011 study found that about 2 percent of a large cohort of DES daughters has developed breast cancer due to their exposure.

DES daughters should be aware of these health risks, share their medical history with their doctors, and get regular physical examinations.

What health problems might women who took DES during pregnancy have?

Women who used DES themselves have a slightly increased risk of breast cancer—approximately 30 percent higher than that of women who did not take DES. Women who used DES also have a 30 percent higher risk of death from breast cancer than unexposed women. This risk has been found to be stable over time—that is, it does not increase as the mothers become older. No evidence exists to suggest that women who took DES are at higher risk for any other type of cancer.

How can people find out if they took DES during pregnancy or were exposed to DES in utero?

It is estimated that 5 to 10 million Americans—pregnant women and the children born to them—were exposed to DES between 1940 and 1971. DES was given widely to pregnant women between 1940 and 1971 to prevent complications during pregnancy. DES was provided under many different product names and also in various forms, such as pills, creams, and vaginal suppositories.

Women who think they used DES during pregnancy, or people who think that their mother used DES during pregnancy, can try contacting the physician or institution where they received their care to request a review of their medical records. If any pills were taken during pregnancy, obstetrical records could be checked to determine the name of the drug.

However, finding medical records after a long period of time can be difficult. If the doctor has retired or died, another doctor may have taken over the practice as well as the records. The county medical society or health department may know where the records have been stored. Some pharmacies keep records for a long time and can be contacted regarding prescription dispensing information. Military medical records are kept for 25 years. In most cases, however, it may be impossible to determine whether DES was used.

What should DES-exposed daughters do?

Women who know or believe they were exposed to DES before birth should be aware of the health effects of DES and inform their doctor about their possible exposure. It has been recommended that exposed women have an annual medical examination to check for the adverse health effects of DES. A thorough examination may include a pelvic examination, Pap test and colposcopy, biopsy, and breast examination.

A routine cervical Pap test is not adequate for DES daughters. The Pap test must gather cells from the cervix and the vagina. It is also good for a clinician to see the cervix and vaginal walls. They may use a colposcope to follow-up if there are any abnormal findings.

It is recommended that DES daughters continue to rigorously follow the routine breast cancer screening recommendations for their age group.

What should DES-exposed mothers do?

A woman who took DES while pregnant or who suspects she may have taken it should inform her doctor. She should try to learn the dosage, when the medication was started, and how it was used. She also should inform her children who were exposed before birth so that this information can be included in their medical records.

It is recommended that DES-exposed mothers have regular breast cancer screenings and yearly medical checkups that include a pelvic examination and a Pap test.

Chapter 18

Environmental Factors and Breast Cancer Risk

In your lifetime, you probably will know several people with breast cancer; an estimated 230,480 women in the United States found out they had the disease in 2011. Throughout their lives, women have experiences and make decisions that can influence their chances of getting breast cancer. We have little control over some of these risk factors. For example, girls who begin menstruating younger than their friends or women who are older at menopause are more likely to develop breast cancer.

But sometimes we can make choices—good or bad—that affect our risk of getting breast cancer.

Avoiding unnecessary or inappropriate exposure to radiation, limiting how much alcohol you drink, avoiding certain kinds of hormone therapy, and minimizing weight gain are steps that might reduce risks for some women. In other cases, it is harder to know what to do. We don't yet know enough about many of the chemicals we encounter to figure out if they are connected to breast cancer.

Many people are concerned that environmental factors are increasing the risk of breast cancer.

In a 2011 report, the Institute of Medicine (IOM) looked at the available evidence and found some answers and many more questions. Obesity, alcohol consumption, and some medical treatments raise the risk of breast cancer at least a little. For other factors, the evidence is not that easy to come by, and sometimes the answers are not as clear as we would like them to be. The IOM also looked at why it's hard to get clear answers and what women can do to reduce their risk.

What does it mean to say one in eight women will get breast cancer?

The one in eight number we often hear is the risk of getting breast cancer during a woman's lifetime. But it does not mean that one in every eight women is diagnosed with breast cancer each year. A breast cancer diagnosis is never good news, and thankfully most women will never get one. In fact, the National Cancer Institute estimates that if a group of 1,000 women were followed for 10 years from their 50th to their 60th birthdays, about 20 to 30 of them would be diagnosed with breast cancer by their 60th birthday.

The other 970 to 980 women in this group would not develop breast cancer during these 10 years—although some of them might develop it later in life.

Age alone is a big factor in who develops breast cancer. Until women reach their thirties, the chance of being diagnosed with breast cancer is very low, and after that the risk begins to rise. The risk of breast cancer is at its highest when women are in their sixties and seventies. Women who begin menstruating later, have a first child at a younger age, or enter menopause earlier will tend to have a relatively lower risk of breast cancer.

Researchers have been studying breast cancer for decades. Why don't we know more about how to prevent it?

For years, breast cancer has been the most common type of invasive cancer among American women, and it's true that millions of dollars have been spent trying to identify its causes. But breast cancer is a complex disease, and the research to understand its causes is as complicated as the disease itself.

A woman's breast changes throughout her entire life. It begins to develop even before a girl is born, and major changes occur during puberty, pregnancy, breastfeeding, and menopause. Hormones, like estrogen, play an important role in changes to the breast, and they also can encourage growth of both normal and abnormal cells. Cancer occurs when abnormal growth of cells cannot be controlled by the body's usual protections. Because the breast changes so much over time, there are a lot of opportunities for cancer to develop in the breast.

Also, many different factors can contribute to breast cancer. A small number of women inherit genes with mutations that make developing breast cancer—and sometimes other cancers too—much more likely. For most women, though, it is what happens during their lifetimes, not the genes they inherited, that contribute most to breast cancer.

Breast cancer can be hard to study. We can't do experiments on women to see if something bad happens to those who are exposed to a chemical or some other agent of concern. That means that studies have to ask women to remember what happened to them in the past, or they have to follow women for many years to see who develops breast cancer and who doesn't, or both. In addition, studies that follow a group of women have to be relatively large (involving many thousands of women) to collect enough cases of breast cancer to do useful analysis of the data.

Researchers are also paying more attention to how experiences as a baby, a child, or an adolescent may influence the risk for breast cancer when women reach middle and older ages. But this gap of many decades between environmental exposures at younger ages and the older ages at which most breast cancers are diagnosed makes research difficult. It can be hard for older women to remember what happened to them when they were much younger or for researchers to follow a large enough group of girls until they reach the older ages at which some of them develop breast cancer.

While research is making progress in understanding breast cancer, we still have many questions.

Should I avoid mammograms?

When you have common medical procedures such as mammograms, dental x-rays, and CT [computed tomography] scans, you are exposed to x-rays. X-rays are a type of ionizing radiation, and exposure to ionizing radiation can increase the risk of breast and other cancers. Children may be especially vulnerable. Because mammograms use a very low dose of radiation and can be helpful in early detection of breast cancer, you should not avoid getting mammograms altogether. Follow your doctor's advice about how often you need them. Some tests—including CT scans—give higher doses of radiation, so it is a good idea to ask questions about these procedures and avoid them when they are not necessary.

Non-ionizing radiation is the kind of energy released by microwave ovens, cell phones, and other products with similar technology. Although ionizing radiation is a risk factor, studies have not found that non-ionizing radiation contributes to women's breast cancer.

What does it mean when I read that something increases risk for breast cancer by 20 percent?

Numbers like this often come from looking at two groups of women: One group exposed to the risk factor and another that is not exposed. A researcher compares the risk of breast cancer in one group relative to the other, giving a "relative risk." (Studies can use other approaches, too, but they all rely on comparing the experience of at least two groups of women.) If the study finds an increase in breast cancer risk, the relative risk will be more than 1.0.

A relative risk of 1.2, for example, means that women with the risk factor are 20 percent more likely to develop breast cancer than women without the risk factor. In the same group of 50-year-old women we considered earlier, an increase in risk of 20 percent would result in about 4 to 6 additional cases among the 1,000 women. That would make a total of 24 to 36 women who would be likely to be diagnosed with breast cancer during the next 10 years, instead of the 20 to 30 who would be diagnosed without that added risk.

How can drinking alcohol be good for the heart and also cause breast cancer?

It is true that just one drink a day of wine or beer makes it slightly more likely for women to develop breast cancer.

But drinking this small amount of alcohol also has been shown to reduce risk of death from heart disease. Of course, drinking a lot of alcohol is unhealthy.

This is an example of how complicated it can be to decide what is good for you. Each individual woman needs to consider how the benefits and risks of alcohol may apply to her. Risks are averages for a whole group or population.

Some women may have higher risks than average, for instance, because they have certain genes or started menstruating at a very young age, while others have lower risks. Talking with your doctor may be helpful.

Is it safe to drink water out of a plastic bottle?

Plastic water bottles have been in the news a lot recently, and you've probably heard about BPA (bisphenol A) and phthalates. Both chemicals are added to plastic products to make them more flexible. They are used in lots of products, ranging from lotion, food packaging, and toys (phthalates) to metal cans, dental appliances, plastic water bottles, and receipt paper (BPA).

Scientists can measure levels of these chemicals in blood or urine but are uncertain what effect these and many other chemicals have on women's risk for breast cancer. In studies in laboratory animals, both BPA and phthalates have been shown to mimic estrogen in the body, potentially changing hormone signals and possibly contributing to breast cancer.

Scientists don't know enough about how these chemicals affect breast cancer risk to know whether avoiding them will reduce that risk. It can be hard to understand and measure the behavior of chemicals like these in humans.

Sometimes tests using animals or cells that were grown in labs are the only tools researchers can use. The results of these tests give us clues about what may happen to people, but we need better tests in animals and cells to predict effects in humans.

What can I do to reduce my risk of developing breast cancer?

While there are many things we don't yet know about breast cancer, some of the risks are clear. Knowing these risks points to some of the ways you can reduce your chance of developing the disease. Ionizing radiation does increase the risk for breast cancer. So do hormone replacement therapies that include both estrogen and progestin. Avoiding medical radiation and hormone therapy, unless they are medically necessary, is a good idea. Drinking alcohol and smoking tobacco appear to slightly increase the risk of developing breast cancer.

Limiting these behaviors can help reduce the risk. Staying fit and avoiding weight gain can also help reduce the risk of breast cancer. Overweight women are more likely to develop breast cancer after menopause, while women who are physically active have lower risk.

Chapter 19

Hormone Replacement Therapy and Breast Cancer Risk

What is menopausal hormone therapy?

Menopausal hormone therapy (MHT) is a treatment that doctors may recommend to relieve common symptoms of menopause and to address long-term biological changes, such as bone loss, that result from declining levels of the natural hormones estrogen and progesterone in a woman's body during and after the completion of menopause.

MHT usually involves treatment with estrogen alone, estrogen plus progesterone, or estrogen plus progestin, which is a synthetic hormone with effects similar to those of progesterone. Women who have had a hysterectomy are generally prescribed estrogen alone. Women who have not had this surgery are prescribed estrogen plus progestin, because estrogen alone is associated with an increased risk of endometrial cancer, whereas research has suggested that estrogen plus progestin may not be.

How do the hormones used in MHT differ from the hormones produced by a woman's body?

The hormones used in MHT come from a variety of plants and animals, or they can be made in a laboratory. The chemical structure of these hormones is similar, although usually not identical, to those of hormones produced by women's bodies.

"Menopausal Hormone Therapy and Cancer," by the National Cancer Institute (NCI, www.cancer.gov), part of the National Institutes of Health, December 5, 2011.

137

The U.S. Food and Drug Administration (FDA) has approved many hormone products for use in MHT. FDA-approved products have undergone extensive testing and are produced under standardized conditions to ensure that every dose—whether in a pill, a skin patch, or a cream—contains the proper amount of the appropriate hormones. These FDA-approved products are available only with a doctor's prescription.

Non-FDA-approved hormone products, sometimes referred to as "bio-identical hormones," are widely promoted and sold without a prescription on the internet. Claims that these products are "safer" or more "natural" than FDA-approved hormonal products are not supported by credible scientific evidence.

Where does evidence about risks and benefits of MHT come from?

The most comprehensive evidence about risks and benefits of MHT comes from two randomized clinical trials that were sponsored by the National Institutes of Health as part of the Women's Health Initiative (WHI):

- The WHI Estrogen-plus-Progestin Study, in which women with a uterus were randomly assigned to receive either a hormone medication containing both estrogen and progestin (Prempro) or a placebo.

- The WHI Estrogen-Alone Study, in which women without a uterus were randomly assigned to receive either a hormone medication containing estrogen alone (Premarin) or a placebo.

More than 27,000 healthy women who were 50 to 79 years of age at the time of enrollment took part in the two trials. Although both trials were stopped early (in 2002 and 2004, respectively) when it was determined that both types of therapy were associated with specific health risks, longer-term follow-up of the participants continues to provide new information about the health effects of MHT.

What are the benefits of menopausal hormone therapy?

Research from the WHI Estrogen-plus-Progestin study has shown that women taking combined hormone therapy had the following benefits:

- One-third fewer hip and vertebral fractures than women taking the placebo: In absolute terms, this meant 10 fractures per 10,000 women per year who took hormone therapy compared with 15 fractures per 10,000 women per year who took the placebo.

- One-third lower risk of colorectal cancer than women taking the placebo: In absolute terms, this meant 10 cases of colorectal cancer per 10,000 women per year who took hormone therapy compared with 16 cases of colorectal cancer per 10,000 women per year who took the placebo.

However, a follow-up study found that neither benefit persisted after the study participants stopped taking combined hormone therapy medication.

Women taking estrogen alone experienced the following benefits:

- One-third lower risk for hip and vertebral fractures than women taking the placebo: In absolute terms, this meant 11 hip and 11 vertebral fractures per 10,000 women per year who took estrogen compared with 17 hip and 17 vertebral fractures per 10,000 women per year who took the placebo.

- A 23 percent reduced risk of breast cancer than women taking the placebo: In absolute terms, this meant 26 cases of invasive breast cancer per 10,000 women per year who took estrogen compared with 33 cases of invasive breast cancer per 10,000 women per year who took the placebo.

After 10.7 years of follow-up, however, the risk of hip fractures was slightly higher in the estrogen-alone group, but the risk of breast cancer remained lower than that among women who took the placebo.

What are the health risks of MHT?

Before the WHI studies began, it was known that MHT with estrogen alone increased the risk of endometrial cancer in women with an intact uterus. It was for this reason that, in the WHI trials, women randomly assigned to receive hormone therapy took estrogen plus progestin if they had a uterus and estrogen alone if they didn't have one.

Research from the WHI studies has shown that MHT is associated with the following harms:

- Urinary incontinence: Use of estrogen plus progestin increased the risk of urinary incontinence.

- Dementia: Use of estrogen plus progestin doubled the risk of developing dementia among postmenopausal women age 65 and older.

- Stroke, blood clots, and heart attack: Women who took either combined hormone therapy or estrogen alone had an increased risk of stroke, blood clots, and heart attack. For women in both groups, however, this risk returned to normal levels after they stopped taking the medication.

- Breast cancer: Women who took estrogen plus progestin were more likely to be diagnosed with breast cancer. The breast cancers in these women were larger and more likely to have spread to the lymph nodes by the time they were diagnosed. The number of breast cancers in this group of women increased with the length of time that they took the hormones and decreased after they stopped taking the hormones. These studies also showed that both combination and estrogen-alone hormone use made mammography less effective for the early detection of breast cancer. Women taking hormones had more repeat mammograms to check on abnormalities found in a screening mammogram and more breast biopsies to determine whether abnormalities detected in mammograms were cancer. The rate of death from breast cancer among those taking estrogen plus progestin was 2.6 per 10,000 women per year, compared with 1.3 per 10,000 women per year among those taking the placebo. The rate of death from any cause after a diagnosis of breast cancer was 5.3 per 10,000 women per year among women taking combined hormone therapy, compared with 3.4 per 10,000 women per year among those taking the placebo.

- Lung cancer: Women who took combined hormone therapy had the same risk of lung cancer as women who took the placebo. However, among those who were diagnosed with lung cancer, women who took estrogen plus progestin were more likely to die of the disease than those who took the placebo. There were no differences in the number of cases or the number of deaths from lung cancer among women who took estrogen alone compared with those among women who took the placebo.

- Colorectal cancer: In the initial study report, women taking combined hormone therapy had a lower risk of colorectal cancer than women who took the placebo. However, the colorectal tumors that arose in the combined hormone therapy group were more advanced at detection than those in the placebo group. There was no difference in either the risk of colorectal cancer or the stage of disease at diagnosis between women who took estrogen alone and those who took the placebo. However, a subsequent analysis of the WHI trials found no strong evidence that either estrogen alone or estrogen plus progestin had any effect on the risk of colorectal cancer, tumor stage at diagnosis, or death from colorectal cancer.

Does hysterectomy affect the cancer risks associated with MHT?

Women who had a hysterectomy and who are prescribed MHT generally take estrogen alone.

In 2004, when the WHI Estrogen-Alone Study was stopped early, women taking estrogen alone had a 23 percent reduced risk of breast cancer compared with those who took the placebo. An analysis conducted after study participants had been followed for an average of 10.7 years found that women who had taken estrogen alone still had a lower risk of breast cancer than women who had taken the placebo.

Do the cancer risks from MHT change over time?

Women who have had a hysterectomy and who use estrogen-alone MHT have a reduced risk of breast cancer that continues for at least five years after they stop taking MHT.

Women who take combined hormone therapy have an increased risk of breast cancer that continues after they stop taking the medication. In the WHI study, where women took the combined hormone therapy for an average of 5.6 years, this increased risk persisted after an average follow-up period of 11 years. Breast cancers diagnosed in this group of women were larger and more likely to have spread to the lymph nodes (a sign of more advanced disease).

Studies have documented a decline in breast cancer diagnoses in the United States after the sharp reduction in the use of MHT that followed publication of the initial results of the Estrogen-plus-Progestin Study in July 2002. Additional factors, such as a reduction in the use of mammography, may also have contributed to this decline.

Is it safe for women who have had a cancer diagnosis to take MHT?

One of the roles of naturally occurring estrogen is to promote the normal growth of cells in the breast and uterus. For this reason, it is generally believed that MHT may promote further tumor growth in women who have already been diagnosed with breast cancer. However, studies of hormone use to treat menopausal symptoms in breast cancer survivors have produced conflicting results, with some showing an increased risk of breast cancer recurrence and others showing no increased risk of recurrence.

What should women do if they have menopausal symptoms but are concerned about taking MHT?

Although MHT provides short-term benefits such as relief from hot flashes and vaginal dryness, several health concerns are associated with its use. Women should discuss whether to take MHT and what alternatives may be appropriate for them with their health care provider. The FDA currently advises women to use MHT for the shortest time and at the lowest dose possible to control menopausal symptoms.

Are there alternatives for women who choose not to take menopausal hormone therapy?

Women who are concerned about the health effects that occur naturally with the decline in hormone production that occurs during menopause can make changes in their lifestyle and diet to reduce certain risks. For example, eating foods that are rich in calcium and vitamin D or taking dietary supplements containing these nutrients may help to prevent osteoporosis. FDA-approved drugs such as alendronate (Fosamax), raloxifene (Evista), and risedronate (Actonel) have been shown in randomized trials to prevent bone loss.

Medications approved by the FDA for treating depression and seizures may help to relieve menopausal symptoms such as hot flashes. Those that have been shown in randomized clinical trials to be effective in treating hot flashes include the following:

- Venlafaxine (Effexor)
- Desvenlafaxine (Pristiq)
- Paroxetine (Paxil)
- Fluoxetine (Prozac)
- Citalopram (Celexa)
- Gabapentin (Neurontin)
- Pregabalin (Lyrica)

Some women seek relief from menopausal symptoms with over-the-counter complementary and alternative therapies. Some of these remedies contain estrogen-like compounds derived from sources such as soy products, whole-grain cereals, oilseeds (primarily flaxseed), legumes, or the plant black cohosh. To date, however, randomized clinical trials have not shown that any of these remedies is superior to a placebo in relieving hot flashes. Trials of other herbal remedies, such as evening primrose oil, ginseng, and wild yam, have also not shown that they effectively reduce menopausal symptoms.

What questions remain in this area of research?

The WHI trials were landmark studies that have transformed our understanding of the health effects of MHT. Follow-up studies have expanded and refined the original findings of these two trials. Many questions, however, remain to be answered, such as the following:

- Are different forms of hormones, lower doses, different hormones, or different methods of administration safer or more effective than those tested in the WHI trials?

- Does hormone use present different risks and benefits for women younger than those studied in the WHI trials?

- Is there an optimal age at which to initiate MHT or an optimal duration of therapy that maximizes benefits and minimizes risks?

It's important to note that women who were enrolled in the WHI trials were, on average, 63 years old, although about 5,000 of them were under age 60, so the results of the study may also apply to younger women. However, women in the study were not using MHT to relieve menopausal symptoms. In addition, the WHI trials tested single-dose strengths of one estrogen-only medication (Premarin) and one estrogen-plus-progestin medication (Prempro).

NIA is sponsoring the Early Versus Late Intervention Trial With Estradiol (ELITE) to try to answer some of these remaining questions. This clinical trial is comparing the effects of estrogen in a group of women who are within six years of menopause and another group of women who are at least 10 years past menopause. Women are randomly assigned to take either estradiol (Estrace) or a placebo for five years. Women with a uterus will also use a progesterone gel or a placebo gel for the last 10 days of each month. This trial has enrolled 643 women and is expected to be completed in the summer of 2013.

NCI is supporting a range of MHT-related research, including studies aimed at understanding the genetic factors that affect women's response to MHT and the role of chronic use of female hormones in the initiation of breast cancer, as well as developing more effective nonhormonal therapies for treating hot flashes.

Chapter 20

Oral Contraceptives and Cancer Risk

What types of oral contraceptives are available in the United States today?

Two types of oral contraceptives (birth control pills) are currently available in the United States. The most commonly prescribed type of oral contraceptive contains man-made versions of the natural female hormones estrogen and progesterone. This type of birth control pill is often called a "combined oral contraceptive." The second type is called the minipill. It contains only progestin, which is the man-made version of progesterone that is used in oral contraceptives.

How could oral contraceptives influence cancer risk?

Naturally occurring estrogen and progesterone have been found to influence the development and growth of some cancers. Because birth control pills contain female hormones, researchers have been interested in determining whether there is any link between these widely used contraceptives and cancer risk.

The results of population studies to examine associations between oral contraceptive use and cancer risk have not always been consistent. Overall, however, the risks of endometrial and ovarian cancer appear to be reduced with the use of oral contraceptives, whereas the risks of breast, cervical, and liver cancer appear to be increased.

Excerpted from "Oral Contraceptives and Cancer Risk: Questions and Answers," by the National Cancer Institute (NCI, www.cancer.gov), part of the National Institutes of Health, March 21, 2012.

How do oral contraceptives affect breast cancer risk?

A woman's risk of developing breast cancer depends on several factors, some of which are related to her natural hormones. Hormonal and reproductive history factors that increase the risk of breast cancer include factors that may allow breast tissue to be exposed to high levels of hormones for longer periods of time, such as the following:

- Beginning menstruation at an early age
- Experiencing menopause at a late age
- Later age at first pregnancy
- Not having children at all

A 1996 analysis of epidemiologic data from more than 50 studies worldwide by the Collaborative Group on Hormonal Factors in Breast Cancer found that women who were current or recent users of birth control pills had a slightly higher risk of developing breast cancer than women who had never used the pill. The risk was highest for women who started using oral contraceptives as teenagers. However, 10 or more years after women stopped using oral contraceptives, their risk of developing breast cancer had returned to the same level as if they had never used birth control pills, regardless of family history of breast cancer, reproductive history, geographic area of residence, ethnic background, differences in study design, dose and type of hormone(s) used, or duration of use. In addition, breast cancers diagnosed in women who had stopped using oral contraceptives for 10 or more years were less advanced than breast cancers diagnosed in women who had never used oral contraceptives.

A recent analysis of data from the Nurses' Health Study, which has been following more than 116,000 female nurses who were 24 to 43 years old when they enrolled in the study in 1989, found that the participants who used oral contraceptives had a slight increase in breast cancer risk. However, nearly all of the increased risk was seen among women who took a specific type of oral contraceptive, a "triphasic" pill, in which the dose of hormones is changed in three stages over the course of a woman's monthly cycle.

Because the association with the triphasic formulation was unexpected, more research will be needed to confirm the findings from the Nurses' Health Study.

How do oral contraceptives affect ovarian cancer risk?

Oral contraceptive use has consistently been found to be associated with a reduced risk of ovarian cancer. In a 1992 analysis of 20 studies, researchers found that the longer a woman used oral contraceptives the more her risk of ovarian cancer decreased. The risk decreased by 10 to 12 percent after 1 year of use and by approximately 50 percent after 5 years of use.

Researchers have studied how the amount or type of hormones in oral contraceptives affects ovarian cancer risk. One study, the Cancer and Steroid Hormone (CASH) study, found that the reduction in ovarian cancer risk was the same regardless of the type or amount of estrogen or progestin in the pill. A more recent analysis of data from the CASH study, however, indicated that oral contraceptive formulations with high levels of progestin were associated with a lower risk of ovarian cancer than formulations with low progestin levels. In another study, the Steroid Hormones and Reproductions (SHARE) Study, researchers investigated new, lower-dose progestins that have varying androgenic (testosterone-like) effects. They found no difference in ovarian cancer risk between androgenic and nonandrogenic pills.

Oral contraceptive use by women at increased risk of ovarian cancer due to a genetic mutation in the BRCA1 or BRCA2 [breast cancer gene 1 or 2] gene has been studied. One study showed a reduction in risk among BRCA1- or BRCA2-mutation carriers who took oral contraceptives, whereas another study showed no effect. A third study, published in 2009, found that women with BRCA1 mutations who took oral contraceptives had about half the risk of ovarian cancer as those who did not.

Chapter 21

Overweight, Obesity, and Cancer Risk

At a time when nearly two thirds of the U.S. population is considered overweight or obese, compelling evidence suggests that excess body weight is a risk factor for many cancers. However, body weight is among many health- and lifestyle-related factors that play a role in cancer risk and survival. The term energy balance describes the complex interaction of diet, physical activity, and genetics, and may play an important role in cancer prevention and control.

What exactly is meant by the term energy balance?

The classic definition of energy balance is the balance between energy taken in, generally by food and drink, and energy expended. Energy expenditure is influenced by genetics, body size and amount of muscle, and by physical activity. In addition, a minor part of energy expenditure is from the thermal effects of food—different foods generate different amounts of energy when you eat them. But it's not just a question of calories in versus calories out. While calories are probably the most critical element in maintaining your energy balance, other factors in your diet such as how much fiber or calcium you eat may influence your energy expenditure and how much muscle and fat you have.

Excerpted from "Striking a Healthy Energy Balance," published in *Benchmarks*, by the National Cancer Institute (NCI, www.cancer.gov), part of the National Institutes of Health, January 30, 2004. Reviewed by David A. Cooke, MD, FACP, February 12, 2012.

How does energy balance relate to cancer risk?

We think it's important to look at this intersection of weight, physical activity, and diet and how we manage those in life, since they all have the potential to influence cancer risk. Rather than focusing solely on diet or physical activity, energy balance is a way of characterizing the important interaction between these behaviors.

We commonly use BMI (body mass index, a measure of body fat based on person's height and weight) to calculate whether a person is overweight or obese.

How have the national averages for BMI changed over the years?

Obesity is defined as a BMI (weight in kilograms divided by height in meters squared) over 30. In the early 1960s, when the government first started tracking BMI in the population, only about 11 percent of men and 16 percent of women had a BMI over 30. Today, close to 30 percent of men and 35 percent of women are obese. Among African-American women, the rate of obesity is 50 percent. There's also evidence that obesity is increasing markedly in adolescents and children. Rates are climbing among African-American and Hispanic populations and among people with lower income, lower education, and fewer resources to address it.

The media are reporting a national obesity epidemic. Is that a fair characterization?

Two thirds of the U.S. adult population have BMIs over 25, and that is the level at which we believe the health risks of cancer and other diseases increase. Actually, you could say obesity is endemic and affects the majority of the population, since two thirds of the U.S. population is experiencing the health problem.

Is there some genetic basis for this increase in obesity?

In the United States today and in other developed countries, people live in an environment of plenty with few undergoing starvation—other than self-imposed dieting. But many thousands of years ago, the first human beings typically lived in an environment where starvation was common and periodic. Changes in the genetic makeup of the most successful humans allowed them to survive during those periods of starvation. We call that genetic trait "the thrifty gene." We think it supports a host of responses that tend to increase the likelihood of people becoming obese in an environment of plenty. The physiological response of the thrifty gene runs counter to remaining lean and has resulted in increases in hypertension, heart disease, diabetes, and many cancers.

What cancers are most associated with a higher BMI or obesity?

Obesity is associated with colon, postmenopausal breast cancer, endometrial cancer, renal cell, esophageal cancer, and thyroid cancer in women. For any cancers, however, our general recommendation is that there's good evidence that avoiding weight gain during adult life and having an active lifestyle can prevent cancer.

Is there a recommended level of activity to reduce cancer risk?

People should be doing moderate to vigorous physical activity at least 30 minutes a day, most days of the week. That's associated with reducing risk for several cancers, particularly colon and breast cancer. However, there's additional benefit observed with being more physically active than that—with benefits observed for up to an hour a day of exercise. Because so few of the population exercises at these much higher levels it is difficult to exactly measure the amount of additional benefit.

Can a person prevent cancer through improved energy balance?

There's good evidence the risk of colon cancer is halved by having an active lifestyle. That's a critical message. The question of what specific diets are most beneficial in avoiding weight gain is less certain, other than eating fewer calories than you burn in a day to avoid weight gain. A plant-based diet is beneficial in decreasing the risk for many cancers, particularly colon cancer. But there are many questions still about the type of carbohydrate in the diet and if the glycemic index of foods may alter risk. Glycemic index is a measure of how rapidly the carbohydrates you eat are converted into simple sugars. Complex carbohydrates with higher amounts of fiber have a lower glycemic index, and may have a more beneficial effect on metabolism than foods with a high glycemic index.

Does obesity ever play a role in preventing cancer?

For some cancers, studies consistently indicate that being heavy is protective or associated with decreased risk. This includes premenopausal breast cancer, head and neck cancers, and lung cancer. However, for the smoking-related cancers—head, neck, and lung—once you control for smoking, which tends to reduce a person's weight, the connection between weight and these cancers is removed.

So obesity may actually prevent breast cancer in premenopausal women?

Studies consistently show heavier women in the premenopausal period are at decreased risk of breast cancer. We think this is the case because heavier women actually have changes in their hormonal metabolism and experience fewer menstrual cycles. These changes result in lower exposure to estrogen and thus lower risk of developing premenopausal breast cancer. Studies also suggest that your weight in your 20s and 30s does not increase your risk for postmenopausal breast cancer. It's the higher weight later in life that increases your risk. However, given the overall evidence, it is best to maintain a healthy weight and avoid excessive weight gain throughout your life to reduce your risk for cancer, as well as many other diseases.

What do we know about obesity and postmenopausal breast cancer?

During menopause, when the ovaries no longer produce estrogen, the source of estrogen is from testosterone and other hormones from the adrenal glands that are converted into estrogen in the fat cells. So it's very dependent on how much fat you have on the body as to how much estrogen you produce. Estrogen is a major factor in postmenopausal breast cancer.

How do obesity and being overweight impact breast cancer prognosis?

Women who are heavier at time of diagnosis and have gained weight during their treatment are more likely to have a reoccurrence of their breast cancer and to have worse survival. This varies by the estrogen receptor status of the cancer. Being heavy, most likely because it increases stimulates estrogen production in the body, appears to increase growth of estrogen receptor positive tumors.

What is the relationship between weight, hormone therapy (HT), and breast cancer?

In the mid-1990s, we began looking at postmenopausal women who were on estrogen, and those who were not, to see if the weight association with breast cancer differed by use of hormone therapy. These studies found women who take estrogen are at an increased risk for breast cancer, but that heavy women in that group did not have further increased risk. The evidence suggests that's because the amount of estrogen from HT is very high, so the modest amount of estrogen contributed by fat cell production of estrogen in the postmenopausal period does not change that risk to a measurable amount.

What about women who do not take HT?

It's a strikingly different picture for these women. Overall, there is a 50 percent increase of breast cancer risk for all women that are heavy in the postmenopausal period. However, for the subgroup of women that have never taken HRT, being heavy results in a 200 to 350 percent increase in risk—a four- to seven-fold increase compared to women overall.

Chapter 22

Myths about Breast Cancer Risk

Chapter Contents

Section 22.1

Having an Abortion or Miscarriage Does Not Increase Breast Cancer Risk

"Abortion, Miscarriage, and Breast Cancer Risk," by the National
Cancer Institute (NCI, www.cancer.gov), part of the National
Institutes of Health, January 12, 2010.

A woman's hormone levels normally change throughout her life for a
variety of reasons, and these hormonal changes can lead to changes in her
breasts. Many such hormonal changes occur during pregnancy, changes
that may influence a woman's chances of developing breast cancer later
in life. As a result, over several decades a considerable amount of research
has been and continues to be conducted to determine whether having an
induced abortion, or a miscarriage (also known as spontaneous abortion),
influences a woman's chances of developing breast cancer later in life.

Current Knowledge

In February 2003, the National Cancer Institute (NCI) convened a workshop of over 100 of the world's leading experts who study pregnancy and
breast cancer risk. Workshop participants reviewed existing population-
based, clinical, and animal studies on the relationship between pregnancy
and breast cancer risk, including studies of induced and spontaneous abortions. They concluded that having an abortion or miscarriage does not
increase a woman's subsequent risk of developing breast cancer.

NCI regularly reviews and analyzes the scientific literature on
many topics, including various risk factors for breast cancer. Considering the body of literature that has been published since 2003, when
NCI held this extensive workshop on early reproductive events and
cancer, the evidence overall still does not support early termination of
pregnancy as a cause of breast cancer.

Background

The relationship between induced and spontaneous abortion and
breast cancer risk has been the subject of extensive research beginning

in the late 1950s. Until the mid-1990s, the evidence was inconsistent. Findings from some studies suggested there was no increase in risk of breast cancer among women who had had an abortion, while findings from other studies suggested there was an increased risk. Most of these studies, however, were flawed in a number of ways that can lead to unreliable results. Only a small number of women were included in many of these studies, and for most, the data were collected only after breast cancer had been diagnosed, and women's histories of miscarriage and abortion were based on their "self-report" rather than on their medical records. Since then, better-designed studies have been conducted. These newer studies examined large numbers of women, collected data before breast cancer was found, and gathered medical history information from medical records rather than simply from self-reports, thereby generating more reliable findings. The newer studies consistently showed no association between induced and spontaneous abortions and breast cancer risk.

Breast Cancer Risk Factors

At present, the factors known to increase a woman's chance of developing breast cancer include age (a woman's chances of getting breast cancer increase as she gets older), a family history of breast cancer, an early age at first menstrual period, a late age at menopause, a late age at the time of birth of her first full-term baby, and certain breast conditions. Obesity is also a risk factor for breast cancer in postmenopausal women.

Identifying Breast Cancer

NCI recommends that, beginning in their 40s, women receive mammography screening every year or two. Women who have a higher than average risk of breast cancer (for example, women with a family history of breast cancer) should seek expert medical advice about whether they should be screened before age 40, and how frequently they should be screened.

Section 22.2

No Link between Antiperspirant and Deodorant Use and Breast Cancer

Excerpted from "Antiperspirants/Deodorants and Breast Cancer:
Questions and Answers," by the National Cancer Institute (NCI, www
.cancer.gov), part of the National Institutes of Health, January 4, 2008.

Can antiperspirants or deodorants cause breast cancer?

Articles in the press and on the internet have warned that underarm antiperspirants (a preparation that reduces underarm sweat) or
deodorants (a preparation that destroys or masks unpleasant odors)
cause breast cancer. The reports have suggested that these products
contain harmful substances, which can be absorbed through the skin or
enter the body through nicks caused by shaving. Some scientists have
also proposed that certain ingredients in underarm antiperspirants or
deodorants may be related to breast cancer because they are applied
frequently to an area next to the breast.

However, researchers at the National Cancer Institute (NCI), a part
of the National Institutes of Health, are not aware of any conclusive
evidence linking the use of underarm antiperspirants or deodorants
and the subsequent development of breast cancer. The U.S. Food and
Drug Administration (FDA), which regulates food, cosmetics, medicines, and medical devices, also does not have any evidence or research
data that ingredients in underarm antiperspirants or deodorants cause
cancer.

*What do scientists know about the ingredients in antiper-
spirants and deodorants?*

Aluminum-based compounds are used as the active ingredient in
antiperspirants. These compounds form a temporary plug within the
sweat duct that stops the flow of sweat to the skin's surface. Some research suggests that aluminum-based compounds, which are applied
frequently and left on the skin near the breast, may be absorbed by the
skin and cause estrogen-like (hormonal) effects. Because estrogen has

the ability to promote the growth of breast cancer cells, some scientists have suggested that the aluminum-based compounds in antiperspirants may contribute to the development of breast cancer.

Some research has focused on parabens, which are preservatives used in some deodorants and antiperspirants that have been shown to mimic the activity of estrogen in the body's cells. Although parabens are used in many cosmetic, food, and pharmaceutical products, according to the FDA, most major brands of deodorants and antiperspirants in the United States do not currently contain parabens. Consumers can look at the ingredient label to determine if a deodorant or antiperspirant contains parabens. Parabens are usually easy to identify by name, such as methylparaben, propylparaben, butylparaben, or benzylparaben. The National Library of Medicine's Household Products Database also has information about the ingredients used in most major brands of deodorants and antiperspirants.

The belief that parabens build up in breast tissue was supported by a 2004 study, which found parabens in 18 of 20 samples of tissue from human breast tumors. However, this study did not prove that parabens cause breast tumors. The authors of this study did not analyze healthy breast tissue or tissues from other areas of the body and did not demonstrate that parabens are found only in cancerous breast tissue. Furthermore, this research did not identify the source of the parabens and cannot establish that the buildup of parabens is due to the use of deodorants or antiperspirants.

More research is needed to specifically examine whether the use of deodorants or antiperspirants can cause the buildup of parabens and aluminum-based compounds in breast tissue. Additional research is also necessary to determine whether these chemicals can either alter the DNA [deoxyribonucleic acid] in some cells or cause other breast cell changes that may lead to the development of breast cancer.

What have scientists learned about the relationship between antiperspirants or deodorants and breast cancer?

In 2002, the results of a study looking for a relationship between breast cancer and underarm antiperspirants/deodorants were reported. This study did not show any increased risk for breast cancer in women who reported using an underarm antiperspirant or deodorant. The results also showed no increased breast cancer risk for women who reported using a blade (nonelectric) razor and an underarm antiperspirant or deodorant, or for women who reported using an underarm antiperspirant or deodorant within one hour of shaving with a blade razor. These conclusions were based on interviews with 813 women with breast cancer and 793 women with no history of breast cancer.

Findings from a different study examining the frequency of un-derarm shaving and antiperspirant/deodorant use among 437 breast cancer survivors were released in 2003. This study found that the age of breast cancer diagnosis was significantly earlier in women who used these products and shaved their underarms more frequently. Further-more, women who began both of these underarm hygiene habits before 16 years of age were diagnosed with breast cancer at an earlier age than those who began these habits later. While these results suggest that underarm shaving with the use of antiperspirants/deodorants may be related to breast cancer, it does not demonstrate a conclusive link between these underarm hygiene habits and breast cancer.

In 2006, researchers examined antiperspirant use and other factors among 54 women with breast cancer and 50 women without breast cancer. The study found no association between antiperspirant use and the risk of breast cancer; however, family history and the use of oral con-traceptives were associated with an increased risk of breast cancer.

Because studies of antiperspirants and deodorants and breast can-cer have provided conflicting results, additional research is needed to investigate this relationship and other factors that may be involved.

Chapter 23

Understanding Your Risk: Genetic Counseling for Cancer

The etiology of cancer is multifactorial, with genetic, environmental, medical, and lifestyle factors interacting to produce a given malignancy. Knowledge of cancer genetics is rapidly improving our understanding of cancer biology, helping to identify at-risk individuals, furthering the ability to characterize malignancies, establishing treatment tailored to the molecular fingerprint of the disease, and leading to the development of new therapeutic modalities. As a consequence, this expanding knowledge base has implications for all aspects of cancer management, including prevention, screening, and treatment.

Genetic information provides a means to identify people who have an increased risk of cancer. Sources of genetic information include biologic samples of DNA [deoxyribonucleic acid], information derived from a person's family history of disease, findings from physical examinations, and medical records. DNA-based information can be gathered, stored, and analyzed at any time during an individual's life span, from before conception to after death. Family history may identify people with a modest to moderately increased risk of cancer or may serve as the first step in the identification of an inherited cancer predisposition that confers a very high lifetime risk of cancer. For an increasing number of diseases, DNA-based testing can be used to identify a specific mutation as the cause of inherited risk and to determine whether family members have inherited the disease-related mutation.

Excerpted from PDQ® Cancer Information Summary. National Cancer Institute; Bethesda, MD. Cancer Genetics Overview (PDQ): Patient version. Updated 03/2012. Available at: www.cancer.gov. Accessed March 21, 2012.

Throughout this text, the term "mutation" will be used to refer to a change in the usual DNA sequence of a particular gene. Mutations can have harmful, beneficial, neutral, or uncertain effects on health and may be inherited as autosomal dominant, autosomal recessive, or X-linked traits. Mutations that cause serious disability early in life are usually rare because of their adverse effect on life expectancy and reproduction. However, if the mutation is autosomal recessive—that is, if the health effect of the mutation is caused only when two copies (one from each parent) of the mutated gene are inherited—mutation carriers (healthy people carrying one copy of the altered gene) may be relatively common in the general population. "Common" in this context refers, by convention, to a prevalence of 1% or more. Mutations that cause health effects in middle and older age, including several mutations known to cause a predisposition to cancer, may also be relatively common. Many cancer-predisposing traits are inherited in an autosomal dominant fashion, that is, the cancer susceptibility occurs when only one copy of the altered gene is inherited. For autosomal dominant conditions, the term "carrier" is often used in a less formal manner to denote people who have inherited the genetic predisposition conferred by the mutation.

Increasingly, the public is turning to the internet for information related both to familial and genetic susceptibility to cancer and to genetic risk assessment and testing. Direct-to-consumer marketing of genetic testing for hereditary breast and colon cancer is also taking place in some communities. This wider availability of information related to inherited cancer risk may raise concerns among persons previously unaware of the implications inherent in their family histories and may lead some of these individuals to consult their primary care physicians for management advice and recommendations. In many instances, the evaluation and advice will be relatively straightforward for physicians with a basic knowledge of familial cancer. In a subset of patients, the evaluation may be more complex, calling for referral to genetics professionals for further evaluation and counseling.

Correctly recognizing and identifying individuals and families at increased risk of developing cancer is one of countless important roles for primary care and other health care providers. Once identified, these individuals can then be appropriately referred for genetic counseling, risk assessment, consideration of genetic testing, and development of a management plan. When medical and family histories reveal cardinal clues to the presence of an underlying familial or genetic cancer susceptibility, further evaluation may be warranted.

In the individual patient, features of hereditary cancer include the following:

- Multiple primary tumors in the same organ
- Multiple primary tumors in different organs
- Bilateral primary tumors in paired organs
- Multifocality within a single organ (e.g., multiple tumors in the same breast, all of which have risen from one original tumor)
- Younger-than-usual age at tumor diagnosis
- Tumors with rare histology
- Tumors occurring in the sex not usually affected (e.g., breast cancer in men)
- Tumors associated with other genetic traits
- Tumors associated with congenital defects
- Tumors associated with an inherited precursor lesion
- Tumors associated with another rare disease
- Tumors associated with cutaneous lesions known to be related to cancer susceptibility disorders (e.g., the genodermatoses)

In the patient's family, features of hereditary cancer include the following:

- One first-degree relative with the same or a related tumor and one of the individual features listed
- Two or more first-degree relatives with tumors of the same site
- Two or more first-degree relatives with tumor types belonging to a known familial cancer syndrome
- Two or more first-degree relatives with rare tumors
- Three or more relatives in two generations with tumors of the same site or etiologically related sites

Concluding that an individual is at increased risk of developing cancer may have important, potentially life-saving management implications and may lead to specific interventions aimed at reducing risk (e.g., tamoxifen for breast cancer, colonoscopy for colon cancer, or risk-reducing salpingo-oophorectomy for ovarian cancer). Information about familial cancer risk may also inform a person's ability to plan for the future (lifestyle and health care decisions, family planning, or other decisions). Genetic information may also provide a direct health benefit by demonstrating the lack of an inherited cancer susceptibility. For example, if a family is known to carry a cancer-predisposing mutation in a particular gene, a family member may experience reduced worry and lower health care costs if his or her genetic test indicates that he or she does not carry the family's disease-related mutation. Conversely, information about familial cancer risk may have psychological effects or social costs (e.g., worry, guilt, or increased health care costs). Family dynamics also may be affected. For instance, the involvement of one or more family members may be required for genetic testing to be informative, and parents may feel guilt about passing inherited risk on to their children.

Knowledge about a cancer-predisposing mutation can be informative not only for the individual tested but also for other family members. Family members who previously had not considered the implications of their family history for their own health may be led to do so, and some will undergo genetic testing, resulting in more definitive information on whether they are at increased genetic risk. Some relatives may learn their mutation status without being directly tested, for example, when a biological parent of a child who is a known mutation carrier is identified as an obligate carrier. Founder effects may result in the recognition that specific ethnic groups have a higher prevalence of certain mutations, knowledge that can be either clinically useful (permitting more rational genetic testing strategies) or potentially stigmatizing. Testing may reveal the presence of nonpaternity in a family. There is the theoretical possibility that genetic information may be misused, and concerns about the potential for insurance and/or employment discrimination may arise. Genetic information may also affect medical and lifestyle decisions.

Genetic Counseling

Genetic counseling is a process of communication between genetics professionals and patients with the goal of providing individuals and families with information on the relevant aspects of their genetic health, available testing and management options, and support as they move toward understanding and incorporating this information into their daily lives. Genetic counseling generally involves the following six steps:

1. Family and medical history assessment
2. Analysis of genetic information
3. Communication of genetic information
4. Education about inheritance, genetic testing, management, risk reduction, resources, and research opportunities

5. Supportive counseling to facilitate informed choices and adaptation to the risk or condition

6. Follow up

Genetic evaluation involves an interaction with a medical geneticist or other genetics professional and may include a physical examination and diagnostic testing, in addition to genetic counseling. The principles of voluntary and informed decision making, nondirective and noncoercive counseling, and protection of client confidentiality and privacy are central to the philosophy of genetic counseling.

From the mid-1990s to the mid-2000s, genetic counseling expanded to include discussion of genetic testing for cancer risk, as more genes associated with inherited cancer risk were discovered. Cancer genetic counseling often involves a multidisciplinary team of health professionals that may include a genetic counselor, an advanced practice genetics nurse, or a medical geneticist; a mental health professional; and various medical experts such as an oncologist, surgeon, or internist. The process of counseling may require a number of visits to address medical, genetic testing, and psychosocial issues. Even when cancer risk counseling is initiated by an individual, inherited cancer risk has implications for the entire family. Because genetic risk affects biological relatives, contact with these relatives is often essential to collect accurate family and medical histories. Cancer genetic counseling may involve several family members, some of whom will have had cancer and others who have not.

The impact of risk assessment and predisposition genetic testing is improved health outcomes. The information derived from risk assessment and/or genetic testing allows the health care provider to tailor an individual approach to health promotion and optimize long-term health outcomes through the identification of at-risk individuals before cancer develops. The health care provider can thus intervene earlier either to reduce the risk or diagnose a cancer at an earlier stage, when the chances for effective treatment are greatest. The information may be used to modify the management approach to an initial cancer, clarify the risks of other cancers, or predict the response of an existing cancer to specific forms of treatment, all of which may alter treatment recommendations and long-term follow-up.

Chapter 24

Breast Cancer Genetic Testing: Understanding BRCA1 and BRCA2

What are BRCA1 and BRCA2?

BRCA1 and BRCA2 [breast cancer gene 1 and breast cancer gene 2] are human genes that belong to a class of genes known as tumor suppressors.

In normal cells, BRCA1 and BRCA2 help ensure the stability of the cell's genetic material (DNA [deoxyribonucleic acid]) and help prevent uncontrolled cell growth. Mutation of these genes has been linked to the development of hereditary breast and ovarian cancer.

The names BRCA1 and BRCA2 stand for breast cancer susceptibility gene 1 and breast cancer susceptibility gene 2, respectively.

How do BRCA1 and BRCA2 gene mutations affect a person's risk of cancer?

Not all gene changes, or mutations, are deleterious (harmful). Some mutations may be beneficial, whereas others may have no obvious effect (neutral). Harmful mutations can increase a person's risk of developing a disease, such as cancer.

A woman's lifetime risk of developing breast and/or ovarian cancer is greatly increased if she inherits a harmful mutation in BRCA1 or BRCA2. Such a woman has an increased risk of developing breast and/

Excerpted from "BRCA1 and BRCA2: Cancer Risk and Genetic Testing," by the National Cancer Institute (NCI, www.cancer.gov), part of the National Institutes of Health, May 29, 2009.

or ovarian cancer at an early age (before menopause) and often has multiple, close family members who have been diagnosed with these diseases. Harmful BRCA1 mutations may also increase a woman's risk of developing cervical, uterine, pancreatic, and colon cancer. Harmful BRCA2 mutations may additionally increase the risk of pancreatic cancer, stomach cancer, gallbladder and bile duct cancer, and melanoma.

Men with harmful BRCA1 mutations also have an increased risk of breast cancer and, possibly, of pancreatic cancer, testicular cancer, and early-onset prostate cancer. However, male breast cancer, pancreatic cancer, and prostate cancer appear to be more strongly associated with BRCA2 gene mutations.

The likelihood that a breast and/or ovarian cancer is associated with a harmful mutation in BRCA1 or BRCA2 is highest in families with a history of multiple cases of breast cancer, cases of both breast and ovarian cancer, one or more family members with two primary cancers (original tumors that develop at different sites in the body), or an Ashkenazi (Central and Eastern European) Jewish background. However, not every woman in such families carries a harmful BRCA1 or BRCA2 mutation, and not every cancer in such families is linked to a harmful mutation in one of these genes. Furthermore, not every woman who has a harmful BRCA1 or BRCA2 mutation will develop breast and/or ovarian cancer.

According to estimates of lifetime risk, about 12.0 percent of women (120 out of 1,000) in the general population will develop breast cancer sometime during their lives compared with about 60 percent of women (600 out of 1,000) who have inherited a harmful mutation in BRCA1 or BRCA2. In other words, a woman who has inherited a harmful mutation in BRCA1 or BRCA2 is about five times more likely to develop breast cancer than a woman who does not have such a mutation.

Lifetime risk estimates for ovarian cancer among women in the general population indicate that 1.4 percent (14 out of 1,000) will be diagnosed with ovarian cancer compared with 15 to 40 percent of women (150–400 out of 1,000) who have a harmful BRCA1 or BRCA2 mutation.

It is important to note, however, that most research related to BRCA1 and BRCA2 has been done on large families with many individuals affected by cancer. Estimates of breast and ovarian cancer risk associated with BRCA1 and BRCA2 mutations have been calculated from studies of these families. Because family members share a proportion of their genes and, often, their environment, it is possible that the large number of cancer cases seen in these families may be due in part to other genetic or environmental factors. Therefore, risk estimates that are based on families with many affected members may not accurately reflect the levels of risk for BRCA1 and BRCA2 mutation carriers in the general population. In addition, no data are available from long-term studies of the general population comparing cancer risk in women who have harmful BRCA1 or BRCA2 mutations with women who do not have such mutations. Therefore, the percentages given above are estimates that may change as more data become available.

Do inherited mutations in other genes increase the risk of breast and/or ovarian tumors?

Yes. Mutations in several other genes, including TP53 [tumor protein 53], PTEN [phosphatase and tensin homolog], STK11/LKB1 [serine/threonine 11], CDH1 [cadherin-1], CHEK2 [checkpoint kinase 2], ATM [ataxia telangiectasia mutated], MLH1 [mutL homolog 1], and MSH2 [mutS homolog 2], have been associated with hereditary breast and/or ovarian tumors. However, the majority of hereditary breast cancers can be accounted for by inherited mutations in BRCA1 and BRCA2. Overall, it has been estimated that inherited BRCA1 and BRCA2 mutations account for 5 to 10 percent of breast cancers and 10 to 15 percent of ovarian cancers among white women in the United States.

Are specific mutations in BRCA1 and BRCA2 more common in certain populations?

Yes. For example, three specific mutations, two in the BRCA1 gene and one in the BRCA2 gene, are the most common mutations found in these genes in the Ashkenazi Jewish population. In one study, 2.3 percent of participants (120 out of 5,318) carried one of these three mutations. This frequency is about five times higher than that found in the general population. It is not known whether the increased frequency of these mutations is responsible for the increased risk of breast cancer in Jewish populations compared with non-Jewish populations.

Other ethnic and geographic populations around the world, such as the Norwegian, Dutch, and Icelandic peoples, also have higher frequencies of specific BRCA1 and BRCA2 mutations.

In addition, limited data indicate that the frequencies of specific BRCA1 and BRCA2 mutations may vary among individual racial and ethnic groups in the United States, including African Americans, Hispanics, Asian Americans, and non-Hispanic whites.

This information about genetic differences between racial and ethnic groups may help health care providers in selecting the most appropriate genetic test(s).

Are genetic tests available to detect BRCA1 and BRCA2 mutations, and how are they performed?

Yes. Several methods are available to test for BRCA1 and BRCA2 mutations. Most of these methods look for changes in BRCA1 and BRCA2 DNA. At least one method looks for changes in the proteins produced by these genes. Frequently, a combination of methods is used.

A blood sample is needed for these tests. The blood is drawn in a laboratory, doctor's office, hospital, or clinic and then sent to a laboratory that specializes in the tests. It usually takes several weeks or longer to get the test results. Individuals who decide to get tested should check with their health care provider to find out when their test results might be available.

Genetic counseling is generally recommended before and after a genetic test. This counseling should be performed by a health care professional who is experienced in cancer genetics. Genetic counseling usually involves a risk assessment based on the individual's personal and family medical history and discussions about the appropriateness of genetic testing, the specific test(s) that might be used and the technical accuracy of the test(s), the medical implications of a positive or a negative test result, the possibility that a test result might not be informative (an ambiguous result), the psychological risks and benefits of genetic test results, and the risk of passing a mutation to children.

How do people know if they should consider genetic testing for BRCA1 and BRCA2 mutations?

Currently, there are no standard criteria for recommending or referring someone for BRCA1 or BRCA2 mutation testing.

In a family with a history of breast and/or ovarian cancer, it may be most informative to first test a family member who has breast or ovarian cancer. If that person is found to have a harmful BRCA1 or BRCA2 mutation, then other family members can be tested to see if they also have the mutation.

Regardless, women who have a relative with a harmful BRCA1 or BRCA2 mutation and women who appear to be at increased risk of breast and/or ovarian cancer because of their family history should consider genetic counseling to learn more about their potential risks and about BRCA1 and BRCA2 genetic tests.

The likelihood of a harmful mutation in BRCA1 or BRCA2 is increased with certain familial patterns of cancer. These patterns include the following:

For women who are not of Ashkenazi Jewish descent:

- two first-degree relatives (mother, daughter, or sister) diagnosed with breast cancer, one of whom was diagnosed at age 50 or younger;

- three or more first-degree or second-degree (grandmother or aunt) relatives diagnosed with breast cancer regardless of their age at diagnosis;

- a combination of first- and second-degree relatives diagnosed with breast cancer and ovarian cancer (one cancer type per person);

- a first-degree relative with cancer diagnosed in both breasts (bilateral breast cancer);

- a combination of two or more first- or second-degree relatives diagnosed with ovarian cancer regardless of age at diagnosis;

- a first- or second-degree relative diagnosed with both breast and ovarian cancer regardless of age at diagnosis; and

- breast cancer diagnosed in a male relative.

For women of Ashkenazi Jewish descent:

- any first-degree relative diagnosed with breast or ovarian cancer; and

- two second-degree relatives on the same side of the family diagnosed with breast or ovarian cancer.

These family history patterns apply to about 2 percent of adult women in the general population. Women who have none of these family history patterns have a low probability of having a harmful BRCA1 or BRCA2 mutation.

How much does BRCA1 and BRCA2 mutation testing cost?

The cost for BRCA1 and BRCA2 mutation testing usually ranges from several hundred to several thousand dollars. Insurance policies vary with regard to whether the cost of testing is covered. People who are considering BRCA1 and BRCA2 mutation testing may want to find out about their insurance company's policies regarding genetic tests.

What does a positive BRCA1 or BRCA2 test result mean?

A positive test result generally indicates that a person has inherited a known harmful mutation in BRCA1 or BRCA2 and, therefore, has an increased risk of developing certain cancers. However, a positive test result provides information only about a person's risk of developing cancer. It cannot tell whether an individual will actually develop cancer or when. Not all women who inherit a harmful BRCA1 or BRCA2 mutation will develop breast or ovarian cancer.

A positive genetic test result may have important health and social implications for family members, including future generations. Unlike most other medical tests, genetic tests can reveal information not only about the person being tested but also about that person's relatives. Both men and women who inherit harmful BRCA1 or BRCA2 mutations, whether they develop cancer themselves or not, may pass the mutations on to their sons and daughters. However, not all children of people who have a harmful mutation will inherit the mutation.

What does a negative BRCA1 or BRCA2 test result mean?

How a negative test result will be interpreted depends on whether someone in the tested person's family is known to carry a harmful BRCA1 or BRCA2 mutation. If someone in the family has a known mutation, testing other family members for the same mutation can provide information about their cancer risk. If a person tests negative for a known mutation in his or her family, it is unlikely that they have an inherited susceptibility to cancer associated with BRCA1 or BRCA2. Such a test result is called a "true negative." Having a true negative test result does not mean that a person will not develop cancer; it means that the person's risk of cancer is probably the same as that of people in the general population.

In cases in which a family has a history of breast and/or ovarian cancer and no known mutation in BRCA1 or BRCA2 has been previously identified, a negative test result is not informative. It is not possible to tell whether an individual has a harmful BRCA1 or BRCA2 mutation that was not detected by testing (a "false negative") or whether the result is a true negative. In addition, it is possible for people to have a mutation in a gene other than BRCA1 or BRCA2 that increases their cancer risk but is not detectable by the test(s) used.

What does an ambiguous BRCA1 or BRCA2 test result mean?

If genetic testing shows a change in BRCA1 or BRCA2 that has not been previously associated with cancer in other people, the person's test result may be interpreted as "ambiguous" (uncertain). One study found that 10 percent of women who underwent BRCA1 and BRCA2 mutation testing had this type of ambiguous result.

Because everyone has genetic differences that are not associated with an increased risk of disease, it is sometimes not known whether a specific DNA change affects a person's risk of developing cancer. As more research is conducted and more people are tested for BRCA1 or BRCA2 changes, scientists will learn more about these changes and cancer risk.

What are the options for a person who has a positive test result?

Several options are available for managing cancer risk in individuals who have a harmful BRCA1 or BRCA2 mutation. However, high-quality data on the effectiveness of these options are limited.

Surveillance: Surveillance means cancer screening, or a way of detecting the disease early. Screening does not, however, change the risk of developing cancer. The goal is to find cancer early, when it may be most treatable.

Surveillance methods for breast cancer may include mammography and clinical breast exams. Studies are currently under way to test the effectiveness of other breast cancer screening methods, such as magnetic resonance imaging (MRI), in women with BRCA1 or BRCA2 mutations. With careful surveillance, many breast cancers will be diagnosed early enough to be successfully treated.

For ovarian cancer, surveillance methods may include transvaginal ultrasound, blood tests for CA–125 antigen [cancer antigen 125], and clinical exams. Surveillance can sometimes find ovarian cancer at an early stage, but it is uncertain whether these methods can help reduce a woman's chance of dying from this disease.

Prophylactic surgery: This type of surgery involves removing as much of the "at-risk" tissue as possible in order to reduce the chance of developing cancer. Bilateral prophylactic mastectomy (removal of healthy breasts) and prophylactic salpingo-oophorectomy (removal of healthy fallopian tubes and ovaries) do not, however, offer a guarantee against developing cancer. Because not all at-risk tissue can be removed by these procedures, some women have developed breast cancer, ovarian cancer, or primary peritoneal carcinomatosis (a type of cancer similar to ovarian cancer) even after prophylactic surgery. In addition, some evidence suggests that the amount of protection salpingo-oophorectomy provides against the development of breast and ovarian cancer may differ between carriers of BRCA1 and BRCA2 mutations.

173

Risk avoidance: Certain behaviors have been associated with breast and ovarian cancer risk in the general population. Research results on the benefits of modifying individual behaviors to reduce the risk of developing cancer among BRCA1 or BRCA2 mutation carriers are limited.

Chemoprevention: This approach involves the use of natural or synthetic substances to reduce the risk of developing cancer or to reduce the chance that cancer will come back. For example, the drug tamoxifen has been shown in numerous clinical studies to reduce the risk of developing breast cancer by about 50 percent in women who are at increased risk of this disease and to reduce the recurrence of breast cancer in women undergoing treatment for a previously diagnosed breast tumor. As a result, tamoxifen was approved by the U.S. Food and Drug Administration (FDA) as a breast cancer treatment and to reduce the risk of breast cancer development in premenopausal and postmenopausal women who are at increased risk of this disease. Few studies, however, have evaluated the effectiveness of tamoxifen in women with BRCA1 or BRCA2 mutations. Data from three studies suggest that tamoxifen may be able to help lower the risk of breast cancer in BRCA1 and BRCA2 mutation carriers. Two of these studies examined the effectiveness of tamoxifen in helping to reduce the development of cancer in the opposite breast of women undergoing treatment for an initial breast cancer.

Another drug, raloxifene, was shown in a large clinical trial sponsored by the National Cancer Institute (NCI) to reduce the risk of developing invasive breast cancer in postmenopausal women at increased risk of this disease by about the same amount as tamoxifen. As a result, raloxifene was approved by the FDA for breast cancer risk reduction in postmenopausal women. Since tamoxifen and raloxifene inhibit the growth of breast cancer cells in similar ways, raloxifene may be able to help reduce breast cancer risk in postmenopausal BRCA1 and BRCA2 mutation carriers. However, this has not been studied directly.

What are some of the benefits of genetic testing for breast and ovarian cancer risk?

There can be benefits to genetic testing, whether a person receives a positive or a negative result. The potential benefits of a negative result include a sense of relief and the possibility that special preventive checkups, tests, or surgeries may not be needed. A positive test result can bring relief from uncertainty and allow people to make informed decisions about their future, including taking steps to reduce their cancer risk. In addition, many people who have a positive test result may be able to participate in medical research that could, in the long run, help reduce deaths from breast cancer.

What are some of the risks of genetic testing for breast and ovarian cancer risk?

The direct medical risks, or harms, of genetic testing are very small, but test results may have an effect on a person's emotions, social relationships, finances, and medical choices.

People who receive a positive test result may feel anxious, depressed, or angry. They may choose to undergo preventive measures, such as prophylactic surgery, that have serious long-term implications and whose effectiveness is uncertain.

People who receive a negative test result may experience "survivor guilt," caused by the knowledge that they likely do not have an increased risk of developing a disease that affects one or more loved ones.

Because genetic testing can reveal information about more than one family member, the emotions caused by test results can create tension within families. Test results can also affect personal choices, such as marriage and childbearing. Issues surrounding the privacy and confidentiality of genetic test results are additional potential risks.

Chapter 25

Preventing Breast Cancer in People Who Are Susceptible

Chapter Contents

177

Section 25.1

Overview of Protective Factors and Interventions

PDQ® Cancer Information Summary. National Cancer Institute; Bethesda, MD. Breast Cancer Prevention (PDQ): Patient version. Updated 09/2011. Available at: www.cancer.gov. Accessed February 14, 2012.

What Is Prevention?

Cancer prevention is action taken to lower the chance of getting cancer. By preventing cancer, the number of new cases of cancer in a group or population is lowered. Hopefully, this will lower the number of deaths caused by cancer.

To prevent new cancers from starting, scientists look at risk factors and protective factors. Anything that increases your chance of developing cancer is called a cancer risk factor; anything that decreases your chance of developing cancer is called a cancer protective factor.

Some risk factors for cancer can be avoided, but many cannot. For example, both smoking and inheriting certain genes are risk factors for some types of cancer, but only smoking can be avoided. Regular exercise and a healthy diet may be protective factors for some types of cancer. Avoiding risk factors and increasing protective factors may lower your risk but it does not mean that you will not get cancer.

Different ways to prevent cancer are being studied, including the following:

- Changing lifestyle or eating habits

- Avoiding things known to cause cancer

- Taking medicines to treat a precancerous condition or to keep cancer from starting

How Breast Cancer Develops

Breast cancer is a disease in which malignant (cancer) cells form in the tissues of the breast.

The breast is made up of lobes and ducts. Each breast has 15 to 20 sections called lobes, which have many smaller sections called lobules. Lobules end in dozens of tiny bulbs that can produce milk. The lobes, lobules, and bulbs are linked by thin tubes called ducts.

Each breast also has blood vessels and lymph vessels. The lymph vessels carry an almost colorless fluid called lymph. Lymph vessels lead to organs called lymph nodes. Lymph nodes are small bean-shaped structures that are found throughout the body. They filter lymph and store white blood cells that help fight infection and disease. Clusters of lymph nodes are found near the breast in the axilla (under the arm), above the collarbone, and in the chest.

Avoiding Risk Factors and Increasing Protective Factors May Help Prevent Cancer

Breast cancer is the second most common type of cancer in American women.

Women in the United States get breast cancer more than any other type of cancer except skin cancer. The number of new cases of breast cancer has stayed about the same since 2003. Breast cancer is second to lung cancer as a cause of cancer death in American women. However, deaths from breast cancer have decreased a little bit every year for the past several years. Breast cancer also occurs in men, but the number of new cases is small.

Risk Factors That May Increase the Risk of Breast Cancer

Estrogen (Endogenous)

Endogenous estrogen is a hormone made by the body. It helps the body develop and maintain female sex characteristics. Being exposed to estrogen over a long time may increase the risk of breast cancer. Estrogen levels are highest during the years a woman is menstruating. A woman's exposure to estrogen is increased in the following ways:

- Early menstruation: Beginning to have menstrual periods at age 11 or younger increases the number of years the breast tissue is exposed to estrogen.

- Late menopause: The more years a woman menstruates, the longer her breast tissue is exposed to estrogen.

- Late pregnancy or never being pregnant: Because estrogen levels are lower during pregnancy, breast tissue is exposed to more estrogen in women who become pregnant for the first time after age 35 or who never become pregnant.

Hormone Replacement Therapy/Hormone Therapy

Hormones that are made outside the body, in a laboratory, are called exogenous hormones. Estrogen, progestin, or both may be given to replace the estrogen no longer produced by the ovaries in postmenopausal women or women who have had their ovaries removed. This is called hormone replacement therapy (HRT) or hormone therapy (HT) and may be given in one of the following ways:

- Combination HRT/HT is estrogen combined with progesterone or progestin. This type of HRT/HT increases the risk of developing breast cancer. Women taking combination HRT/HT also may be more likely to have an abnormal mammogram. Studies show that when women stop taking estrogen combined with progesterone, the risk of getting breast cancer decreases.

- Estrogen-only therapy may be given to women who have had a hysterectomy. Clinical trials studying whether estrogen-only therapy affects the risk of breast cancer have had mixed results. In women who have a uterus, estrogen-only therapy increases the risk of uterine cancer.

Exposure to Radiation

Radiation therapy to the chest for the treatment of cancers increases the risk of breast cancer, starting 10 years after treatment and lasting for a lifetime. The risk of developing breast cancer depends on the dose of radiation and the age at which it is given. The risk is highest if radiation treatment was used during puberty. For example, radiation therapy used to treat Hodgkin disease by age 16, especially radiation to the chest and neck, increases the risk of breast cancer.

Radiation therapy to treat cancer in one breast does not appear to increase the risk of developing cancer in the other breast.

For women who are at risk of breast cancer due to inherited changes in the BRCA1 and BRCA2 (breast cancer genes 1 and 2), exposure to radiation, such as that from chest x-rays, may further increase the risk of breast cancer, especially in women who were x-rayed before 20 years of age.

Obesity

Obesity increases the risk of breast cancer in postmenopausal women who have not used hormone replacement therapy.

Alcohol

Drinking alcohol increases the risk of breast cancer. The level of risk rises as the amount of alcohol consumed rises.

Inherited Risk

Women who have inherited certain changes in the BRCA1 and BRCA2 genes have a higher risk of breast cancer, and the breast cancer may develop at a younger age.

Risk Factors That May Decrease the Risk of Breast Cancer

Exercise

Exercising four or more hours a week may decrease hormone levels and help lower breast cancer risk. The effect of exercise on breast cancer risk may be greatest in premenopausal women of normal or low weight. Care should be taken to exercise safely, because exercise carries the risk of injury to bones and muscles.

Estrogen (Decreased Exposure)

Decreasing the length of time a woman's breast tissue is exposed to estrogen may help prevent breast cancer. Exposure to estrogen is reduced in the following ways:

- Pregnancy: Estrogen levels are lower during pregnancy. The risk of breast cancer appears to be lower if a woman has her first full-term pregnancy before she is 20 years old.

- Breastfeeding: Estrogen levels may remain lower while a woman is breastfeeding.

- Ovarian ablation: The amount of estrogen made by the body can be greatly reduced by removing one or both ovaries, which make estrogen. Also, drugs may be taken to lower the amount of estrogen made by the ovaries.

- Late menstruation: Beginning to have menstrual periods at age 14 or older decreases the number of years the breast tissue is exposed to estrogen.

- Early menopause: The fewer years a woman menstruates, the shorter the time her breast tissue is exposed to estrogen.

Selective Estrogen Receptor Modulators

Selective estrogen receptor modulators (SERMs) are drugs that act like estrogen on some tissues in the body, but block the effect of estrogen on other tissues. Tamoxifen is a SERM that belongs to the family of drugs called antiestrogens. Antiestrogens block the effects of the hormone estrogen in the body. Tamoxifen lowers the risk of breast cancer in women who are at high risk for the disease. This effect lasts for several years after drug treatment is stopped.

Taking tamoxifen increases the risk of developing other serious conditions, including endometrial cancer, stroke, cataracts, and blood clots, especially in the lungs and legs. The risk of developing these conditions increases with age. Women younger than 50 years who have a high risk of breast cancer may benefit the most from taking tamoxifen. Talk with your doctor about the risks and benefits of taking this drug.

Raloxifene is another SERM that helps prevent breast cancer. In postmenopausal women with osteoporosis (decreased bone density), raloxifene lowers the risk of breast cancer for women at both high risk and low risk of developing the disease. It is not known if raloxifene would have the same effect in women who do not have osteoporosis. Like tamoxifen, raloxifene may increase the risk of blood clots, especially in the lungs and legs, but does not appear to increase the risk of endometrial cancer.

Other SERMs are being studied in clinical trials.

Aromatase Inhibitors

Aromatase inhibitors lower the risk of new breast cancers in postmenopausal women with a history of breast cancer. In postmenopausal women, taking aromatase inhibitors decreases the amount of estrogen made by the body. Before menopause, estrogen is made by the ovaries and other tissues in a woman's body, including the brain, fat tissue, and skin. After menopause, the ovaries stop making estrogen, but the other tissues do not. Aromatase inhibitors block the action of an enzyme called aromatase, which is used to make all of the body's estrogen. Possible harms from taking aromatase inhibitors include osteoporosis and effects on brain function (such as talking, learning, and memory).

Prophylactic Mastectomy

Some women who have a high risk of breast cancer may choose to have a prophylactic mastectomy (the removal of both breasts when there are no signs of cancer). The risk of breast cancer is lowered in these women. However, it is very important to have a cancer risk assessment and counseling about all options for possible prevention before making this decision. In some women, prophylactic mastectomy may cause anxiety, depression, and concerns about body image.

Prophylactic Oophorectomy

Some women who have a high risk of breast cancer may choose to have a prophylactic oophorectomy (the removal of both ovaries when there are no signs of cancer). This decreases the amount of estrogen made by the body and lowers the risk of breast cancer. However, it is very important to have a cancer risk assessment and counseling before making this decision. The sudden drop in estrogen levels may cause the onset of symptoms of menopause, including hot flashes, trouble sleeping, anxiety, and depression. Long-term effects include decreased sex drive, vaginal dryness, and decreased bone density. These symptoms vary greatly among women.

Fenretinide

Fenretinide is a type of vitamin A called a retinoid. When given to premenopausal women who have a history of breast cancer, fenretinide may lower the risk of forming a new breast cancer. Taken over time, fenretinide may cause night blindness and skin disorders. Women must avoid pregnancy while taking this drug because it could harm a developing fetus.

Factors Not Proven to Increase Risk of Breast Cancer

Abortion

There does not appear to be a link between abortion and breast cancer.

Oral Contraceptives

Taking oral contraceptives ("the pill") may slightly increase the risk of breast cancer in current users. This risk decreases over time. The most commonly used oral contraceptive contains estrogen.

Progestin-only contraceptives that are injected or implanted do not appear to increase the risk of breast cancer.

Environment

Studies have not proven that being exposed to certain substances in the environment (such as chemicals, metals, dust, and pollution) increases the risk of breast cancer.

Diet

Diet is being studied as a risk factor for breast cancer. It is not proven that a diet low in fat or high in fruits and vegetables will prevent breast cancer.

Active and Passive Cigarette Smoking

It has not been proven that either active cigarette smoking or passive smoking (inhaling secondhand smoke) increases the risk of developing breast cancer.

Statins

Studies have not found that taking statins (cholesterol-lowering drugs) affects the risk of breast cancer.

Section 25.2

Reducing the Risk of Breast Cancer with Medication

Excerpted from "Reducing the Risk of Breast Cancer with
Medicine," by the Agency for Healthcare Research and Quality
(AHRQ, www.ahrq.gov), January 2010.

Two different medicines can reduce the risk of breast cancer for
women who have never had breast cancer before.

- Raloxifene: It is only approved for use after menopause.
- Tamoxifen: It is approved for use before and after menopause.

To reduce the risk of breast cancer, tamoxifen or raloxifene must
be taken once every day for up to five years.

How They Work

Estrogen is a natural hormone found in the body. Some breast cancers use estrogen to grow. There is a place on some breast cancer cells,
called a receptor, where estrogen can attach. This type of breast cancer
is called estrogen-receptor positive cancer.

Tamoxifen and raloxifene work by blocking estrogen. They attach
to the receptor, so estrogen can't. Without estrogen, this type of breast
cancer cell can't multiply and grow.

Some breast cancers do not have estrogen receptors. This type of
breast cancer is called estrogen-receptor negative cancer. It is not as
common, but it is harder to treat.

Raloxifene and tamoxifen reduce the risk of breast cancers that
have estrogen receptors.

They do not reduce the risk of breast cancers without estrogen
receptors.

Possible Benefits

For women who have never had breast cancer, both tamoxifen and
raloxifene reduce invasive breast cancer risk by about 50 percent.

Raloxifene does not lower the risk of non-invasive breast cancers (LCIS [lobular carcinoma in situ] and DCIS [ductal carcinoma in situ]). Research can't tell us yet about tamoxifen and non-invasive breast cancers.

Possible Problems

Both tamoxifen and raloxifene have common side effects. They both can cause hot flashes. Tamoxifen can cause vaginal symptoms, like itching, dryness, or discharge. Raloxifene can cause leg cramps.

Some women who have taken tamoxifen or raloxifene have had a stroke. Research studies have found that the number of strokes in women taking these medicines is about the same as in women not taking these medicines. Talk with your doctor or nurse about your risk for stroke.

Other serious and life-threatening side effects can also happen:

- Blood clots in the lungs and legs: Tamoxifen and raloxifene raise the risk of blood clots. Blood clots happen more often with tamoxifen than raloxifene.

- Endometrial cancer (cancer of the uterus lining): Tamoxifen raises the risk of endometrial cancer. Raloxifene does not. For every 100 women who take tamoxifen or raloxifene for five years, the medicine will cause a blood clot or endometrial cancer in about one woman.

Taking raloxifene or tamoxifen reduces a woman's risk of some kinds of breast cancer. Some women who take these medicines will still get breast cancer.

Taking the medicines does not reduce the risk of dying from breast cancer. It also does not mean a woman will live longer. It is not clear why this is the case. Maybe the medicines reduce the kinds of breast cancers that are easiest to treat.

Thinking about the Decision

Most women will never get breast cancer. But some women are at higher risk than others. Talk with your doctor or nurse about your risk of breast cancer.

Tamoxifen and raloxifene can lower the risk of getting some kinds of breast cancer. These medicines also can raise the risk of serious problems. Talk with your doctor or nurse about your risk for serious problems from these medicines.

Think about these questions:

• Do I have a high or a low risk for breast cancer? Do I have a high or low risk for serious problems from the medicine? The risk of side effects should not be higher than the benefit of the medicine.

• Can I stick with it? These medicines need to be taken every day for up to five years. They often can cause hot flashes.

• Does the cost of the medicines affect my decision? The cost of the medicines may be important to you. They need to be taken for a long time, and the cost can add up. Check to see if your insurance covers using these medicines to lower breast cancer risk.

Section 25.3

Preventive Mastectomy

"Preventive Mastectomy," by the National Cancer Institute (NCI, www .cancer.gov), part of the National Institutes of Health, July 27, 2006. Reviewed by David A. Cooke, MD, FACP, February 12, 2012.

What is preventive mastectomy, and what types of procedures are used in preventive mastectomy?

Preventive mastectomy (also called prophylactic or risk-reducing mastectomy) is the surgical removal of one or both breasts in an effort to prevent or reduce the risk of breast cancer. Preventive mastectomy involves one of two basic procedures: total mastectomy and subcutaneous mastectomy. In a total mastectomy, the doctor removes the entire breast and nipple. In a subcutaneous mastectomy, the doctor removes the breast tissue but leaves the nipple intact. Doctors most often recommend a total mastectomy because it removes more tissue than a subcutaneous mastectomy. A total mastectomy provides the greatest protection against cancer developing in any remaining breast tissue.

Why would a woman consider undergoing preventive mastectomy?

Women who are at high risk of developing breast cancer may consider preventive mastectomy as a way of decreasing their risk of this disease. Some of the factors that increase a woman's chance of developing breast cancer include the following:

- **Previous breast cancer:** A woman who has had cancer in one breast is more likely to develop a new cancer in the opposite breast. Occasionally, such women may consider preventive mastectomy to decrease the chance of developing a new breast cancer.

- **Family history of breast cancer:** Preventive mastectomy may be an option for a woman whose mother, sister, or daughter had breast cancer, especially if they were diagnosed before age 50. If multiple family members have breast or ovarian cancer, then a woman's risk of breast cancer may be even higher.

- **Breast cancer-causing gene alteration:** A woman who tests positive for changes, or mutations, in certain genes that increase the risk of breast cancer (such as the BRCA1 or BRCA2 [breast cancer gene 1 or 2]) may consider preventive mastectomy.

- **Lobular carcinoma in situ:** Preventive mastectomy is sometimes considered for a woman with lobular carcinoma in situ, a condition that increases the risk of developing breast cancer in either breast.

- **Diffuse and indeterminate breast microcalcifications or dense breasts:** Rarely, preventive mastectomy may be considered for a woman who has diffuse and indeterminate breast microcalcifications (tiny deposits of calcium in the breast) or for a woman whose breast tissue is very dense. Dense breast tissue is linked to an increased risk of breast cancer and also makes diagnosing breast abnormalities difficult. Multiple biopsies, which may be necessary for diagnosing abnormalities in dense breasts, cause scarring and further complicate examination of the breast tissue, by both physical examination and mammography.

- **Radiation therapy:** A woman who had radiation therapy to the chest (including the breasts) before age 30 is at an increased risk of developing breast cancer throughout her life. This includes women treated for Hodgkin lymphoma.

It is important for a woman who is considering preventive mastectomy to talk with a doctor about her risk of developing breast cancer (with or without a mastectomy), the surgical procedure, and potential complications. All women are different, so preventive mastectomy should be considered in the context of each woman's unique risk factors and her level of concern.

How effective is preventive mastectomy in preventing or reducing the risk of breast cancer?

Existing data suggest that preventive mastectomy may significantly reduce (by about 90 percent) the chance of developing breast cancer in moderate- and high-risk women. However, no one can be certain that this procedure will protect an individual woman from breast cancer. Breast tissue is widely distributed on the chest wall, and can sometimes be found in the armpit, above the collarbone, and as far down as the abdomen. Because it is impossible for a surgeon to remove all breast tissue, breast cancer can still develop in the small amount of remaining tissue.

What are the possible drawbacks of preventive mastectomy?

Like any other surgery, complications such as bleeding or infection can occur. Preventive mastectomy is irreversible and can have psychological effects on a woman due to a change in body image and loss of normal breast functions. A woman should discuss her feelings about mastectomy, as well as alternatives to surgery, with her health care providers. Some women obtain a second medical opinion to help with the decision.

What alternatives to surgery exist for preventing or reducing the risk of breast cancer?

Doctors do not always agree on the most effective way to manage the care of women who have a strong family history of breast cancer and/or have other risk factors for the disease. Some doctors may advise very close monitoring (periodic mammograms, regular checkups that include a clinical breast examination performed by a health care professional, and monthly breast self-examinations) to increase the chance of detecting breast cancer at an early stage. Some doctors may recommend preventive mastectomy, while others may prescribe tamoxifen or raloxifene, medications that have been shown to decrease the chances of getting breast cancer in women at high risk of the disease.

Doctors may also encourage women at high risk to limit their consumption of alcohol, eat a low-fat diet, engage in regular exercise, and avoid menopausal hormone use. Although these lifestyle recommendations make sense and are part of an overall healthy way of living, we do not yet have clear and convincing proof that they specifically reduce the risk of developing breast cancer.

What is breast reconstruction?

Breast reconstruction is a plastic surgery procedure in which the shape of the breast is rebuilt. Many women who choose to have preventive mastectomy also decide to have breast reconstruction, either at the time of the mastectomy or at some later time.

Before performing breast reconstruction, the plastic surgeon carefully examines the breasts and discusses the reconstruction options. In one type of reconstructive procedure, the surgeon inserts an implant (a balloon-like device filled with saline or silicone) under the skin and the chest muscles. Another procedure, called tissue flap reconstruction, uses skin, fat, and muscle from the woman's abdomen, back, or buttocks to create the breast shape. The surgeon will discuss with the patient any limitations on exercise or arm motion that might result from these operations.

What type of follow-up care is needed after reconstructive surgery?

Women who have reconstructive surgery are monitored carefully to detect and treat complications, such as infection, movement of the implant, or contracture (the formation of a firm, fibrous shell or scar tissue around the implant caused by the body's reaction to the implant). Women who have tissue flap reconstruction may want to ask their surgeon about physical therapy, which can help them adjust to limitations in activity and exercise after surgery. Routine screening for breast cancer is also part of the postoperative follow-up, because the risk of cancer cannot be completely eliminated. When women with breast implants have mammograms, they should tell the radiology technician about the implant. Special procedures may be necessary to improve the accuracy of the mammogram and to avoid damaging the implant. However, women who have had reconstructive surgery on both breasts should ask their doctors whether mammograms are still necessary.

Section 25.4

Prophylactic Oophorectomy

Excerpted from PDQ® Cancer Information Summary. National Cancer
Institute; Bethesda, MD. Ovarian Cancer Prevention (PDQ): Patient version.
Updated 02/2012. Available at: www.cancer.gov. Accessed March 1, 2012.

Some women who have a high risk of ovarian cancer may choose to
have a prophylactic oophorectomy (surgery to remove both ovaries when
there are no signs of cancer). This includes women who have inherited
certain changes in the BRCA1 and BRCA2 [breast cancer 1 and 2] genes or
in the genes linked to hereditary nonpolyposis colon cancer (HNPCC).

It is very important to have a cancer risk assessment and counseling before making this decision. These and other factors should be discussed:

- Risk of ovarian cancer in the peritoneum: Women who have had
  a prophylactic oophorectomy continue to have a small risk of ovarian cancer in the peritoneum (thin layer of tissue that lines the
  inside of the abdomen). This may occur if ovarian cancer cells
  had already spread to the peritoneum before the surgery or if
  some ovarian tissue remains after surgery.

- Early menopause: The drop in estrogen levels caused by remov-
  ing the ovaries can cause early menopause. Symptoms of meno-
  pause include the following:
  - Hot flashes
  - Night sweats
  - Trouble sleeping
  - Mood changes
  - Decreased sex drive
  - Heart disease
  - Vaginal dryness
  - Osteoporosis (decreased bone density)

These symptoms may not be the same in all women. Hormone replacement therapy (HRT) may be needed to lessen these symptoms.

Part Four

Screening, Diagnosis, and Stages of Breast Cancer

Chapter 26

Breast Cancer Screening and Exams

Chapter Contents

Section 26.1

Overview of Breast Cancer Screening

Excerpted from PDQ® Cancer Information Summary. National Cancer Institute; Bethesda, MD. Breast Cancer Screening (PDQ): Patient version. Updated 08/2011. Available at: www.cancer.gov. Accessed February 7, 2012.

Screening is looking for cancer before a person has any symptoms. This can help find cancer at an early stage. When abnormal tissue or cancer is found early, it may be easier to treat. By the time symptoms appear, cancer may have begun to spread.

Scientists are trying to better understand which people are more likely to get certain types of cancer. They also study the things we do and the things around us to see if they cause cancer. This information helps doctors recommend who should be screened for cancer, which screening tests should be used, and how often the tests should be done.

It is important to remember that your doctor does not necessarily think you have cancer if he or she suggests a screening test. Screening tests are given when you have no cancer symptoms.

If a screening test result is abnormal, you may need to have more tests done to find out if you have cancer. These are called diagnostic tests.

Some screening tests are used because they have been shown to be helpful both in finding cancers early and in decreasing the chance of dying from these cancers. Other tests are used because they have been shown to find cancer in some people; however, it has not been proven in clinical trials that use of these tests will decrease the risk of dying from cancer.

Scientists study screening tests to find those with the fewest risks and most benefits. Cancer screening trials also are meant to show whether early detection (finding cancer before it causes symptoms) decreases a person's chance of dying from the disease. For some types of cancer, the chance of recovery is better if the disease is found and treated at an early stage.

Clinical trials that study cancer screening methods are taking place in many parts of the country.

Two tests are commonly used by health care providers to screen for breast cancer:

- Mammogram: A mammogram is an x-ray of the breast. This test may find tumors that are too small to feel. A mammogram may also find ductal carcinoma in situ, abnormal cells in the lining of a breast duct, which may become invasive cancer in some women. The ability of a mammogram to find breast cancer may depend on the size of the tumor, the density of the breast tissue, and the skill of the radiologist. Mammograms are less likely to find breast tumors in women younger than 50 years than in older women. This may be because younger women have denser breast tissue that appears white on a mammogram. A tumor also appears white on a mammogram, which makes it hard to find.

- Clinical breast exam (CBE): A clinical breast exam is an exam of the breast by a doctor or other health professional. The doctor will carefully feel the breasts and under the arms for lumps or anything else that seems unusual.

It is important to know how your breasts usually look and feel. If you feel any lumps or notice any other changes, talk to your doctor.

If a lump or anything else that seems abnormal is found using one of these two tests, ultrasound may be used to learn more. Ultrasound is not used by itself as a screening test for breast cancer. This is a procedure in which high-energy sound waves (ultrasound) are bounced off internal tissues or organs and make echoes. The echoes form a picture of body tissues called a sonogram.

Other screening tests are being studied in clinical trials. MRI [magnetic resonance imaging] is a procedure that uses a magnet, radio waves, and a computer to make a series of detailed pictures of areas inside the body. This procedure is also called nuclear magnetic resonance imaging (NMRI). MRI does not use any x-rays.

In women with a high inherited risk of breast cancer, screening trials of MRI breast scans have shown that MRI is more sensitive than mammography for finding breast tumors. It is common for MRI breast scan results to appear abnormal even though no cancer is present. Screening studies of breast MRI in women at high inherited risk are ongoing.

In women at average risk for breast cancer, MRI scans may be done to help with diagnosis. MRI may be used to do the following:

- Study lumps in the breast that remain after surgery or radiation therapy

- Study breast lumps or enlarged lymph nodes found during a clinical breast exam or a breast self-exam that were not seen on mammography or ultrasound

- Plan surgery for patients with known breast cancer

Breast tissue sampling is taking cells from breast tissue to examine under a microscope. Abnormal cells in breast fluid have been linked to an increased risk of breast cancer in some studies. Scientists are studying whether breast tissue sampling can be used to find breast cancer at an early stage or predict the risk of developing breast cancer. Three methods of tissue sampling are under study:

- Fine-needle aspiration: A thin needle is inserted into the breast tissue around the areola (darkened area around the nipple) to withdraw cells and fluid.

- Nipple aspiration: This procedure involves the use of gentle suction to collect fluid through the nipple. This is done with a device similar to the breast pumps used by nursing women.

- Ductal lavage: A hair-size catheter (tube) is inserted into the nipple and a small amount of salt water is released into the duct. The water picks up breast cells and is removed.

Screening clinical trials are taking place in many parts of the country.

Risks of Breast Cancer Screening

Decisions about screening tests can be difficult. Not all screening tests are helpful and most have risks. Before having any screening test, you may want to discuss the test with your doctor. It is important to know the risks of the test and whether it has been proven to reduce the risk of dying from cancer.

The risks of breast cancer screening tests include the following:

Finding breast cancer may not improve health or help a woman live longer.

Screening may not help you if you have fast-growing breast cancer or if it has already spread to other places in your body. Also, some breast cancers found on a screening mammogram may never cause symptoms or become life-threatening. When such cancers are found, treatment would not help you live longer and may instead cause serious treatment-related side effects. At this time, it is not possible to be sure which breast cancers found by screening will cause symptoms and which breast cancers will not.

False-negative test results can occur.

Screening test results may appear to be normal even though breast cancer is present. A woman who receives a false-negative test result (one that shows there is no cancer when there really is) may delay seeking medical care even if she has symptoms.

One in five cancers may be missed by mammography. False-negatives occur more often in younger women than in older women because the breast tissue of younger women is more dense. The size of the tumor, the rate of tumor growth, the level of hormones, such as estrogen and progesterone, in the woman's body, and the skill of the radiologist can also affect the chance of a false-negative result.

False-positive test results can occur.

Screening test results may appear to be abnormal even though no cancer is present. A false-positive test result (one that shows there is cancer when there really isn't) can cause anxiety and is usually followed by more tests (such as biopsy), which also have risks.

Most abnormal test results turn out not to be cancer. False-positives are more common in younger women, women who have had previous breast biopsies, women with a family history of breast cancer, and women who take hormones, such as estrogen and progesterone. The skill of the doctor also can affect the chance of a false-positive result.

Mammograms expose the breast to radiation.

Being exposed to radiation is a risk factor for breast cancer. The risk of developing breast cancer from radiation exposure, such as screening mammograms or x-rays, is greater with higher doses of radiation and in younger women. For women older than 40 years, the benefits of an annual screening mammogram may be greater than the risks from radiation exposure.

The risks and benefits of screening for breast cancer may be different for different groups of people.

The benefits of breast cancer screening may vary among age groups:

- In women who have a life expectancy of five years or less, finding and treating early stage breast cancer may reduce their quality of life without helping them live longer.

- In women older than 65 years, the results of a screening test may lead to more diagnostic tests and anxiety while waiting for the test results. Also, the breast cancers found are usually not life-threatening.

- It has not been shown that women benefit from starting mammography at younger than 40 years.

Routine breast cancer screening is advised for women who have had radiation treatment to the chest, especially at a young age. The benefits and risks of mammograms and MRIs for these women are not known. There is no information on the benefits or risks of breast cancer screening in men.

No matter how old you are, if you have risk factors for breast cancer you should ask for medical advice about when to begin having mammograms and how often to be screened.

Section 26.2

Breast Self-Exam

A breast self-exam is when a woman examines her own breasts for changes or problems.

Many women feel that doing this is important to their health. It helps them learn how their breasts normally feel, so that if they find a lump they will know if they should call their doctor or nurse.

However, there is not agreement among experts about recommending breast self-exams. It is not known for sure what role breast self-exams play in finding breast cancer or saving lives.

Talk to your health care provider about whether breast self-exams are right for you.

Information

If you decide to do breast self-exams, make sure you do so about three to five days after your period starts. Your breasts are not as tender or lumpy during this time of month.

If you have gone through menopause, do your exam on the same day every month.

- First, lie on your back. It is easier to examine all breast tissue if you are lying down.

- Place your right hand behind your head. With the middle fingers of your left hand, gently yet firmly press down using small motions to examine the entire right breast.

- Next, sit or stand. Feel your armpit, because breast tissue goes into that area.

- Gently squeeze the nipple, checking for discharge. Repeat the process on the left breast.

- Make sure that you are covering all of the breast tissue.

Next, stand in front of a mirror with your arms by your side.

- Look at your breasts directly and in the mirror. Look for changes in skin texture, such as dimpling, puckering, indentations, or skin that looks like an orange peel.

- Also note the shape and contour of each breast.

- Check to see if the nipple turns inward.

Do the same with your arms raised above your head.

Most women have some lumps. Your goal is to find anything new or different. If you do, call your health care provider right away.

Section 26.3

Recommendations for Mammography and Breast Self-Exams: How and Why Have They Changed?

"Independent Task Force Updates Recommendations on Breast Cancer Screening," by the National Cancer Institute (NCI, www.cancer.gov), part of the National Institutes of Health, November 17, 2009.

In November 2009, the United States Preventive Services Task Force (USPSTF) updated recommendations on breast cancer screening, suggesting that women ages 50 to 74 who are at average risk for getting the disease undergo a routine screening mammogram every two years. The recommendations were published in the November 17, 2009, *Annals of Internal Medicine*.

"When women are screened every other year instead of every year, you see a large reduction in the harms caused by false-positive screening results, and the reduction in breast cancer mortality remains high—between 70 and 99 percent of what you see with annual screening," explained Dr. Diana Petitti, vice chair of the USPSTF committee that issued the recommendations. False-positive screening results can cause harms including unnecessary biopsies and emotional distress.

The USPSTF is a panel of independent primary care physicians from around the country that periodically reviews the evidence for preventive health services, including screening, medication, and counseling. The panel's earlier recommendations for breast cancer screening, last updated in 2002, advised mammography with or without clinical breast exam every one to two years for women ages 40 and older.

The new recommendations do not advise routine mammography for average-risk women ages 40 to 49. Instead, they advocate for "individualized informed decision making based on specific benefits and harms for women who consider screening before age 50 years," noted Dr. Karla Kerlikowske of the San Francisco Veterans Affairs Medical Center in an accompanying editorial.

The updated 2009 recommendations also advise against teaching breast self-exam(BSE). The 2002 recommendations did not advise either for or against teaching BSE, but because no clinical trials to date have shown that widespread teaching of the technique reduces the number of deaths from breast cancer, the task force now recommends against systematic teaching of BSE.

However, explained Dr. Stephen Taplin, senior scientist in the National Cancer Institute's Division of Cancer Control and Population Sciences' Applied Research Program (ARP), a recommendation against routine teaching of BSE "certainly does not mean that women shouldn't respond to lumps and bumps or other troublesome changes in their breasts that they discover on their own. Women should go to their health care provider when they have a concern."

The task force based the updated recommendations, in part, on two commissioned evidence reports that synthesized data that had accumulated since the USPSTF's last revision seven years ago. One of these was performed by the Oregon Evidence-based Practice Center (EPC) at Oregon Health and Science University and was intended to find and summarize all the high-quality, pertinent studies that could help answer the questions about optimizing breast cancer screening.

To this end, the EPC reviewed new studies and new data from published trials of screening mammography that had been reviewed by the task force in 2002, including the Age trial from the United Kingdom, the only clinical trial to specifically evaluate the effectiveness of screening mammography in women in their 40s. This set of data allowed the task force to more precisely estimate the reduction in deaths from breast cancer with mammography in this age group.

The EPC also analyzed data on more than 600,000 women ages 40 or older that had been collected by the Breast Cancer Surveillance Consortium. These data indicated that false-positive results on a mammogram are most common among women ages 40 to 49.

The second evidence report was prepared by NCI-funded members of the Cancer Intervention and Surveillance Modeling Network (CISNET). For this new study of mammography, six modeling teams examined the hypothetical outcomes of 20 different mammography screening strategies that differed in the ages when screening began and ended and in the number of years between scheduled screenings.

The models developed by these teams showed that screening every other year produced an average of 81 percent of the mortality reduction of yearly screening, but with nearly 50 percent fewer false-positive results. Screening women ages 50 to 69 every other year would provide a median reduction in breast cancer mortality of 16.5 percent compared with no screening. When compared with screening from ages 50 to 69, beginning screening every other year at age 40 produced a small additional reduction in mortality but increased the number of false-positive results by more than 50 percent.

"Everything about breast cancer screening is a trade-off, within the ages for which it has been shown to be beneficial," explained Dr. Petitti. "All of these lines of evidence indicate that women ages 40 to 49 would have a small improvement in breast cancer mortality but also a large set of harms related to false-positive results."

"It is important for women to understand that these results come from analyses of women who were drawn from the general U.S. population," added Dr. Taplin, "and as such, they do not account for all variations in breast cancer risk and do not apply to women at very high risk for breast cancer."

Section 26.4

Breast Cancer Screening for Women with Cosmetic Breast Implants

Getting breast implants does not increase a woman's breast cancer risks or prevent her from getting accurate mammogram test results.

"The question of how implants affect breast cancer risk and screening tests, like the mammogram, is a question that many women ask," says Therese Bevers, MD, medical director of the Cancer Prevention Center at M. D. Anderson. "The good news is that implants do not increase breast cancer risks. But, they also don't decrease them because women with implants still have their natural breast tissue."

Breast Awareness with Implants

If you have implants, M. D. Anderson recommends paying special attention to your breasts and promptly reporting any changes to your doctor. Getting used to how breasts look and feel after implants may take women a little while to get used to, but that doesn't mean they can't notice the signs of breast cancer.

"The person most likely to find a lump in the breast is the woman herself," Bevers says. "With implants, becoming familiar with your breasts is more difficult at first because the breast will have a different texture. It also will have new folds or dimples. But after a woman knows her new breasts, having implants should not get in the way of her noticing a change that might be cancer."

Women with implants might even be more likely to notice changes to their breasts.

"Noticing breast changes can sometimes be easier for women with implants because the implants push the natural breast tissue to the outside of the breast, making a lump easier to feel," says Elisabeth Beahm, MD, FACS, a professor in the Department of Plastic Surgery at MD Anderson. "Also, most women with implants are more aware of their breasts and changes to their body."

For any woman, checking your breasts regularly can lead to early detection.

Screening Guidelines for Women with Breast Implants

While being familiar with your breasts is good advice for women with natural breasts and for women with implants, the way that breast cancer screening exams are done for each are different. During a mammogram, images are collected by flattening the breast between two mammogram plates. Implants can get in the way of this flattening, which makes it difficult to see the breast as clearly. This doesn't mean that women with implants can't be screened for breast cancer. It just means that women with implants need additional pictures taken during the mammogram.

"We do the standard views with the implants," Bevers says. "Then, we push the implants out of the way so that we can get views of the flattened breast tissue. Although it is a more complex process, we can still get good images of the breast."

Women also should be aware that the size of their implants can affect breast cancer testing.

"Very large implants can be more difficult to image with mammography," Beahm says. "So we suggest that women concerned about breast cancer not get extremely large implants. Stick with implants that fit your body type."

If You Get Implants, Educate Yourself about Breast Cancer

Women should get a mammogram before and after they get implants. They also should talk to their doctor about their family history of cancer. They should protect themselves by being aware of their own breasts, talking to their doctor about their family history and following current breast cancer screening guidelines.

"If you get implants, get a mammogram before your reconstructive surgery," Beahm says. "Also, get a mammogram six months after to serve as a baseline for future tests. There can be changes in the breast after any surgery. It may seem like a lot of time, trouble, and money, but it is well worth it."

When getting a mammogram, women should remind their doctor, radiologist, and gynecologist that they have implants at every appointment.

Chapter 27

Mammograms

Chapter Contents

Section 27.1

Questions and Answers about Mammograms

Excerpted from "Mammograms," by the National Cancer Institute (NCI, www .cancer.gov), part of the National Institutes of Health, September 22, 2010.

What is a mammogram?

A mammogram is an x-ray picture of the breast.

Mammograms can be used to check for breast cancer in women who have no signs or symptoms of the disease. This type of mammogram is called a screening mammogram. Screening mammograms usually involve two x-ray pictures, or images, of each breast. The x-ray images make it possible to detect tumors that cannot be felt. Screening mammograms can also find microcalcifications (tiny deposits of calcium) that sometimes indicate the presence of breast cancer.

Mammograms can also be used to check for breast cancer after a lump or other sign or symptom of the disease has been found. This type of mammogram is called a diagnostic mammogram. Signs of breast cancer may include pain, skin thickening, nipple discharge, or a change in breast size or shape; however, these signs may also be indicators of benign conditions. A diagnostic mammogram can also be used to evaluate changes found during a screening mammogram or to view breast tissue when it is difficult to obtain a screening mammogram because of special circumstances, such as the presence of breast implants.

How are screening and diagnostic mammograms different?

Diagnostic mammography takes longer than screening mammography because more x-rays are needed to obtain views of the breast from several angles. The technician may magnify a suspicious area to produce a detailed picture that can help the doctor make an accurate diagnosis.

What are the benefits of screening mammograms?

Early detection of breast cancer with screening mammography means that treatment can be started earlier in the course of the disease, possibly before it has spread. Results from randomized clinical trials and other studies show that screening mammography can help reduce the number of deaths from breast cancer among women ages 40 to 74, especially for those over age 50. However, studies conducted to date have not shown a benefit from regular screening mammography in women under age 40 or from baseline screening mammograms (mammograms used for comparison) taken before age 40.

What are some of the potential harms of screening mammograms?

Finding cancer does not always mean saving lives: Even though mammograms can detect malignant tumors that cannot be felt, treating a small tumor does not always mean that a woman's life will be saved. A fast-growing or aggressive cancer may have already spread to other parts of the body before it is detected. In addition, screening mammograms may not help a woman who is suffering from other, more life-threatening health conditions.

False-negative results: False-negative results occur when mammograms appear normal even though breast cancer is present. Overall, screening mammograms miss up to 20 percent of breast cancers that are present at the time of screening.

The main cause of false-negative results is high breast density. Breasts contain both dense tissue (i.e., glandular tissue and connective tissue, together known as fibroglandular tissue) and fatty tissue. Fatty tissue appears dark on a mammogram, whereas dense tissue and tumors appear as white areas. Because fibroglandular tissue and tumors have similar density, tumors can be harder to detect in women with denser breasts.

False-negative results occur more often among younger women than among older women because younger women are more likely to have dense breasts. As a woman ages, her breasts usually become more fatty, and false-negative results become less likely. False-negative results can lead to delays in treatment and a false sense of security for affected women.

False-positive results: False-positive results occur when radiologists decide mammograms are abnormal but no cancer is actually present. All abnormal mammograms should be followed up with additional testing (diagnostic mammograms, ultrasound, and/or biopsy) to determine whether cancer is present.

False-positive results are more common for younger women, women who have had previous breast biopsies, women with a family history of breast cancer, and women who are taking estrogen (for example, menopausal hormone therapy).

False-positive mammogram results can lead to anxiety and other forms of psychological distress in affected women. The additional testing required to rule out cancer can also be costly and time consuming and can cause physical discomfort.

Overdiagnosis and overtreatment: Screening mammograms can find cancers and cases of ductal carcinoma in situ (DCIS, a noninvasive lesion in which abnormal cells that may become cancerous form in the lining of breast ducts) that need to be treated. However, they can also find cancers and cases of DCIS that will never cause symptoms or threaten a woman's life, leading to "overdiagnosis" of breast cancer. Treatment of these latter cancers and cases of DCIS is not needed, leading to "overtreatment." Overtreatment exposes women unnecessarily to the adverse effects associated with cancer therapy.

Because doctors cannot currently distinguish cancers and cases of DCIS that need to be treated from those that do not, they are all treated.

Radiation exposure: Mammograms require very small doses of radiation. The risk of harm from this radiation exposure is low, but repeated x-rays have the potential to cause cancer. The benefits, however, nearly always outweigh the risk.

Women should talk with their health care providers about the need for each x-ray. In addition, they should always let their health care provider and the technician know if there is any possibility that they are pregnant.

What are the National Cancer Institute's (NCI) recommendations for screening mammograms?

Women age 40 and older should have mammograms every one to two years.

Women who are at higher than average risk of breast cancer should talk with their health care providers about whether to have mammograms before age 40 and how often to have them.

What factors increase a woman's risk of breast cancer?

The strongest risk factor for breast cancer is age. A woman's risk of developing this disease increases as she gets older. The risk of breast cancer, however, is not the same for all women in a given age group.

Research has shown that women with the following risk factors have an increased chance of developing breast cancer.

Personal history of breast cancer: Women who have had breast cancer are more likely to develop a second breast cancer.

Family history: A woman's chance of developing breast cancer increases if her mother, sister, and/or daughter have been diagnosed with the disease, especially if they were diagnosed before age 50. Having a close male blood relative with breast cancer also increases a woman's risk of developing the disease.

Genetic alterations (changes): Inherited changes in certain genes (for example, BRCA1 [breast cancer gene 1], BRCA2 [breast cancer gene 2], and others) increase the risk of breast cancer. These changes are estimated to account for no more than 10 percent of all breast cancers. However, women who carry certain changes in these genes have a much higher risk of breast cancer than women who do not carry these changes.

Breast density: Women who have a high percentage of dense breast tissue have a higher risk of breast cancer than women of similar age who have little or no dense tissue in their breasts. Some of this increase may reflect the "masking" effect of fibroglandular tissue on the ability to detect tumors on mammograms.

Certain breast changes found on biopsy: Looking at breast tissue under a microscope allows doctors to determine whether cancer or another type of breast change is present. Most breast changes are not cancer, but some may increase the risk of developing breast cancer. Changes associated with an increased risk of breast cancer include atypical hyperplasia (a noncancerous condition in which cells have abnormal features and are increased in number), lobular carcinoma in situ (LCIS) (abnormal cells are found in the lobules of the breast), and DCIS. Because some cases of DCIS will eventually become cancer, this type of breast change is actively treated. Women with atypical hyperplasia or LCIS are usually monitored carefully and not actively treated. In addition, women who have had two or more breast biopsies for other noncancerous conditions also have an increased risk of developing breast cancer. This increased risk is due to the conditions that led to the biopsies and not to the biopsy procedures.

Reproductive and menstrual history: Women who had their first menstrual period before age 12 or who went through menopause after age 55 are at increased risk of developing breast cancer. Women who had their first full-term pregnancy after age 30 or who have never had a full-term pregnancy are also at increased risk of breast cancer.

Long-term use of menopausal hormone therapy: Women who use combined estrogen and progestin menopausal hormone therapy for more than five years have an increased chance of developing breast cancer.

Radiation therapy: Women who had radiation therapy to the chest (including the breasts) before age 30 have an increased risk of developing breast cancer throughout their lives. This includes women treated for Hodgkin lymphoma. Studies show that the younger a woman was when she received treatment, the higher her risk of developing breast cancer later in life.

Alcohol: Studies indicate that the more alcohol a woman drinks, the greater her risk of breast cancer.

DES (diethylstilbestrol): The drug DES was given to some pregnant women in the United States between 1940 and 1971 to prevent miscarriage. Women who took DES during pregnancy may have a slightly increased risk of breast cancer. The effects of DES exposure on breast cancer risk in their daughters are unclear and still under study.

Body weight: Studies have found that the chance of getting breast cancer after menopause is higher in women who are overweight or obese.

Physical activity level: Women who are physically inactive throughout life may have an increased risk of breast cancer. Being active may help reduce risk by preventing weight gain and obesity.

What are the chances that a woman in the United States might develop breast cancer?

Age is the most important risk factor for breast cancer. The older a woman is, the greater her chance of developing the disease. Most breast cancers occur in women over the age of 50. The number of cases is especially high for women over age 60. Breast cancer is relatively uncommon in women under age 40.

What is the best method of detecting breast cancer as early as possible?

Getting a high-quality screening mammogram and having a clinical breast exam (an exam done by a health care provider) on a regular basis are the most effective ways to detect breast cancer early. As with any screening test, screening mammograms have both benefits and limitations. For example, some cancers cannot be detected by a screening mammogram but may be found by a clinical breast exam.

Checking one's own breasts for lumps or other unusual changes is called a breast self-exam, or BSE. This type of exam cannot replace regular screening mammograms or clinical breast exams. In clinical trials, BSE alone was not found to help reduce the number of deaths from breast cancer.

Although regular BSE is not specifically recommended for breast cancer screening, many women choose to examine their own breasts. Women who do so should remember that breast changes can occur because of pregnancy, aging, menopause, during menstrual cycles, or when taking birth control pills or other hormones. It is normal for breasts to feel a little lumpy and uneven. Also, it is common for breasts to be swollen and tender right before or during a menstrual period. If a woman notices any unusual changes in her breasts, she should contact her health care provider.

How much does a mammogram cost?

The cost of screening mammograms varies by state and by facility, and can depend on insurance coverage. However, most states have laws that require health insurance companies to reimburse all or part of the cost of screening mammograms. Women are encouraged to contact their mammography facility or their health insurance company for information about cost and coverage.

All women age 40 and older with Medicare can get a screening mammogram each year. Medicare will also pay for one baseline mammogram for female beneficiaries between the ages of 35 and 39. There is no deductible requirement for this benefit, but Medicare beneficiaries have to pay 20 percent of the Medicare-approved amount. Information about Medicare coverage is available at www.medicare.gov on the internet, or through the Medicare Hotline at 800-MEDICARE (800-633-4227). For the hearing impaired, the telephone number is 877-486-2048.

How can uninsured or low-income women obtain a free or low-cost screening mammogram?

Some state and local health programs and employers provide mammograms free or at low cost. For example, the Centers for Disease Control and Prevention (CDC) coordinates the National Breast and Cervical

Cancer Early Detection Program. This program provides screening services, including clinical breast exams and mammograms, to low-income, uninsured women throughout the United States and in several U.S. territories. Contact information for local programs is available on the CDC's website at apps.nccd.cdc.gov/cancercontacts/nbccedp/contacts.asp or by calling the CDC at 800-CDC-INFO (800-232-4636).

Information about low-cost or free mammography screening programs is also available through NCI's Cancer Information Service (CIS) at 800-4-CANCER (800-422-6237). Women can also check with their local hospital, health department, women's center, or other community groups to find out how to access low-cost or free mammograms.

What should women with breast implants do about screening mammograms?

Women with breast implants should continue to have mammograms. (A woman who had an implant following a mastectomy should ask her doctor whether a mammogram of the reconstructed breast is necessary.) It is important to let the mammography facility know about breast implants when scheduling a mammogram. The technician and radiologist must be experienced in performing mammography on women who have breast implants. Implants can hide some breast tissue, making it more difficult for the radiologist to detect an abnormality on the mammogram. If the technician performing the procedure is aware that a woman has breast implants, steps can be taken to make sure that as much breast tissue as possible can be seen on the mammogram. A special technique called implant displacement views may be used.

What is digital mammography? How is it different from conventional (film) mammography?

Digital and conventional mammography both use x-rays to produce an image of the breast; however, in conventional mammography, the image is stored directly on film, whereas in digital mammography, an electronic image of the breast is stored as a computer file. This digital information can be enhanced, magnified, or manipulated for further evaluation more easily than information stored on film. Except for the difference in how the image is recorded and stored, there is no other difference between the two types of mammography.

Because digital mammography allows a radiologist to adjust, store, and retrieve digital images electronically, digital mammography may offer the following advantages over conventional mammography:

- Health care providers can share image files electronically, making long-distance consultations between radiologists and breast surgeons easier.

- Subtle differences between normal and abnormal tissues may be more easily noted.

- Fewer follow-up procedures may be needed.

- Fewer repeat images may be needed, reducing the exposure to radiation.

The U.S. Food and Drug Administration (FDA) approved the use of digital mammography in January 2000. In September 2005, preliminary results from a large clinical trial that compared digital mammography with film mammography were published. These results showed no difference between digital and film mammograms in detecting breast cancer in the general population of women in the trial. However, the researchers concluded that digital mammography may be more accurate than conventional film mammography in women with dense breasts who are premenopausal or perimenopausal (i.e., women who had their last menstrual period within 12 months of their mammograms) or who are younger than age 50. Whether this improved accuracy will translate into a reduced risk of breast cancer death is not yet known.

Some health care providers recommend that women who have a very high risk of breast cancer, such as those with BRCA1 or BRCA2 gene alterations, have digital mammograms instead of conventional mammograms; however, no studies have shown that digital mammograms are superior to conventional mammograms for these women.

Digital mammography can be done only in facilities that are certified to practice conventional mammography and have received FDA approval to offer digital mammography. The procedure for having a mammogram with a digital system is the same as with conventional mammography.

Section 27.2

Digital Mammography

One of the most recent advances in x-ray mammography is digital mammography. Digital (computerized) mammography is similar to standard mammography in that x-rays are used to produce detailed images of the breast. Digital mammography uses essentially the same mammography system as conventional mammography, but the system is equipped with a digital receptor and a computer instead of a film cassette. Several studies have demonstrated that digital mammography is at least as accurate as standard mammography.

Digital spot view mammography allows faster and more accurate stereotactic biopsy. This results in shorter examination times and significantly improved patient comfort and convenience since the time the patient must remain still is much shorter. With digital spot-view mammography, images are acquired digitally and displayed immediately on the system monitor. Spot-view digital systems have been approved by the U.S. Food and Drug Administration (FDA) for use in guiding breast biopsy. Traditional stereotactic biopsy requires a mammogram film be exposed, developed, and then reviewed, greatly increasing the time before the breast biopsy can be completed.

In addition to spot-view digital mammography, the FDA has approved a "full-field" digital mammography system to screen for and diagnose breast cancer. With continued improvements, the "full-field" mammography systems may eventually replace traditional mammography.

How Does Digital Mammography Differ from Standard Mammography?

In standard mammography, images are recorded on film using an x-ray cassette. The film is viewed by the radiologist using a "light box" and then stored in a jacket in the facility's archives. With digital mammography, the breast image is captured using a special electronic x-ray detector, which converts the image into a digital picture for review

216

on a computer monitor. The digital mammogram is then stored on a computer. With digital mammography, the magnification, orientation, brightness, and contrast of the image may be altered after the exam is completed to help the radiologist more clearly see certain areas.

To date, studies of digital mammography and standard film mammography have shown that digital mammography is "comparable" to film mammography in terms of detecting breast cancer. In a 2004 article published in the journal, *Radiologic Clinics of North America Radiology,* researchers admit that early studies of digital mammography have been somewhat disappointing because they have not shown a significant advantage over standard film mammography. However, the researchers reiterate that digital mammography is in its infancy and can expect to improve more rapidly than standard film mammography. Small studies have shown that digital mammography may provide additional benefits, such as lower radiation doses and higher sensitivity to abnormalities. For example, a study reported in the March 2001 issue of *Radiology* found that the use of digital mammography can lead to fewer "recalls" (repeat mammograms) than film mammography. Other data from German researchers suggest that the radiation dose can be reduced by up to 50% with digital mammography and still detect breast cancer as well as the standard radiation dose of film mammography. However, the radiation dose of standard film mammography is still extremely low and does not pose a risk to women.

The largest U.S. federally-funded clinical trial on medical imaging is currently underway determine whether digital mammography is equal or superior to standard film mammography in helping to detect breast cancer. The study, called the Digital Mammographic Screening Trial (DMIST), is being coordinated by the American College of Radiology Imaging Network. Nearly 50,000 women have been recruited to participate in several locations throughout the United States. Preliminary results released in September 2005 show that digital mammography is not more accurate for the majority of women. However, the study found that women with dense breasts, those who are pre- or perimenopausal (women who had a last menstrual period within 12 months of their mammograms), or those who are younger than age 50 may benefit from having a digital rather than a film mammogram. Further results are expected as researchers continue to analyze the study's findings.

Digital mammography systems cost approximately 1.5 to 4 times as much as standard film mammography systems. While procedural time saved by using digital mammography over standard film mammography justifies part of the cost for facilities that perform several thousand mammograms each year, the study will determine whether

217

the high cost of digital mammography is justifiable in terms of its benefits in detecting breast cancer.

From the patient's perspective, a digital mammogram is the same as a standard film-based mammogram in that breast compression and radiation are necessary to create clear images of the breast. The time needed to position the patient is the same for each method. However, conventional film mammography requires several minutes to develop the film while digital mammography provides the image on the computer monitor in less than a minute after the exposure/data acquisition. Thus, digital mammography provides a shorter exam for the woman and may possibly allow mammography facilities to conduct more mammograms in a day. Digital mammography can also be manipulated to correct for under- or over-exposure after the exam is completed, eliminating the need for some women to undergo repeat mammograms before leaving the facility.

With digital mammography, the magnification, orientation, brightness, and contrast of the mammogram image may also be altered after the exam is completed to help the radiologist more clearly see certain areas of the breast.

In the near future, digital mammography may provide many benefits over standard film mammography. These benefits include:

- improved contrast between dense and non-dense breast tissue;

- faster image acquisition (less than a minute);

- shorter exam time (approximately half that of film-based mammography);

- easier image storage;

- physician manipulation of breast images for more accurate detection of breast cancer;

- ability to correct under- or over-exposure of films without having to repeat mammograms;

- transmittal of images over phone lines or a network for remote consultation with other physicians.

Promising Developments in Digital Mammography

As stated earlier, preliminary results of the Digital Mammographic Screening Trial (DMIST), released in September 2005, show that digital mammography may be more accurate at detecting breast cancer in some women than standard film mammography. According to the study results, digital and standard film mammography had similar accuracy rates for many women. However, digital mammography was significantly better at screening women in any of the following categories:

- Under age 50, regardless of what level of breast tissue density they had

- Of any age with very dense or extremely dense breasts

- Pre- or perimenopausal women of any age (defined as women who had a last menstrual period within 12 months of their mammograms)

The study showed no benefit for postmenopausal women over age 50 who did not have dense breast tissue.

The FDA approved the first "full-field" digital mammography scanner to screen for and diagnose breast cancer in February 2000. Before applying for FDA certification, data was gathered from 662 patients at four institutions: The University of Colorado, the University of Massachusetts Medical Center, Massachusetts General Hospital, and the Hospital of the University of Pennsylvania. The data compared hard copies of digital breast images on film to conventional mammography films finding that digital mammography is as effective at detecting breast cancer as standard film mammograms. A separate study revealed that the digital mammography scanner showed a slight advantage in the visibility of breast tissue at the skin line.

Disadvantages to Digital Mammography

While digital mammography is quite promising, it still has additional hurdles to undergo before it replaces conventional mammography. Digital mammography must:

- provide higher detail resolution (as standard mammography does);

- become less expensive (digital mammography is currently several times more costly than conventional mammography);

- provide a method to efficiently compare digital mammogram images with existing mammography films on computer monitors.

Standard mammography using film cassettes has the benefit of providing very high detail resolution (image sharpness), which is especially useful for imaging microcalcifications (tiny calcium deposits) and very small abnormalities that may indicate early breast cancer. While full-field digital mammography may lack the spatial resolution of film,

219

clinical trials have shown digital mammography to be at least equivalent to standard film screening mammography. This is because digital mammography has the benefit of providing improved contrast resolution, which may make abnormalities easier to see. Various manufacturers are trying to develop digital mammography systems with detail resolution equivalent to standard film mammography while also providing the benefits of digital mammography noted in the preceding text.

The high cost of digital mammography is a major obstacle. Digital mammography systems cost roughly 1.5 to 4 times as much as standard mammography equipment. Standard mammography systems are currently installed in over 10,000 locations across the United States. It may take years for this current equipment to be updated or replaced and for digital mammography to become widespread.

Section 27.3

Ductography: A Special Type of Mammogram

What is ductography/galactography and why is it performed?

Ductography (also called galactography or ductogalactography) is a special type of contrast enhanced mammography used for imaging the breast ducts. Ductography can aid in diagnosing the cause of an abnormal nipple discharge and is valuable in diagnosing intraductal papillomas and other conditions. Papillomas are wart-like, non-cancerous tumors with branchings or stalks that have grown inside the breast duct; they are the most common cause of nipple discharge.

Nipple discharge can be caused by non-cancerous tumors (such as papillomas) or cancer (such as ductal carcinoma in situ, DCIS). However, the majority of nipple discharges are due to benign (non-cancerous) causes. In particular, discharges that are yellow, green, blue, or black in color are usually categorized as less suspicious. For example, blue or black discharges are often associated with benign cysts. Discharges that are bloody, colorless, or clear in color are categorized as more suspicious, but further investigation usually results in a benign diagnosis. Bilateral nipple discharge (discharge occurring from both breasts) is usually benign and does not typically require investigation with ductography or other procedures. However, all persistent discharges should be reported to a physician for evaluation.

Most women are able to undergo ductography. However, it may be more difficult to perform ductography in [the following]:

- Women who have severe allergies to the contrast media used during the procedure (In some cases, it may be possible to perform ductography with premedication and non-ionic contrast since little contrast is actually absorbed during the procedure.)

- Women who have had previous nipple surgery that has completely disconnected the nipple pores from the underlying ducts (This may be a limited study but it may still be valuable in detecting abnormalities in the small segment of duct just beneath the nipple.)

- Women with severe nipple retraction (turning inward) that would make the procedure difficult to perform (However, the procedure may be worth attempting in select cases.)

Screening mammography and diagnostic mammography differ from ductography in that they do not use contrast injection. Ductography is a specialized procedure and is only performed at select centers and hospitals by radiologists with significant experience with ductography. Many healthcare locations that perform screening or diagnostic mammography do not perform ductography.

How is ductography performed?

The ductography procedure takes between 30 minutes to an hour. Patients referred for ductography most always have nipple discharge at the time of the study. Before performing the procedure, the nipple is usually cleaned and sterilized with an alcohol swab or other material to remove any dried discharge. The radiologist then applies manual pressure to the breast to elicit a fluid discharge. In patients who experience nipple discharge, there is often a "trigger" spot that causes discharge from the nipple when pressure is applied to it. After identifying the discharging duct, the radiologist feeds a small hollow needle (called a blunt-tipped cannula) into this area of the nipple while stabilizing the nipple between his or her thumb and forefinger. Usually, no force, only downward guidance, is needed to insert the cannula into the patient's breast duct.

Once the cannula has been gently fed down the duct, a small amount of radiopaque substance (contrast media) is injected into the breast through a syringe that is connected to the cannula. The breast is then imaged with mammography; the radiopaque contrast helps enhance the duct anatomy on the resulting images. After the procedure is completed, a bandage is typically placed over the nipple to prevent fluid or dye from staining the patient's clothes.

The radiopaque contrast media is a pharmaceutical liquid made up of substances that weaken (attenuate) x-rays as they pass through the organ containing the contrast (in this case, the breast duct). The breast duct filled with contrast is then seen more clearly on the resulting mammogram image and allows the radiologist to better visualize intraductal papillomas or other abnormalities that may be present. The abnormality in the breast appears as a black nodule in the middle of the white duct.

If the radiologist has difficulty feeding the cannula into the breast duct, a local anesthetic gel or warm compress or washcloth is often used before reattempting the procedure. Some physicians coat the tip of the cannula with anesthetic gel and also dab it on the surface of the nipple. If the cannula is still unable to be thread into the breast duct after three attempts, the procedure is typically canceled and rescheduled for one to two weeks later.

Is ductography painful?

A ductogram procedure can be mildly uncomfortable but is not usually painful. A ductogram is likely to be more uncomfortable when there is not a significant quantity of nipple discharge, making it difficult for the physician to find the opening of the discharging duct. This may require probing to find the right duct. If there is significant fluid discharge, the needle (cannula) insertion into the breast duct is usually much easier to perform and less uncomfortable for the patient.

The syringe is used to slowly instill the contrast material through the needle (cannula) into the breast duct. This is not painful but may cause a full sensation similar to when the breast fills with milk during lactation (breastfeeding). If the patient feels fullness or pain during the injection of contrast, she should tell the radiologist. The goal is to completely fill the duct with contrast to get the best image possible. A sensation of pressure or fullness is a good sign that the duct is full and distended (enlarged). However, care should be taken to avoid overfilling because this can hide abnormalities.

In some cases, extravasation may occur during ductography. Extravasation is the flow of contrast media from the breast duct out into the surrounding breast tissue. If extravasation occurs, the cannula is removed from the breast and the patient may be treated with a pain reliever (such as ibuprofen) if necessary. The procedure is usually rescheduled for a later date, typically one to two weeks later. To help minimize the occurrence of extravasation, ductography should be performed by radiologists with significant experience with the procedure.

What treatment may follow ductography?

The ductogram (also called galactogram) may or may not identify the cause of the nipple discharge. The majority of patients who undergo ductography ultimately need surgery to treat the discharge. Surgery may involve removing a papilloma or other nodule in the breast duct. In some cases, removal of the entire ductal system may be required. For example, some patients with duct ectasia (widening and hardening of the duct) may need surgery to remove the affected duct if other treatments, such as heat compresses, do not help.

Even if the cause of discharge remains unknown after ductography, the ductogram can still help the surgeon find the affected duct so that only that duct needs to be removed. This is accomplished by mixing blue dye with the radiographic contrast so the surgeon can see the abnormal duct as blue.

Some surgeons feel that ductography is unnecessary since the patient will likely need surgery anyway. However, identifying the type of abnormality, the number of abnormalities, and their extent in the breast can be very helpful in aiding the surgeon in either removing as little tissue as necessary or in making sure to remove all of the involved tissue associated with extensive abnormalities.

Chapter 28

Other Breast Imaging Procedures

Chapter Contents

Section 28.1

Breast Magnetic Resonance Imaging (MRI)

A breast MRI (magnetic resonance imaging) scan is an imaging test that uses powerful magnets and radio waves to create pictures of the breast and surrounding tissue. It does not use radiation (x-rays).

A breast MRI may be done in combination with mammography or ultrasound. However, it is not a replacement for mammography.

How the Test Is Performed

You will lie on your stomach with your breasts hanging down into cushioned openings. The narrow table slides into the MRI scanner, which is shaped like a tunnel.

You may be asked to wear a hospital gown or clothing without metal fasteners (such as sweatpants and a t-shirt). Certain types of metal can cause blurry images.

Some exams require a special dye (contrast). The dye is usually given before the test through a vein (IV [intravenous]) in your hand or forearm. The dye helps the radiologist see certain areas more clearly.

During the MRI, the person who operates the machine will watch you from another room. The test most often lasts 30–60 minutes, but may take longer.

How to Prepare for the Test

You may be asked not to eat or drink anything for four to six hours before the scan.

Tell your doctor if you are afraid of close spaces (have claustrophobia). You may be given a medicine to help you feel sleepy and less anxious, or your doctor may suggest an open MRI, in which the machine is not as close to the body.

Before the test, tell your health care provider if you have:

• brain aneurysm clips;

- certain types of artificial heart valves;
- heart defibrillator or pacemaker;
- inner ear (cochlear) implants;
- kidney disease or dialysis (you may not be able to receive contrast);
- recently placed artificial joints;
- certain types of vascular stents;
- worked with sheet metal in the past (you may need tests to check for metal pieces in your eyes).

Because the MRI contains strong magnets, metal objects are not allowed into the room with the MRI scanner:

- Pens, pocketknives, and eyeglasses may fly across the room.
- Items such as jewelry, watches, credit cards, and hearing aids can be damaged.
- Pins, hairpins, metal zippers, and similar metallic items can distort the images.
- Removable dental work should be taken out just before the scan.

How the Test Will Feel

An MRI exam causes no pain. If you have difficulty lying still or are very nervous, you may be given a medicine to relax you. Too much movement can blur MRI images and cause errors.

The table may be hard or cold, but you can request a blanket or pillow. The machine produces loud thumping and humming noises when turned on. You can wear ear plugs to help reduce the noise.

An intercom in the room allows you to speak to someone at any time. Some MRIs have televisions and special headphones that you can use to help the time pass.

There is no recovery time, unless you were given a medicine to relax. After an MRI scan, you can resume your normal diet, activity, and medications.

Why the Test Is Performed

MRI provides detailed pictures of the breast. It also provides clear pictures of parts of the breast that are difficult to see clearly on ultrasound or mammogram.

Breast MRI may also be performed to:

- check for more cancer in the same breast or the other breast after breast cancer has been diagnosed;
- distinguish between scar tissue and tumors in the breast;
- evaluate a breast lump (usually after biopsy);
- evaluate an abnormal result on a mammogram or breast ultrasound;
- evaluate for possible rupture of breast implants;
- find any cancer that remains after surgery or chemotherapy;
- guide a biopsy (rare);
- screen for cancer in women at very high risk for breast cancer (such as those with a strong family history);
- screen for cancer in women with very dense breast tissue.

An MRI of the breast can also show:

- blood flow through the breast area;
- blood vessels in the breast area.

What Abnormal Results Mean

Abnormal results may be due to:

- breast cancer;
- cysts;
- leaking or ruptured breast implants.

Consult your health care provider with any questions and concerns.

Risks

MRI contains no radiation. To date, no side effects from the magnetic fields and radio waves have been reported.

The most common type of contrast (dye) used is gadolinium. It is very safe. Allergic reactions to the substance rarely occur. However, gadolinium can be harmful to patients with kidney problems who require dialysis. If you have kidney problems, please tell your health care provider before the test.

The strong magnetic fields created during an MRI can cause heart pacemakers and other implants to not work as well. It can also cause a piece of metal inside your body to move or shift.

Considerations

Breast MRI is more sensitive than mammogram, especially when it is performed using contrast dye. However, breast MRI may not always be able to distinguish breast cancer from noncancerous breast growths. This can lead to a false positive result.

MRI also cannot pick up tiny pieces of calcium (microcalcifications), which mammogram can detect.

A biopsy is needed to confirm the results of a breast MRI.

Section 28.2

Scintimammography (Nuclear Medicine Breast Imaging)

Nuclear medicine breast imaging (also called scintimammography) is a supplemental breast exam that may be used in some patients to investigate a breast abnormality. A nuclear medicine test is not a primary investigative tool for breast cancer but can be helpful in selected cases after diagnostic mammography has been performed. Nuclear medicine breast imaging involves injecting a radioactive tracer (dye) into the patient. Since the dye accumulates differently in cancerous and non-cancerous tissues, scintimammography can help physicians determine whether cancer is present.

Currently, only the Miraluma Tc-99m sestamibi compound, manufactured by DuPont Pharmaceuticals, is approved by the Food and Drug Administration (FDA) for breast imaging in the United States. Therefore, the nuclear medicine breast imaging test may be referred to as a "Miraluma." Nuclear medicine may be appropriate in patients who have dense breast tissue that makes their mammograms difficult to interpret or in patients with palpable abnormalities (i.e., those able to be physically felt) but whose mammograms do not reveal any abnormalities.

Who Is a Candidate for Nuclear Medicine Breast Imaging?

Nuclear medicine breast imaging is not a screening tool for breast cancer. However, after a physical breast exam, mammography, and ultrasound are performed, nuclear medicine breast imaging may be appropriate for certain patients. Supplemental breast imaging helps determine whether a patient has a suspicious breast abnormality that would require a biopsy to confirm the presence of breast cancer.

Nuclear medicine breast imaging may be appropriate for patients with [the following]:

• Dense breast tissue

• Large, palpable (able to be felt) abnormalities that cannot be imaged well with mammography or ultrasound

• Breast implants

• When multiple tumors are suspected

• A lump at the surgical site after mastectomy (breast removal) since scar tissue may be difficult to distinguish from other tumors with other breast imaging exams

• To check the axillary (underarm) lymph nodes to determine whether they contain cancer cells (sentinel lymph node biopsy)

Like magnetic resonance imaging (MRI) of the breast, nuclear medicine may also be helpful to determine if multiple breast tumors are present. For instance, a mammogram or ultrasound (sonogram) of the breast may reveal breast cancer in one area. However, a nuclear medicine breast imaging test may show that the cancer is in fact multifocal; tumors are present in several areas of the breast. Determining the extent of breast cancer with nuclear medicine can help indicate treatment: Breast conserving surgery (lumpectomy) or breast removal (mastectomy). Mastectomy is indicated if there are multiple tumors.

Studies show that nuclear medicine breast imaging is only 40% to 60% accurate in imaging small breast abnormalities but more than 90% accurate in detecting abnormalities over 1 cm. However, mammography and physical exams are often very useful for detecting large abnormalities. It is the small abnormalities that tend to need additional imaging. Therefore, in this respect, nuclear medicine breast imaging is often of limited value.

How Is Nuclear Medicine Breast Imaging Performed?

The nuclear medicine breast imaging test takes approximately 45 minutes to one hour to perform and costs approximately $200 to $600 per exam. Nuclear medicine involves the use of radiation, but the dose is very low and is not harmful to patients. Most of the drug leaves the body within a few hours of the test.

To perform the exam, a radioactive tracer (Tc-99m sestamibi) is injected in the patient's arm opposite of the breast being studied. Patients may experience a brief metallic taste after the tracer is injected. The radioactive tracer travels throughout the body, including to the breast that needs to be imaged. Normal tissue will only accumulate a small amount of the radioactive tracer (dye). However, cancer cells tend to take up more of the dye.

After the radioactive tracer has been injected, the patient is instructed to lie face down on a special table while the breast hangs down through a hole in the table. Approximately five minutes after the injection, a special gamma camera is used to capture images of the breast from several angles. This takes several minutes for each image that is taken. During this time, the patient should try to lie as still as possible. After all of the images are taken while the patient is lying face down on the table, she may be asked to sit up or raise her arms while additional images of her breast are taken. Unlike mammography, no breast compression is necessary during a nuclear medicine test (although mammography is performed prior to the recommendation of a nuclear medicine breast imaging test).

Recent Research on Nuclear Medicine Breast Imaging

In a recent study conducted by Italian researchers, mammography and nuclear medicine breast imaging were compared in 134 women aged 32 to 78. While the overall accuracy of the two tests were similar, mammography was less likely to identify breast cancer in the younger women than the nuclear medicine test. This suggests that nuclear medicine may be effective in women with dense breast tissue. The researchers concluded that nuclear medicine may help in surgical planning because of its high specificity and could be considered complementary to mammography, especially in younger women. A Turkish study also found that nuclear medicine breast imaging may be helpful in detecting breast cancer that had spread to the axillary (armpit) lymph nodes. In fact, nuclear medicine imaging is sometimes used with sentinel lymph node biopsy to help determine if the lymph nodes contain cancer cells.

In another study by researchers from the Los Robles Regional Medical Center in California, nuclear medicine breast imaging was evaluated in 75 patients with signs on either mammography or physical exam that might or might not have indicated breast cancer. Of the 30 diagnosed cancers, 27 were positively identified with nuclear medicine. Eight of those 27 cancers were not identified with mammography or physical exam, and 11 of the cancers were smaller than 1 cm. The researchers concluded that nuclear medicine is a useful method of evaluating patients with indeterminate (difficult to read) mammograms or physical exams and may help detect additional small breast tumors. However, further research is needed to confirm the results of this study, especially since previous studies have shown that nuclear medicine may not be helpful in detecting small breast abnormalities.

Section 28.3

Thermogram No Substitute for Mammogram

From the U.S. Food and Drug Administration (FDA, www.fda.gov),
September 9, 2011.

Despite widely publicized claims to the contrary, thermography should not be used in place of mammography for breast cancer screening or diagnosis.

The Food and Drug Administration (FDA) says mammography—an x-ray of the breast—is still the most effective way of detecting breast cancer in its earliest, most treatable stages. Thermography produces an infrared image that shows the patterns of heat and blood flow on or near the surface of the body.

The agency has sent several warning letters to health care providers and a thermography manufacturer who claim that the thermal imaging can take the place of mammography.

Websites have been touting thermography as a replacement for mammography and claim that thermography can find breast cancer years before it would be detected by mammography.

The problem is that FDA has no evidence to support these claims. "Mammography is still the most effective screening method for detecting breast cancer in its early, most treatable stages," said Helen Barr, MD, director of the Division of Mammography Quality and Radiation Programs in the FDA's Center for Devices and Radiological Health. "Women should not rely solely on thermography for the screening or diagnosis of breast cancer."

"While there is plenty of evidence that mammography is effective in breast cancer detection, there is simply no evidence that thermography can take its place," said Barr.

Thermography devices have been cleared by the FDA for use as an adjunct, or additional, tool for detecting breast cancer. Toni Stifano, a consumer safety officer in FDA's Center for Devices and Radiological Health, explains that this means thermography should not be used by itself to screen for or to diagnose breast cancer.

The National Cancer Institute (NCI), part of the National Institutes of Health, estimates that about one in eight women will be diagnosed with breast cancer sometime in her life.

The greatest danger, says Stifano, a breast cancer survivor herself, is that patients who substitute thermography for mammography may miss the chance to detect cancer at its earliest stage. There has been a steady decline in breast cancer deaths and one of the reasons is early detection through mammography, says FDA.

As for concerns about exposure to radiation from a mammogram, evidence shows that the benefits outweigh the risks of harm, especially when compared to the danger of breast cancer.

FDA is advising patients to continue to have regular mammograms according to screening guidelines or as recommended by their health care professional.

Patients are also advised to follow their health care professional's recommendations for additional diagnostic procedures, such as other mammographic views, clinical breast exam, breast ultrasound, MRI [magnetic resonance imaging], or biopsy. Additional procedures could include thermography.

Section 28.4

Breast Ultrasound

Breast ultrasound uses sound waves that cannot be heard by humans to look at the breast.

How the Test Is Performed

You will be asked to undress from the waist up and put on a medical gown. During the test, you will lie on your back on the examining table.

A water-soluble gel is placed on the skin of the breast. A hand-held device (transducer) directs the sound waves to the breast tissue. The transducer is moved over the skin of the breast to create a picture that can be seen on a screen.

Breast ultrasound may also be used to guide a needle during a breast biopsy.

How to Prepare for the Test

Because you need to remove your clothing from the waist up, it may be helpful to wear a two-piece outfit. On the day of the test, do not use any lotions or powders on your breasts or wear deodorant under your arms.

How the Test Will Feel

The number of people involved in the test will be limited to protect your privacy.

You will be asked to raise your arms above your head and turn to the left or right as needed.

There is no discomfort from the ultrasound.

Why the Test Is Performed

If a breast lump is found during an exam or something abnormal is seen on your mammogram, an ultrasound can help show whether it is a solid mass or a cyst. It can also be used to check for a growth in the breast if a woman has clear or bloody nipple discharge.

Normal Results

Normally, the breast tissue will look the same and will not have any suspicious growths.

What Abnormal Results Mean

Ultrasound can help show noncancerous growths such as:

- cysts—fluid-filled sacs;
- fibroadenomas—noncancerous solid growths;
- lipomas—noncancerous fatty lumps that can occur anywhere in the body, including the breasts.

Breast cancers can also be seen with ultrasound.

Risks

There are no risks associated with breast ultrasound. There is no radiation exposure.

Chapter 29

Breast Biopsy

Chapter Contents

237

Section 29.1

Breast Biopsy Basics

Excerpted from "Having a Breast Biopsy: A Guide for Women and Their Families," by the Agency for Healthcare Research and Quality (AHRQ, www.ahrq.gov), April 2010.

Screening for breast cancer increases the chance of surviving breast cancer. Screening tests can find cancers before they cause symptoms and when they are most treatable. Two common tests are used to screen for breast cancer.

- Mammogram: A mammogram is a breast x-ray. It looks for suspicious changes in breast tissue. It can detect cancers even when they are too small to be felt. A mammogram is the best screening test for breast cancer.

- Breast exam by your doctor or nurse: This is usually part of a woman's yearly exam. But if you find a breast lump or another change that worries you, don't wait. Make an appointment with your doctor or nurse to have it checked.

When a suspicious area on a mammogram or a lump is found, your doctor will probably send you for more tests. Your doctor might send you for another mammogram or a breast ultrasound. These tests tell your doctor if you need a biopsy. Most women who have further tests do not need a biopsy.

If the test results are still suspicious, your doctor will recommend a biopsy.

What Is a Breast Biopsy?

A biopsy is the only test that can tell for sure if a suspicious area is cancer. During a breast biopsy, the doctor removes a small amount of tissue from the breast.

There are two main kinds of breast biopsies. One is called surgical biopsy. The other is called core-needle biopsy.

The kind of breast biopsy a doctor recommends may depend on what the suspicious area looks like. It also might depend on the size and where it is located in the breast.

After the biopsy, the tissue is sent to a doctor who will look at the tissue under a microscope. This doctor, called a pathologist, looks for tissue changes. The pathology report tells if there is cancer or not. It takes about a week to get the report.

Kinds of Breast Biopsy

Surgical Biopsy

A surgical biopsy is usually done using local anesthesia. Local anesthesia means that the breast will be numbed.

You will have an IV [intravenous therapy] and may have medicine to make you drowsy. The surgeon makes a one- to two-inch cut on the breast and removes part or all of the suspicious tissue. Some of the tissue around it also may be taken out.

A radiologist is a doctor who specializes in medical imaging (like x-rays and mammograms). If the suspicious area can be seen on mammogram or ultrasound but can't be felt, a radiologist usually inserts a thin wire to mark the spot for the surgeon before the biopsy.

Core-Needle Biopsy

A core-needle biopsy is done using local anesthesia. The doctor inserts a hollow needle into the breast and removes a small amount of suspicious tissue. The doctor may place a tiny marker inside the breast. It marks the spot where the biopsy was done.

Radiologists or surgeons usually do core-needle biopsies using special imaging equipment.

Ultrasound-guided core-needle biopsy uses ultrasound to guide the needle to the suspicious area. Ultrasound uses sound waves to create a picture of the inside of the breast. It is like what is used to look at the baby when a woman is pregnant. You will lie on your back or side for this procedure. The doctor will hold the ultrasound device against your breast to guide the needle.

Stereotactic-guided core-needle biopsy uses x-ray equipment and a computer to guide the needle. Usually for this kind of biopsy, you lie on your stomach on a special table. The table will have an opening for your breast. Your breast will be compressed like it is for a mammogram.

Freehand core-needle biopsy does not use ultrasound or x-ray equipment. It is used less often and only for lumps that can be felt through the skin.

Research about Breast Biopsy

Accuracy

Surgical biopsies and core-needle biopsies both work well for finding breast cancer. But biopsies are not 100-percent accurate. In a few cases, a biopsy can miss breast cancer.

Surgical biopsies and ultrasound or stereotactic-guided core-needle biopsies have about the same accuracy. Freehand core-needle biopsies are less accurate.

Out of every 100 women who have breast cancer, the following are true:

- Surgical biopsies will find 98 to 99 of those breast cancers.

- Ultrasound or stereotactic-guided biopsies will find 97 to 99 of those breast cancers.

- Freehand biopsies will find about 86 of those breast cancers.

Side Effects

Bleeding, bruising, and infection can happen after a biopsy. Core-needle biopsies have a much lower risk of these problems than surgical biopsies.

Side effects are rare with any kind of core-needle biopsy.

- Less than 1 out of 100 women who have a core-needle biopsy have a problem like severe bruising, bleeding, or infection. Side effects happen more often with surgical biopsy.

- Up to 10 out of 100 women who have surgical biopsy get severe bruising.

- About 5 out of 100 women who have surgical biopsy get an infection.

Some medicines, including aspirin, increase the risk of bleeding and bruising. Your doctor will ask you about the medicines you take. You may need to stop some medicines a few days before the biopsy.

Pain

Women who have a surgical biopsy sometimes need prescription pain medicine to control pain after the procedure. Women who have a core-needle biopsy rarely need prescription pain medicine.

Biopsy Results

After the biopsy, the pathologist who looked at the tissue will send the pathology report to your doctor. It will tell if the suspicious area is cancer or not. Your doctor will go over the report with you.

Waiting for these results can be difficult. It can take about a week to get the results.

If No Cancer Is Found

If no cancer is found, the biopsy result is called benign. Benign means it is not cancer. Some benign results need follow-up or treatment. Talk to your doctor or nurse about what they recommend.

If Cancer Is Found

If cancer is found, the report will tell you the kind of cancer. It will help you and your doctor talk about the next steps. Usually, you will be referred to a breast cancer specialist. You may need more imaging tests or surgery. All this information will help you and your doctor think through your treatment options.

Take time to think. Most women with breast cancer have time to consider their options.

Make sure to ask your doctor if you don't understand your test results. After going over the results with your doctor, ask for a copy of the pathology report for your records.

Questions for Your Doctor or Nurse

Deciding on a Biopsy

- What kind of biopsy are you recommending?

- Why are you recommending this kind of biopsy?

- Are there any other options?

- What are the possible side effects from my biopsy?

- How long will it take?

Preparing for a Biopsy

- How many days before my biopsy should I stop taking aspirin? Are there other medicines to avoid?
- Can I have someone in the room with me?
- Do I need someone to drive me home?
- Who will give me the results?
- When will I get the results?

When Your Biopsy Is Benign

- What kind of follow-up do I need?
- When should I have my next mammogram?

When Your Biopsy Finds Cancer

- What are the next steps?
- What are my options for treatment?
- Can you tell me about support groups for breast cancer?

Section 29.2

MRI Breast Biopsy

A MRI [magnetic resonance imaging] breast biopsy uses computer-guided imagery to precisely position a biopsy needle within the breast. In this special type of biopsy, the radiologist samples breast tissue so that the patient may avoid surgery.

Note: Medications containing aspirin, Advil (ibuprofen), Aleve (naproxen), Vitamin E, and Fish Oil should be stopped for at least four days before the biopsy. If you are taking anticoagulants (blood-thinning medications) you must ask your prescribing doctor when to stop taking the medication before the procedure.

On the Day of Your Procedure

* Eat lightly before the procedure.
* Arrive 30 minutes before your scheduled appointment.
* You can come alone or bring family and/or friends. They can wait in the waiting room during the procedure.
* You may not drive yourself home after the procedure. Make sure someone can pick you up after your biopsy.
* You sign a consent form stating that you understand the procedure.

During Your Procedure

* A staff member shows you to a private room where you change from the waist up.

- The nurse puts an IV (intravenous needle) in your arm.

- You lie face down on a table.

- The MRI scanner takes pictures of the breast. Then, contrast dye is put into your arm through the IV and more pictures are taken. These scans help the radiologist find the area to be sampled.

- The radiologist gives you a shot to numb your breast and then makes a quarter-inch cut so that the biopsy needle can be guided easily into your breast.

- Using the MRI pictures as a guide, the radiologist takes several tissue samples through the needle. A tiny clip made may be inserted through the biopsy needle to mark the area being sampled. The procedure is painless for most women, although you may feel some vibration or pressure when the samples are taken.

- After the biopsy is done, the nurse applies antibiotic ointment, Steri-Strips (incision tapes), a Band-Aid, and an ice pack.

After Your Procedure

- You must have someone drive you home after the procedure.

- Before you go, your nurse will discuss how to care for yourself at home and give you written instructions and supplies, if needed.

- A nurse may call you the afternoon of the biopsy to schedule a mammogram and follow-up appointment.

- Your biopsy results will be available in two to four days. You get the results from a nurse, the radiologist, or from your referring doctor.

Caring for Yourself at Home

- Keep the ice pack on your skin for 20 minutes, then remove it and place it in the freezer for 10 minutes, repeating for 3 hours. Placing the pack within your bra is the easiest way to keep it in place.

- Go home and rest for the remainder of the day. Avoid strenuous activities for 24 hours.

Section 29.3

Sentinel Lymph Node Biopsy

Excerpted from "Sentinel Lymph Node Biopsy," National
Cancer Institute (NCI, www.cancer.gov), part of the National
Institutes of Health, August 11, 2011.

What are lymph nodes?

Lymph nodes are small round organs that are part of the body's
lymphatic system. They are found widely throughout the body and
are connected to one another by lymph vessels. Groups of lymph
nodes are located in the neck, underarms, chest, abdomen, and
groin. A clear fluid called lymph flows through lymph vessels and
lymph nodes.

Lymph originates from a fluid, known as interstitial fluid, that
has diffused, or leaked, out of small blood vessels called capillaries.
This fluid contains many substances, including blood plasma, proteins,
glucose, and oxygen. It bathes most of the body's cells, providing them
with the oxygen and nutrients they need for growth and survival. Interstitial fluid also picks up waste products from cells as well as other
materials, such as bacteria and viruses, to help remove them from the
body's tissues. Interstitial fluid eventually collects in lymph vessels,
where it becomes known as lymph. Lymph flows through the body's
lymph vessels to reach two large ducts at the base of the neck, where
it is emptied into the bloodstream.

Lymph nodes are important parts of the body's immune system.
They contain B lymphocytes, T lymphocytes, and other types of immune system cells. These cells monitor lymph for the presence of foreign substances, such as bacteria and viruses. If a foreign substance
is detected, some of the cells will become activated and an immune
response will be triggered.

Lymph nodes are also important in helping to determine whether
cancer cells have developed the ability to spread to other parts of the
body. Many types of cancer spread through the lymphatic system,
and one of the earliest sites of spread for these cancers is nearby
lymph nodes.

What is a sentinel lymph node?

A sentinel lymph node is defined as the first lymph node to which cancer cells are most likely to spread from a primary tumor. Sometimes, there can be more than one sentinel lymph node.

What is a sentinel lymph node biopsy?

A sentinel lymph node biopsy (SLNB) is a procedure in which the sentinel lymph node is identified, removed, and examined to determine whether cancer cells are present.

A negative SLNB result suggests that cancer has not developed the ability to spread to nearby lymph nodes or other organs. A positive SLNB result indicates that cancer is present in the sentinel lymph node and may be present in other nearby lymph nodes (called regional lymph nodes) and, possibly, other organs. This information can help a doctor determine the stage of the cancer (extent of the disease within the body) and develop an appropriate treatment plan.

What happens during an SLNB?

A surgeon injects a radioactive substance, a blue dye, or both near the tumor to locate the position of the sentinel lymph node. The surgeon then uses a device that detects radioactivity to find the sentinel node or looks for lymph nodes that are stained with the blue dye. Once the sentinel lymph node is located, the surgeon makes a small incision (about half an inch) in the overlying skin and removes the node.

The sentinel node is then checked for the presence of cancer cells by a pathologist. If cancer is found, the surgeon may remove additional lymph nodes, either during the same biopsy procedure or during a follow-up surgical procedure. SLNBs may be done on an outpatient basis or may require a short stay in the hospital.

SLNB is usually done at the same time the primary tumor is removed. However, the procedure can also be done either before or after removal of the tumor.

What are the benefits of SLNB?

In addition to helping doctors stage cancers and estimate the risk that tumor cells have developed the ability to spread to other parts of the body, SLNB may help some patients avoid more extensive lymph node surgery. Removing additional nearby lymph nodes to look for cancer cells may not be necessary if the sentinel node is negative for cancer. All lymph node surgery can have adverse effects, and some of these effects may be reduced or avoided if fewer lymph nodes are removed.

Lymphedema, or tissue swelling, is a potential adverse effect of lymph node surgery. During SLNB or more extensive lymph node surgery, lymph vessels leading to and from the sentinel node or group of nodes are cut, thereby disrupting the normal flow of lymph through the affected area. This disruption may lead to an abnormal buildup of lymph fluid. In addition to swelling, patients with lymphedema may experience pain or discomfort in the affected area, and the overlying skin may become thickened or hard. In the case of extensive lymph node surgery in an armpit or groin, the swelling may affect an entire arm or leg. In addition, there is an increased risk of infection in the affected area or limb. Very rarely, chronic lymphedema due to extensive lymph node removal may cause a cancer of the lymphatic vessels called lymphangiosarcoma.

Other potential adverse effects of lymph node surgery include the following:

- Seroma, or the buildup of lymph fluid at the site of the surgery
- Numbness, tingling, or pain at the site of the surgery
- Difficulty moving the affected body part

Is SLNB associated with other harms?

SLNB, like other surgical procedures, can cause short-term pain, swelling, and bruising at the surgical site and increase the risk of infection. In addition, some patients may have skin or allergic reactions to the blue dye used in SLNB. Another potential harm is a false-negative biopsy result—that is, cancer cells are not seen in the sentinel lymph node although they are present and may have already spread to other regional lymph nodes or other parts of the body. A false-negative biopsy result gives the patient and the doctor a false sense of security about the extent of cancer in the patient's body.

Is SLNB used to help stage all types of cancer?

No. SLNB is most commonly used to help stage breast cancer and melanoma. However, it is being studied with other cancer types, including colorectal cancer, gastric cancer, esophageal cancer, head and neck cancer, thyroid cancer, and non-small cell lung cancer.

What has research shown about the use of SLNB in breast cancer?

Breast cancer cells are most likely to spread first to lymph nodes located in the axilla, or armpit area, next to the affected breast. However, in breast cancers close to the center of the chest (near the breastbone), cancer cells may spread first to lymph nodes inside the chest (under the breastbone) before they can be detected in the axilla.

The number of lymph nodes in the axilla varies from person to person but usually ranges from 20 to 40. Historically, removal of these lymph nodes (in an operation called axillary lymph node dissection, or ALND) was done for two reasons: To help stage breast cancer and to help prevent a regional recurrence of the disease. (Regional recurrence of breast cancer occurs when breast cancer cells that have migrated to nearby lymph nodes give rise to a new tumor.)

Because removing multiple lymph nodes at the same time has been associated with adverse effects, the possibility that SLNB alone might be sufficient for staging breast cancer in women who have no clinical signs of axillary lymph node metastasis, such as swollen or matted (clumped or stuck together) nodes, was investigated.

In a phase III trial involving 5,611 women with breast cancer and no clinical signs of axillary metastasis, researchers from the National Surgical Adjuvant Breast and Bowel Project, which is a National Cancer Institute (NCI) clinical trials cooperative group, randomly assigned participants to receive SLNB alone or SLNB plus ALND. The women in the two groups whose sentinel lymph node(s) were negative for cancer (a total of 3,989 women) were then followed for an average of 8 years. Most of the women (87.5 percent) had a lumpectomy, and the rest had a mastectomy. Nearly 88 percent of the women also received adjuvant systemic therapy (chemotherapy, hormonal therapy, or both), and 82 percent had external-beam radiation therapy to the affected breast.

The researchers found no differences in overall survival and disease-free survival between the two groups of women. Based on these results, it was concluded that ALND might not be necessary for women with clinically negative axillary lymph nodes and a negative SLNB whose breast cancer is treated with surgery, adjuvant systemic therapy, and external-beam radiation therapy.

Subsequently, the American College of Surgeons Oncology Group, which is another NCI clinical trials cooperative group, reported findings from an additional phase III clinical trial, this one testing whether women with a positive sentinel lymph node but no clinical evidence of axillary lymph node metastasis could be safely treated with tumor removal and no further lymph node surgery other than the SLNB. In this trial, 891 women were randomly assigned to SLNB only or ALND after SLNB. All of the women were treated with lumpectomy. More than 95 percent of them also received adjuvant systemic therapy (chemotherapy, hormone therapy, or both), and about 90 percent received external-beam radiation therapy to the affected breast.

When the results of this trial were reported, the patients had been followed for a median of 6.3 years. The two groups of women had similar 5-year overall survival (92.5 percent in the SLNB-only group versus 91.8 percent in the SLNB plus ALND group) and 5-year disease-free survival (83.9 percent in the SLNB-only group and 82.2 percent in the SLNB plus ALND group). The researchers concluded that SLNB alone is safe and does not affect the survival of women who have sentinel lymph node metastasis but no clinical signs of other lymph node involvement and whose breast cancer is treated with surgery, systemic therapy, and external-beam radiation therapy. The excellent outcome in this trial for women treated with SLNB without ALND is likely due, at least in part, to the ability of local radiation therapy and modern systemic treatments to effectively treat breast cancer cells that may have spread to other axillary lymph nodes besides the sentinel node or to other parts of the body.

Section 29.4

Stereotactic Breast Biopsy

A breast biopsy is the removal of breast tissue to examine it for signs of breast cancer or other disorders. Several different types of biopsy may be done. This text discusses stereotactic breast biopsy. A stereotactic breast biopsy uses mammography to help pinpoint the spot in the breast that needs to be removed.

How the Test Is Performed

You will be asked to undress from the waist up.

You will most likely be asked to lie facing down on the biopsy table. The breast that is being biopsied will hang through an opening in the table. The table is raised and the doctor will perform the biopsy from underneath. In some cases, stereotactic breast biopsy is done while the woman sits in an upright position.

A stereotactic biopsy includes the following steps:

- The health care provider will first clean the area on your breast, and will then inject a numbing medicine. This may sting a little bit.

- The breast is pressed down to hold it in position during the procedure. You need to hold still while the biopsy is being performed.

- The doctor will make a very small cut on your breast over the area that needs to be biopsied.

- Using a special machine, a needle or sheath is guided to the exact location of the abnormal area. Up to six or more tissue samples are taken.

- A small metal clip or needle may be placed into the breast in the biopsy area to mark it for biopsy, if needed.

The biopsy itself is done using one of the following:

- Fine needle aspiration

- Hollow needle (called a core needle)
- Vacuum-powered device
- Both a needle and vacuum-powered device

The procedure usually takes about one hour, including the time it takes for the x-rays. The actual biopsy only takes several minutes.

After the tissue sample has been taken, the catheter or needle is removed. Ice and pressure are applied to the site to stop any bleeding. A bandage will be applied to absorb any fluid. You will not need stitches after the needle is taken out. Steri-Strips may be placed over any wound, if needed.

How to Prepare for the Test

The health care provider will ask questions about your medical history and perform a manual breast exam.

You must sign an informed consent form. If you are going to have general anesthesia, you may be asked not to eat or drink anything for 8–12 hours before the test.

If you take medications (including aspirin or herbal medications), ask your doctor whether you need to stop taking these before the biopsy.

Tell your doctor if you may be pregnant before having an open biopsy.

Do not wear lotion, perfume, powder, or deodorant underneath your arms or on your breasts.

How the Test Will Feel

You may feel a sharp, stinging sensation when the local anesthetic is injected. During the procedure, you may feel slight discomfort or light pressure.

Lying on your stomach for up to one hour may be uncomfortable. Using cushions or pillows may help. Some patients are given a pill to help relax them before the procedure.

After the test, the breast may be sore and tender to the touch for several days. Do not do any heavy lifting or work with your arms for 24 hours after the biopsy. You can use acetaminophen (Tylenol) for pain relief.

Why the Test Is Performed

This test may be done if your doctor suspects cancer due to abnormal findings on a mammogram or ultrasound of the breast, or during a physical exam.

251

To identify whether someone has breast cancer, a biopsy must be done. Tissue and fluid from the abnormal area are removed and examined with a microscope.

Stereotactic breast biopsy is often used when a small growth or calcifications are seen on a mammogram, but cannot be seen using an ultrasound of the breast.

Normal Results

A normal result means there is no sign of cancer.

Your doctor or nurse will let you know when you need a follow-up mammogram or other tests.

What Abnormal Results Mean

A biopsy can identify a number of breast conditions that are not cancer or precancer, including:

- adenofibroma;
- fibrocystic breast disease;
- mammary fat necrosis.

Biopsy results may show precancerous breast conditions, including:

- atypical ductal hyperplasia;
- atypical lobular hyperplasia;
- intraductal papilloma.

Two main types of breast cancer may be found:

- Ductal carcinoma starts in the tubes (ducts) that move milk from the breast to the nipple. Most breast cancers are of this type.
- Lobular carcinoma starts in parts of the breast called lobules, which produce milk.

Depending on the results of the biopsy, you may need further surgery or treatment.

Risks

There is a slight chance of infection at the injection or surgical cut site.

Excessive bleeding is rare, but may require draining or re-bandaging. Bruising is common.

Chapter 30

Testing for Hormone Receptor Status

At a Glance

Why get tested?: To determine whether a breast cancer tumor is positive for estrogen and/or progesterone receptors, which helps to guide treatment and determine prognosis.

When to get tested?: When you have been diagnosed with breast cancer and your doctor wants to determine whether the tumor's growth is influenced by the hormones estrogen and/or progesterone.

Sample required?: A sample of breast cancer tissue obtained during a biopsy or a tumor removed surgically during a lumpectomy or mastectomy.

Test preparation needed?: Your doctor may have you discontinue taking hormones for a time period before your sample is collected.

The Test Sample

What is being tested?

Estrogen receptors (ER) and progesterone receptors (PR) are specialized proteins found within certain cells throughout the body. These receptors bind to estrogen and progesterone, female hormones that circulate in the blood, and promote new cell growth and division.

Many breast cancer tumors have receptors for estrogen and/or progesterone, often in large numbers. These tumors are said to be hormone-dependent, and estrogen and/or progesterone feed their growth. Breast cancer tissue can be tested to see if it is positive for these receptors.

How is the sample collected for testing?

A sample of breast cancer tissue is obtained by doing a fine needle aspiration, needle biopsy, or surgical biopsy or when a tumor removed surgically during a lumpectomy or mastectomy is tested.

Is any test preparation needed to ensure the quality of the sample?

Your doctor may have you discontinue taking hormones for a time period before your sample is collected.

The Test

How is it used?

Estrogen and progesterone hormone receptor status tests are typically performed on all invasive breast cancers. Hormone receptor status is used as a prognostic marker, and used to help guide the treatment of people with primary or recurrent breast cancer.

Those who have ER-positive and PR-positive tumors tend to have a better prognosis for disease-free survival and overall survival than those with ER-negative or PR-negative tumors. They are also much more likely to respond to endocrine therapy (anti-hormone treatments such as tamoxifen).

When is it ordered?

Hormone receptor status testing is recommended as part of an initial workup of invasive breast cancer. It is not diagnostic but helps the doctor to determine treatment options and to understand more about the tumor's characteristics.

What does the test result mean?

In general, if a person's cancer is ER-positive and PR-positive, the patient will have a better-than-average prognosis, and their cancer is likely to respond to endocrine therapy (anti-hormone treatments).

The more receptors present and the more intense their reaction, the more likely the response. If a person's cancer is ER-negative but PR-positive, or ER-positive but PR-negative, then she may still benefit from endocrine therapy but may have a diminished response.

If the cancer is both ER-negative and PR-negative, then the person will probably not benefit from endocrine therapy.

An individual's response to endocrine therapy will depend on a variety of factors, but typical response rates include:

- ER positive, PR positive: 75–80%;

- ER positive, PR negative: 40–50%;

- ER negative, PR positive: 25–30%;

- ER negative, PR negative: 10% or less.

Is there anything else I should know?

Her-2 [human epidermal growth factor receptor 2]/neu testing may be done at the same time as hormone receptor status testing. A patient with a positive estrogen and/or progesterone receptor status may find their response to endocrine therapy diminished if they are also Her-2/neu-positive.

Hormone receptor status testing is not available in every laboratory. It requires experience and special training to perform and interpret. Your doctor will probably send your sample to a reference laboratory and it may take several weeks before your results are available.

It takes a small amount of cancer tissue to perform hormone receptor status testing. If a sufficient sample is not available, your doctor may make an assumption that your cancer is ER-positive and PR-positive in order to broaden your treatment options.

Common Questions

Is there a blood test that can be done to check my hormone receptor status?

No. The cancer cells do not "shed" the receptors, so they are not detectable in the blood. They must be evaluated in the cancer tissue itself.

Would this testing also be performed on a man?

Yes. Men do not get breast cancer as frequently as women, but it does occur and their cancer may also be ER or PR positive.

Chapter 31

Understanding Your Breast Pathology Report

What is a pathology report?

A pathology report is a document that contains the diagnosis determined by examining cells and tissues under a microscope. The report may also contain information about the size, shape, and appearance of a specimen as it looks to the naked eye. This information is known as the gross description.

A pathologist is a doctor who does this examination and writes the pathology report. Pathology reports play an important role in cancer diagnosis and staging (describing the extent of cancer within the body, especially whether it has spread), which helps determine treatment options.

How is tissue obtained for examination by the pathologist?

In most cases, a doctor needs to do a biopsy or surgery to remove cells or tissues for examination under a microscope.

Some common ways a biopsy can be done are as follows:

- A needle is used to withdraw tissue or fluid.

- An endoscope (a thin, lighted tube) is used to look at areas inside the body and remove cells or tissues.

Excerpted from "Pathology Reports," by the National Cancer Institute (NCI, www.cancer.gov), part of the National Institutes of Health, September 23, 2010.

- Surgery is used to remove part of the tumor or the entire tumor. If the entire tumor is removed, typically some normal tissue around the tumor is also removed.

Tissue removed during a biopsy is sent to a pathology laboratory, where it is sliced into thin sections for viewing under a microscope. This is known as histologic (tissue) examination and is usually the best way to tell if cancer is present. The pathologist may also examine cytologic (cell) material. Cytologic material is present in urine, cerebrospinal fluid (the fluid around the brain and spinal cord), sputum (mucus from the lungs), peritoneal (abdominal cavity) fluid, pleural (chest cavity) fluid, cervical/vaginal smears, and in fluid removed during a biopsy.

How is tissue processed after a biopsy or surgery? What is a frozen section?

The tissue removed during a biopsy or surgery must be cut into thin sections, placed on slides, and stained with dyes before it can be examined under a microscope. Two methods are used to make the tissue firm enough to cut into thin sections: Frozen sections and paraffin-embedded (permanent) sections. All tissue samples are prepared as permanent sections, but sometimes frozen sections are also prepared.

Permanent sections are prepared by placing the tissue in fixative (usually formalin) to preserve the tissue, processing it through additional solutions, and then placing it in paraffin wax. After the wax has hardened, the tissue is cut into very thin slices, which are placed on slides and stained. The process normally takes several days. A permanent section provides the best quality for examination by the pathologist and produces more accurate results than a frozen section.

Frozen sections are prepared by freezing and slicing the tissue sample. They can be done in about 15 to 20 minutes while the patient is in the operating room. Frozen sections are done when an immediate answer is needed; for example, to determine whether the tissue is cancerous so as to guide the surgeon during the course of an operation.

How long after the tissue sample is taken will the pathology report be ready?

The pathologist sends a pathology report to the doctor within 10 days after the biopsy or surgery is performed. Pathology reports are written in technical medical language. Patients may want to ask their doctors to give them a copy of the pathology report and to explain the report to them. Patients also may wish to keep a copy of their pathology report in their own records.

What information does a pathology report usually include?

The pathology report may include the following information:

- Patient information, including name, birth date, biopsy date
- Gross description, including color, weight, and size of tissue as seen by the naked eye
- Microscopic description, such as how the sample looks under the microscope and how it compares with normal cells
- Diagnosis, or the type of tumor/cancer and grade (how abnormal the cells look under the microscope and how quickly the tumor is likely to grow and spread)
- Tumor size, measured in centimeters (cm)
- Other information, usually notes about samples that have been sent for other tests or a second opinion
- Pathologist's signature and name and address of the laboratory

The report may also include information on tumor margins. There are three possible findings when the biopsy sample is the entire tumor:

- Positive margins mean that cancer cells are found at the edge of the material removed.
- Negative, not involved, clear, or free margins mean that no cancer cells are found at the outer edge.
- Close margins are neither negative nor positive.

What might the pathology report say about the physical and chemical characteristics of the tissue?

After identifying the tissue as cancerous, the pathologist may perform additional tests to get more information about the tumor that cannot be determined by looking at the tissue with routine stains, such as hematoxylin and eosin (also known as H&E), under a microscope. The pathology report will include the results of these tests. For example, the pathology report may include information obtained from immunochemical stains (IHC). IHC uses antibodies to identify specific antigens on the surface of cancer cells. IHC can often be used to determine where the cancer started, distinguish among different cancer types, such as carcinoma, melanoma, and lymphoma, and help diagnose and classify leukemias and lymphomas.

The pathology report may also include the results of flow cytometry. Flow cytometry is a method of measuring properties of cells in a sample, including the number of cells, percentage of live cells, cell size and shape, and presence of tumor markers on the cell surface. (Tumor markers are substances produced by tumor cells or by other cells in the body in response to cancer or certain noncancerous conditions.) Flow cytometry can be used in the diagnosis, classification, and management of cancers such as acute leukemia, chronic lymphoproliferative disorders, and non-Hodgkin lymphoma.

Finally, the pathology report may include the results of molecular diagnostic and cytogenetic studies. Such studies investigate the presence or absence of malignant cells, and genetic or molecular abnormalities in specimens.

What information about the genetics of the cells might be included in the pathology report?

Cytogenetics uses tissue culture and specialized techniques to provide genetic information about cells, particularly genetic alterations. Some genetic alterations are markers or indicators of a specific cancer. For example, the Philadelphia chromosome is associated with chronic myelogenous leukemia (CML). Some alterations can provide information about prognosis, which helps the doctor make treatment recommendations.

Can individuals get a second opinion about their pathology results?

Although most cancers can be easily diagnosed, sometimes patients or their doctors may want to get a second opinion about the pathology results. Patients interested in getting a second opinion should talk with their doctor. They will need to obtain the slides and/or paraffin block from the pathologist who examined the sample or from the hospital where the biopsy or surgery was done.

Many institutions provide second opinions on pathology specimens. National Cancer Institute (NCI)-designated cancer centers or academic institutions are reasonable places to consider. Contact information for NCI-designated cancer centers can be found in the NCI-Designated Cancer Centers database at https://cissecure.nci.nih.gov/factsheet/FactSheetSearch1_2.aspx on the internet. Patients should contact the facility in advance to determine if this service is available, the cost, and shipping instructions.

Chapter 32

Breast Cancer Diagnosis: Questions to Ask

After you receive a breast cancer diagnosis, your doctor will order various diagnostic tests that provide important details about your type and stage of breast cancer. The results of these tests help guide his or her treatment recommendations. If you have early-stage breast cancer, you may also be a candidate for newer tests that can estimate your risk of recurrence and/or predict how likely it is that you will benefit from the hormonal therapy tamoxifen.

The following are questions you may want to ask your doctor about the results of your diagnostic tests:

Is my tumor invasive or noninvasive?

Invasive breast tumors have started growing into nearby healthy breast tissues. Noninvasive or in situ tumors are confined to the milk ducts; this is the earliest stage of breast cancer. As is true for most cancers, breast cancer in the earliest stage usually has the best chance of being cured.

What stage is my tumor?

A tumor's stage refers to its size and extent of spread in the body—e.g., whether it has spread to lymph nodes or other organs. Cancer confined to the breast may be called localized cancer. Cancer that has

"After a Breast Cancer Diagnosis: Questions to Ask Your Doctor," reprinted with permission of www.cancercare.org and Cancer Care, Inc. © 2011. For more information about Cancer*care*'s free, professional support services for people facing cancer, visit the website or call 800-813-HOPE (4673).

spread to other organs is called metastatic cancer. A cancer's stage is often denoted by a Roman numeral (I, II, III, or IV). The higher the numeral, the more the cancer has spread within the body.

What grade is my tumor?

A tumor's grade refers to how the tumor cells look under a microscope. The more different they look from healthy cells, the higher the grade and the more quickly the cancer is likely to grow.

What is my hormone receptor status?

Some breast tumors are stimulated to grow by the hormone estrogen. Tumors take in estrogen via structures on tumor cell surfaces called estrogen or progesterone receptors. Tumor cells with many of these receptors on their surfaces are said to be estrogen or progesterone receptor positive. These tumors are often successfully treated with hormonal therapy (e.g., tamoxifen and aromatase inhibitors).

What is my HER2/neu status?

HER2 [human epidermal growth factor receptor 2]/neu is a substance that is overproduced by about 25% of breast tumors. Tumors that overproduce HER2/neu are called HER2 positive and may respond to treatment with drugs like trastuzumab (Herceptin) which target HER2/neu.

How likely is my cancer to spread or to come back?

To estimate the likelihood that the cancer will spread or come back (recur), doctors usually look at tumor features such as size, stage, and grade, as well as hormone receptor and HER2/neu status. Today, there are also new tests that can estimate risk of recurrence for women with early-stage breast cancer. Such prognostic tests are performed on samples of tumor tissue removed during surgery. They analyze the activity of various genes to predict how the tumor will behave—that is, whether it is likely to come back or spread. Two tests now on the market, Oncotype DX and MammaPrint, can estimate the risk that certain early-stage breast tumors will recur.

Is a prognostic test right for me?

Currently, there are only two such tests approved, and each is appropriate only for women with a specific type of early-stage breast cancer. Oncotype DX is approved for use in women with recently diagnosed stage I or II, node-negative (has not spread to the lymph nodes), hormone receptor positive breast cancer, who are or will be receiving hormonal therapy. MammaPrint is approved for patients aged 61 or younger with stage I or II breast cancer that is node-negative, whose tumors are less than five centimeters (two inches) in diameter. Your doctor can give you more information about whether one of these tests may be a good option for you.

What can a prognostic test tell me about my chance of recurrence?

Tests like Oncotype DX and MammaPrint tests cannot say with certainty whether your cancer will come back or not. They can measure, for example, whether the risk of your cancer coming back is low, intermediate, or high. The test results may provide additional information to help you and your doctor decide on the best way to treat your cancer.

Will I need to have chemotherapy?

If you are diagnosed with early-stage breast cancer, chemotherapy could reduce the risk that your cancer will come back, but it may also cause long-lasting side effects. In addition to estimating risk of recurrence, Oncotype DX identifies patients who may be successfully treated with tamoxifen alone and may not need chemotherapy. Oncotype DX is the only such test currently on the market, but more may be available in the future. Check with your doctor about whether this type of test might be right for you.

Chapter 33

Breast Cancer Staging

Cancer Staging

What is staging?

Staging describes the severity of a person's cancer based on the extent of the original (primary) tumor and whether or not cancer has spread in the body. Staging is important for several reasons:

- Staging helps the doctor plan the appropriate treatment.

- The stage can be used to estimate the person's prognosis.

- Knowing the stage is important in identifying clinical trials that may be suitable for a particular patient.

Staging helps health care providers and researchers exchange information about patients; it also gives them a common terminology for evaluating the results of clinical trials and comparing the results of different trials.

Staging is based on knowledge of the way cancer progresses. Cancer cells grow and divide without control or order, and they do not die when they should. As a result, they often form a mass of tissue called a tumor. As the tumor grows, it can invade nearby tissues and organs.

This chapter contains text from "Cancer Staging," by the National Cancer Institute (NCI, www.cancer.gov), part of the National Institutes of Health, September 22, 2010, and excerpted from "What You Need to Know about Breast Cancer," by the NCI, October 15, 2009.

Cancer cells can also break away from the tumor and enter the bloodstream or the lymphatic system. By moving through the bloodstream or lymphatic system, cancer cells can spread from the primary site to lymph nodes or to other organs, where they may form new tumors. The spread of cancer is called metastasis.

What are the common elements of staging systems?

Staging systems for cancer have evolved over time. They continue to change as scientists learn more about cancer. Some staging systems cover many types of cancer; others focus on a particular type. The common elements considered in most staging systems are as follows:

- Site of the primary tumor

- Tumor size and number of tumors

- Lymph node involvement (spread of cancer into lymph nodes)

- Cell type and tumor grade (how closely the cancer cells resemble normal tissue cells)

- The presence or absence of metastasis

What is the TNM system?

The TNM system is one of the most widely used staging systems. This system has been accepted by the International Union Against Cancer (UICC) and the American Joint Committee on Cancer (AJCC). Most medical facilities use the TNM system as their main method for cancer reporting. PDQ®, NCI's comprehensive cancer information database, also uses the TNM system.

The TNM system is based on the extent of the tumor (T), the extent of spread to the lymph nodes (N), and the presence of distant metastasis (M). A number is added to each letter to indicate the size or extent of the primary tumor and the extent of cancer spread. See Tables 33.1, 33.2, and 33.3.

For example, breast cancer classified as T3 N2 M0 refers to a large tumor that has spread outside the breast to nearby lymph nodes but not to other parts of the body. Prostate cancer T2 N0 M0 means that the tumor is located only in the prostate and has not spread to the lymph nodes or any other part of the body.

For many cancers, TNM combinations correspond to one of five stages. Criteria for stages differ for different types of cancer. For example, bladder cancer T3 N0 M0 is stage III, whereas colon cancer T3 N0 M0 is stage II. See Table 33.4.

Table 33.1. Primary Tumor (T)

TX	Primary tumor cannot be evaluated
T0	No evidence of primary tumor
Tis	Carcinoma in situ (CIS; abnormal cells are present but have not spread to neighboring tissue; although not cancer, CIS may become cancer and is sometimes called preinvasive cancer.)
T1, T2, T3, T4	Size and/or extent of the primary tumor

Table 33.2. Regional Lymph Nodes (N)

NX	Regional lymph nodes cannot be evaluated
N0	No regional lymph node involvement
N1, N2, N3	Involvement of regional lymph nodes (number of lymph nodes and/or extent of spread)

Table 33.3. Distant Metastasis (M)

MX	Distant metastasis cannot be evaluated
M0	No distant metastasis
M1	Distant metastasis is present

Table 33.4. Criteria for Stages

Stage	Definition
Stage 0	Carcinoma in situ
Stage I, Stage II, and Stage III	Higher numbers indicate more extensive disease: Larger tumor size and/or spread of the cancer beyond the organ in which it first developed to nearby lymph nodes and/or organs adjacent to the location of the primary tumor.
Stage IV	The cancer has spread to another organ(s).

Are all cancers staged with TNM classifications?

Most types of cancer have TNM designations, but some do not. For example, cancers of the brain and spinal cord are staged according to their cell type and grade. Different staging systems are also used for many cancers of the blood or bone marrow, such as lymphomas. The Ann Arbor staging classification is commonly used to stage lymphomas and has been adopted by both the AJCC and the UICC. However, other cancers of the blood or bone marrow, including most types of leukemia, do not have a clear-cut staging system. Another staging system, developed by the International Federation of Gynecology and Obstetrics, is used to stage cancers of the cervix, uterus, ovary, vagina, and vulva. This system uses the TNM format. Additionally, childhood cancers are staged using either the TNM system or the staging criteria of the Children's Oncology Group, which conducts pediatric clinical trials.

Many cancer registries, such as NCI's Surveillance, Epidemiology, and End Results Program (SEER), use summary staging. This system is used for all types of cancer. It groups cancer cases into five main categories:

- In situ: Abnormal cells are present only in the layer of cells in which they developed.

- Localized: Cancer is limited to the organ in which it began, without evidence of spread.

- Regional: Cancer has spread beyond the primary site to nearby lymph nodes or organs and tissues.

- Distant: Cancer has spread from the primary site to distant organs or distant lymph nodes.

- Unknown: There is not enough information to determine the stage.

What types of tests are used to determine stage?

The types of tests used for staging depend on the type of cancer.

Physical exams are used to gather information about the cancer. The doctor examines the body by looking, feeling, and listening for anything unusual. The physical exam may show the location and size of the tumor(s) and the spread of the cancer to the lymph nodes and/or to other organs.

Imaging studies produce pictures of areas inside the body. These studies are important tools in determining stage. Procedures such as x-rays, computed tomography (CT) scans, magnetic resonance imaging (MRI) scans, and positron emission tomography (PET) scans can show the location of the cancer, the size of the tumor, and whether the cancer has spread.

Laboratory tests are studies of blood, urine, other fluids, and tissues taken from the body. For example, tests for liver function and tumor markers (substances sometimes found in increased amounts if cancer is present) can provide information about the cancer.

Pathology reports may include information about the size of the tumor, the growth of the tumor into other tissues and organs, the type of cancer cells, and the grade of the tumor. A biopsy may be performed to provide information for the pathology report. Cytology reports also describe findings from the examination of cells in body fluids.

Surgical reports tell what is found during surgery. These reports describe the size and appearance of the tumor and often include observations about lymph nodes and nearby organs.

What You Need to Know about Breast Cancer Staging

If the biopsy shows that you have breast cancer, your doctor needs to learn the extent (stage) of the disease to help you choose the best treatment. The stage is based on the size of the cancer, whether the cancer has invaded nearby tissues, and whether the cancer has spread to other parts of the body.

Staging may involve blood tests and other tests:

- Bone scan: The doctor injects a small amount of a radioactive substance into a blood vessel. It travels through the bloodstream and collects in the bones. A machine called a scanner detects and measures the radiation. The scanner makes pictures of the bones. The pictures may show cancer that has spread to the bones.

- CT (computed tomography) scan: Doctors sometimes use CT scans to look for breast cancer that has spread to the liver or lungs. An x-ray machine linked to a computer takes a series of detailed pictures of your chest or abdomen. You may receive contrast material by injection into a blood vessel in your arm or hand. The contrast material makes abnormal areas easier to see.

- Lymph node biopsy: The stage often is not known until after surgery to remove the tumor in your breast and one or more lymph nodes under your arm. Surgeons use a method called sentinel lymph node biopsy to remove the lymph node most likely to have breast cancer cells. The surgeon injects a blue dye, a radioactive substance, or both near the breast tumor. Or the surgeon may inject a radioactive substance under the nipple. The surgeon then uses a scanner to find the sentinel lymph node containing the radioactive substance or looks for the lymph node stained with dye. The sentinel node is removed and checked for cancer cells. Cancer cells may appear first in the sentinel node before spreading to other lymph nodes and other places in the body.

These tests can show whether the cancer has spread and, if so, to what parts of your body. When breast cancer spreads, cancer cells are often found in lymph nodes under the arm (axillary lymph nodes). Also, breast cancer can spread to almost any other part of the body, such as the bones, liver, lungs, and brain.

When breast cancer spreads from its original place to another part of the body, the new tumor has the same kind of abnormal cells and the same name as the primary (original) tumor. For example, if breast cancer spreads to the bones, the cancer cells in the bones are actually breast cancer cells. The disease is metastatic breast cancer, not bone cancer. For that reason, it is treated as breast cancer, not bone cancer. Doctors call the new tumor "distant" or metastatic disease.

These are the stages of breast cancer:

- Stage 0 is sometimes used to describe abnormal cells that are not invasive cancer. For example, Stage 0 is used for ductal carcinoma in situ (DCIS). DCIS is diagnosed when abnormal cells are in the lining of a breast duct, but the abnormal cells have not invaded nearby breast tissue or spread outside the duct. Although many doctors don't consider DCIS to be cancer, DCIS sometimes becomes invasive breast cancer if not treated.

- Stage I is an early stage of invasive breast cancer. Cancer cells have invaded breast tissue beyond where the cancer started, but the cells have not spread beyond the breast. The tumor is no more than 2 centimeters, or cm (three-quarters of an inch) across.

- Stage II is one of the following:

  - The tumor is no more than two cm (three-quarters of an inch) across. The cancer has spread to the lymph nodes under the arm.

  - The tumor is between two and five cm (three-quarters of an inch to two inches). The cancer has not spread to the lymph nodes under the arm.

  - The tumor is between two and five cm (three-quarters of an inch to two inches). The cancer has spread to the lymph nodes under the arm.

  - The tumor is larger than five cm (two inches). The cancer has not spread to the lymph nodes under the arm.

- Stage III is locally advanced cancer. It is divided into Stage IIIA, IIIB, and IIIC. Stage IIIA is one of the following:

  - The tumor is no more than five cm (two inches) across. The cancer has spread to underarm lymph nodes that are attached to each other or to other structures. Or the cancer may have spread to lymph nodes behind the breastbone.

- The tumor is more than five cm across. The cancer has spread to underarm lymph nodes that are either alone or attached to each other or to other structures. Or the cancer may have spread to lymph nodes behind the breastbone.

- Stage IIIB is a tumor of any size that has grown into the chest wall or the skin of the breast. It may be associated with swelling of the breast or with nodules (lumps) in the breast skin:

  - The cancer may have spread to lymph nodes under the arm.

  - The cancer may have spread to underarm lymph nodes that are attached to each other or other structures. Or the cancer may have spread to lymph nodes behind the breastbone. Inflammatory breast cancer is a rare type of breast cancer. The breast looks red and swollen because cancer cells block the lymph vessels in the skin of the breast. When a doctor diagnoses inflammatory breast cancer, it is at least Stage IIIB, but it could be more advanced.

- Stage IIIC is a tumor of any size. It has spread in one of the following ways:

  - The cancer has spread to the lymph nodes behind the breastbone and under the arm.

  - The cancer has spread to the lymph nodes above or below the collarbone.

- Stage IV is distant metastatic cancer. The cancer has spread to other parts of the body, such as the bones or liver.

- Recurrent cancer is cancer that has come back after a period of time when it could not be detected. Even when the cancer seems to be completely destroyed, the disease sometimes returns because undetected cancer cells remained somewhere in your body after treatment. It may return in the breast or chest wall. Or it may return in any other part of the body, such as the bones, liver, lungs, or brain.

Part Five

Breast Cancer Treatments

Chapter 34

How to Find a Doctor or Treatment Facility If You Have Cancer

If you have been diagnosed with cancer, finding a doctor and treatment facility for your cancer care is an important step to getting the best treatment possible. Although the health care system is complex, resources are available to guide you in finding a doctor, getting a second opinion, and choosing a treatment facility.

Physician Training and Credentials

When choosing a doctor for your cancer care, you may find it helpful to know some of the terms used to describe a doctor's training and credentials. Most physicians who treat people with cancer are medical doctors (they have an MD degree) or osteopathic doctors (they have a DO degree). The basic training for both types of physicians includes four years of premedical education at a college or university, four years of medical school to earn an MD or DO degree, and postgraduate medical education through internships and residences. This training usually lasts three to seven years. Physicians must pass an exam to become licensed (legally permitted) to practice medicine in their state. Each state or territory has its own procedures and general standards for licensing physicians.

Specialists are physicians who have completed their residency training in a specific area, such as internal medicine. Independent

"How to Find a Doctor or Treatment Facility If You Have Cancer," by the National Cancer Institute (NCI, www.cancer.gov), June 29, 2009.

275

specialty boards certify physicians after they have fulfilled certain requirements. These requirements include meeting specific education and training criteria, being licensed to practice medicine, and passing an examination given by the specialty board. Doctors who have met all of the requirements are given the status of "Diplomate" and are board-certified as specialists. Doctors who are board-eligible have obtained the required education and training, but have not completed the specialty board examination.

After being trained and certified as a specialist, a physician may choose to become a subspecialist. A subspecialist has at least one additional year of full-time education in a particular area of a specialty. This training is designed to increase the physician's expertise in a specific field. Specialists can be board-certified in their subspecialty as well.

The following are some specialties and subspecialties that pertain to cancer treatment:

- Medical oncology is a subspecialty of internal medicine. Doctors who specialize in internal medicine treat a wide range of medical problems. Medical oncologists treat cancer and manage the patient's course of treatment. A medical oncologist may also consult with other physicians about the patient's care or refer the patient to other specialists.

- Hematology is a subspecialty of internal medicine. Hematologists focus on diseases of the blood and related tissues, including the bone marrow, spleen, and lymph nodes.

- Radiation oncology is a subspecialty of radiology. Radiology is the use of x-rays and other forms of radiation to diagnose and treat disease. Radiation oncologists specialize in the use of radiation to treat cancer.

- Surgery is a specialty that pertains to the treatment of disease by surgical operation. General surgeons perform operations on almost any area of the body. Physicians can also choose to specialize in a certain type of surgery; for example, thoracic surgeons are specialists who perform operations specifically in the chest area, including the lungs and the esophagus.

The American Board of Medical Specialties (ABMS) is a not-for-profit organization that assists medical specialty boards with the development and use of standards for evaluation and certification of physicians. Information about other specialties that treat cancer is available from the ABMS website (www.abms.org).

Almost all board-certified specialists are members of their medical specialty society. Physicians can attain Fellowship status in a specialty society, such as the American College of Surgeons (ACS), if they demonstrate outstanding achievement in their profession. Criteria for Fellowship status may include the number of years of membership in the specialty society, years practicing in the specialty, and professional recognition by peers.

Finding a Doctor

One way to find a doctor who specializes in cancer care is to ask for a referral from your primary care physician. You may know a specialist yourself, or through the experience of a family member, coworker, or friend.

The following resources may also be able to provide you with names of doctors who specialize in treating specific diseases or conditions. However, these resources may not have information about the quality of care that the doctors provide.

- Your local hospital or its patient referral service may be able to provide you with a list of specialists who practice at that hospital.

- Your nearest National Cancer Institute (NCI)-designated cancer center can provide information about doctors who practice at that center. The NCI is a component of the National Institutes of Health (NIH). The NCI-Designated Cancer Centers database (https://cissecure.nci.nih.gov/factsheet/FactSheetSearch1_2.aspx) provides contact information for NCI-designated cancer centers located throughout the United States. Users can select all cancer centers or search by location, type of cancer center, or cancer center name.

- The ABMS has a list of doctors who have met certain education and training requirements and have passed specialty examinations. *Is Your Doctor Board Certified* (https://www .certificationmatters.org/is-your-doctor-board-certified/search-now .aspx) lists doctors' names along with their specialty and their educational background. Users must register to use this online self-serve resource, which allows users to conduct searches by a physician's name or area of certification and a state name. The directory is available in most libraries.

- The American Medical Association (AMA) DoctorFinder database (https://extapps.ama-assn.org/doctorfinder/recaptcha.jsp) provides

277

basic information on licensed physicians in the United States. Users can search for physicians by name or by medical specialty.

- The American Society of Clinical Oncology (ASCO) provides an online list of doctors who are members of ASCO. The member database (www.cancer.net/patient/Publications+and+Resources/Find+an+Oncologist/Find+an+Oncologist+Database) has the names and affiliations of nearly 30,000 oncologists worldwide. It can be searched by doctor's name, institution, location, oncology specialty, and/or type of board certification.

- The American College of Surgeons (ACS) membership database (web3.facs.org/acsdir/default_public.cfm) is an online list of surgeons who are members of the ACS. The list can be searched by doctor's name, geographic location, or medical specialty. The ACS can be contacted by telephone at 800-621-4111.

- The American Osteopathic Association (AOA) Find a Doctor database (www.osteopathic.org/osteopathic-health/find-a-do/Pages/default.aspx) provides an online list of practicing osteopathic physicians who are AOA members. The information can be searched by doctor's name, geographic location, or medical specialty. The AOA can be contacted by telephone at 800-621-1773.

- Local medical societies may maintain lists of doctors in each specialty.

- Public and medical libraries may have print directories of doctors' names listed geographically by specialty.

- Your local Yellow Pages or Yellow Book may have doctors listed by specialty under "Physicians."

If you are a member of a health insurance plan, your choice may be limited to doctors who participate in your plan. Your insurance company can provide you with a list of participating primary care doctors and specialists. It is important to ask your insurance company if the doctor you choose is accepting new patients through your health plan. You also have the option of seeing a doctor outside your health plan and paying the costs yourself. If you have a choice of health insurance plans, you may first wish to consider which doctor or doctors you would like to use, and then choose a plan that includes your chosen physician(s).

If you are using a federal or state health insurance program such as Medicare or Medicaid, you may want to ask the doctor about accepting patients who use these programs.

You will have many factors to consider when choosing a doctor. To make an informed decision, you may wish to speak with several doctors before choosing one. When you meet with each doctor, you might want to consider the following:

- Does the doctor have the education and training to meet my needs?
- Does the doctor use the hospital that I have chosen?
- Does the doctor listen to me and treat me with respect?
- Does the doctor explain things clearly and encourage me to ask questions?
- What are the doctor's office hours?
- Who covers for the doctor when he or she is unavailable? Will that person have access to my medical records?
- How long does it take to get an appointment with the doctor?

If you are choosing a surgeon, you may wish to ask additional questions about the surgeon's background and experience with specific procedures. These questions may include:

- Is the surgeon board-certified?
- Has the surgeon been evaluated by a national professional association of surgeons, such as the ACS?
- At which treatment facility or facilities does the surgeon practice?
- How often does the surgeon perform the type of surgery I need?
- How many of these procedures has the surgeon performed? What was the success rate?

It is important for you to feel comfortable with the specialist that you choose because you will be working closely with that person to make decisions about your cancer treatment. Trust your own observations and feelings when deciding on a doctor for your medical care.

Getting a Second Opinion

Once you receive your doctor's opinion about the diagnosis and treatment plan, you may want to get another doctor's advice before you begin treatment. This is known as getting a second opinion. You can do this by asking another specialist to review all of the materials related to your case. A second opinion can confirm or suggest modifications to your doctor's proposed treatment plan, provide reassurance that you have explored all of your options, and answer any questions you may have.

Getting a second opinion is done frequently, and most physicians welcome another doctor's views. In fact, your doctor may be able to recommend a specialist for this consultation. However, some people find it uncomfortable to request a second opinion. When discussing this issue with your doctor, it may be helpful to express satisfaction with your doctor's decision and care and to mention that you want your decision about treatment to be as thoroughly informed as possible. You may also wish to bring a family member along for support when asking for a second opinion. It is best to involve your doctor in the process of getting a second opinion, because your doctor will need to make your medical records (such as your test results and x-rays) available to the specialist.

Some health care plans require a second opinion, particularly if a doctor recommends surgery. Other health care plans will pay for a second opinion if the patient requests it. If your plan does not cover a second opinion, you can still obtain one if you are willing to cover the cost.

If your doctor is unable to recommend a specialist for a second opinion, or if you prefer to choose one on your own, the following resources can help:

- Many of the resources listed above for finding a doctor can also help you find a specialist for a consultation.

- The NIH Clinical Center in Bethesda, Maryland, is the research hospital for the NIH, including NCI. Several branches of the NCI provide second opinion services.

- The R. A. Bloch Cancer Foundation, Inc., can refer cancer patients to institutions that are willing to provide multidisciplinary second opinions. A list of these institutions is available on the organization's website (blochcancer.org/resources/multidisciplinary-second-opinion-centers/). You can also contact the R. A. Bloch Cancer Foundation, Inc., by telephone at 816-854-5050 or 800-433-0464.

Finding a Treatment Facility for Patients Living in the United States

Choosing a treatment facility is another important consideration for getting the best medical care possible. Although you may not be able to choose which hospital treats you in an emergency, you can choose a facility for scheduled and ongoing care. If you have already found a doctor for your cancer treatment, you may need to choose a facility based on where your doctor practices. Your doctor may be able to recommend a facility that provides quality care to meet your needs. You may wish to ask the following questions when considering a treatment facility:

- Has the facility had experience and success in treating my condition?

- Has the facility been rated by state, consumer, or other groups for its quality of care?

- How does the facility check on and work to improve its quality of care?

- Has the facility been approved by a nationally recognized accrediting body, such as the ACS Commission on Cancer and/or The Joint Commission?

- Does the facility explain patients' rights and responsibilities? Are copies of this information available to patients?

- Does the treatment facility offer support services, such as social workers and resources, to help me find financial assistance if I need it?

- Is the facility conveniently located?

If you are a member of a health insurance plan, your choice of treatment facilities may be limited to those that participate in your plan. Your insurance company can provide you with a list of approved facilities. Although the costs of cancer treatment can be very high, you have the option of paying out-of-pocket if you want to use a treatment facility that is not covered by your insurance plan. If you are considering paying for treatment yourself, you may wish to discuss the possible costs with your doctor beforehand. You may also want to speak with the person who does the billing for the treatment facility. In some instances, nurses and social workers can provide you with more information about coverage, eligibility, and insurance issues.

The following resources may help you find a hospital or treatment facility for your care:

- The NCI-Designated Cancer Centers database (https://cissecure. nci.nih.gov/factsheet/FactSheetSearch1_2.aspx) provides contact information for NCI-designated cancer centers around the country.

- The ACS's Commission on Cancer (CoC) accredits cancer programs at hospitals and other treatment facilities. More than

1,430 programs in the United States have been designated by the CoC as Approved Cancer Programs. The ACS website offers a searchable database (datalinks.facs.org/cpm/cpmapproved hospitals_search.htm) of these programs. The CoC can be contacted by telephone at 312-202-5085.

• The Joint Commission is an independent, not-for-profit organization that evaluates and accredits health care organizations and programs in the United States. It also offers information for the general public about choosing a treatment facility. The Joint Commission is available online (www.jointcommission.org) and can be contacted by telephone at 630-792-5000. The Joint Commission offers an online Quality Check service that patients can use to determine whether a specific facility has been accredited by the Joint Commission and to view the organization's performance reports.

Finding a Treatment Facility for Patients Living Outside the United States

If you live outside the United States, facilities that offer cancer treatment may be located in or near your country. Cancer information services are available in many countries to provide information and answer questions about cancer; they may also be able to help you find a cancer treatment facility close to where you live. A list of these cancer information services is available on the International Cancer Information Service Group's (ICISG) website (www.icisg.org/meet_memberslist.htm).

The ICISG is an independent international organization composed of cancer information services. Its mission is to provide high-quality cancer information services and resources to those concerned about, or affected by, cancer throughout the world.

The Union for International Cancer Control (UICC) is another resource for people living outside the United States who want to find a cancer treatment facility. The UICC consists of international cancer-related organizations devoted to the worldwide fight against cancer. UICC membership includes research facilities and treatment centers and, in some countries, ministries of health. Other members include volunteer cancer leagues, associations, and societies. These organizations serve as resources for the public and may have helpful information about cancer and treatment facilities. To find a resource in or near your country, contact the Geneva, Switzerland-based Union for International Cancer Control (UICC) at + 41 22 809 1811 or www.uicc.org.

Some people living outside the United States may wish to obtain a second opinion or have their cancer treatment in this country. Many facilities in the United States offer these services to international cancer patients. These facilities may also provide support services, such as language interpretation, assistance with travel, and guidance in finding accommodations near the treatment facility for patients and their families.

If you live outside the United States and would like to obtain cancer treatment in this country, you should contact cancer treatment facilities directly to find out whether they have an international patient office. The NCI-Designated Cancer Centers database (https://cissecure.nci.nih .gov/factsheet/FactSheetSearch1_2.aspx) offers contact information for NCI-designated cancer centers throughout the United States.

Citizens of other countries who are planning to travel to the United States for cancer treatment generally must first obtain a nonimmigrant visa for medical treatment from the U.S. Embassy or Consulate in their home country. Visa applicants must demonstrate that the purpose of their trip is to enter the United States for medical treatment; that they plan to remain for a specific, limited period; that they have funds to cover expenses in the United States; that they have a residence and social and economic ties outside the United States; and that they intend to return to their home country.

To determine the specific fees and documentation required for the nonimmigrant visa and to learn more about the application process, contact the U.S. Embassy or Consulate in your home country. A list of links to the websites of U.S. Embassies and Consulates worldwide can be found on the U.S. Department of State's website (www.usembassy.gov).

Chapter 35

Making Breast Cancer Treatment Decisions

Chapter Contents

Section 35.1

Considerations before Undergoing Breast Cancer Treatment

Now What? First Steps in Making Decisions

When you are first diagnosed, you may feel as if you will do anything to get rid of the breast cancer. Remember, breast cancer is rarely a medical emergency, although it can feel like an emotional emergency. Living with a new diagnosis and worries about your future can be very difficult.

Right now, you and your provider know very little about the cancer. Tests will tell you what makes the cancer grow, how fast it is growing, and whether it has traveled to other areas of your body. The results help your doctors select the treatments most likely to benefit you.

You are unlikely to make treatment decisions overnight. Instead, you, your healthcare team, and key family or friends will go through a process together. It may take several weeks to gather the information you need. This is safe.

Take the time you need to get your questions answered. Ask your doctor how much time is reasonable to take.

Treating Breast Cancer Today

Just 20 or 30 years ago, doctors viewed breast cancer as a single disease. There were very few treatment choices, and providers typically told women what to do without talking about their options, needs, or lifestyle.

Today, that has changed. Treatment is no longer "one size fits all." We now know there are many different types of breast cancer, each with its own features. Breakthroughs in breast cancer research have helped doctors learn who is most likely to benefit from certain treatments.

You may be surprised to learn that your treatment could be very different from the treatment your friend, family member, or coworker received. This does not mean you are not getting the best treatment for you.

Your treatment plan should be based on the unique features of the cancer, your overall health and health history, and other issues you discuss with your healthcare team.

Creating Personalized Treatment Plans

To tailor treatment, doctors will do tests on tissue taken from the cancer. The results explain what makes the cancer grow and how it behaves. This information makes up your pathology report, a profile of the cancer that guides your healthcare team in choosing the best treatments for you.

Sometimes the pathology report makes the best course of treatment very clear. In other cases, it may show you have several equally good options. Deciding among them may be a matter of what makes most sense for you.

If you are having trouble making a decision or feel "stuck," we encourage you to speak with your providers and to call the LBBC Survivors' Helpline at 888-753-LBBC (753-5222). Sometimes asking a different question, or thinking in a slightly different way, may be all you need to do to take your next steps.

Getting Started: Surgery and the Pathology Report

To plan treatment, your doctors need to learn about the makeup of the breast cancer. This process began with your biopsy, when a doctor removed a small amount of your breast tissue with a needle or through an incision (a cut). This sample was sent to a pathologist, a doctor who diagnoses diseases by looking at tissues under a microscope. After seeing cancer cells in the sample, your pathologist diagnosed breast cancer.

This diagnosis was included in your first pathology report. Yet many questions remain. To learn more, you will have one or more surgeries to take out all the breast cancer and to check for cancer in one or several sentinel lymph nodes, the first nodes the breast cancer is most likely to travel.

Breast Cancer Surgery

Surgery reduces the risk for local recurrence, a return of the cancer to the same area of the breast or lymph nodes.

After diagnosis, you will need at least one surgery to remove the breast cancer. Your doctor could call this surgery excisional biopsy, lumpectomy, breast-conserving surgery, partial mastectomy, or segmental mastectomy. These terms all mean the same thing: Surgery to remove only the cancer or the part of your breast with cancer, plus a small rim of healthy tissue around it, called the margin.

Your pathology report will say whether the doctor got all the cancer. If it reports negative margins, you should not need further breast surgery. But if it shows positive or close margins, you will need either a second lumpectomy, also called a re-excision, or a mastectomy, a surgery to remove the whole breast.

Sometimes mastectomy is the only option. Other times doctors can offer lumpectomy or mastectomy. This option should be given if your chances of distant recurrence, the cancer coming back in an area away from the breast, are about the same whether you do one surgery or the other. In past clinical trials, lumpectomy and mastectomy worked equally well in women with tumors less than five cm across who had radiation therapy and negative margins after lumpectomy.

If you have a choice of surgeries, it may be a relief, or it might feel nerve-racking and uncertain. Please know that either response is normal. Many, many women stood in your place before, not knowing what to do. If you feel uncertain at all, it is OK to ask why you have both options. This is also the best time to discuss options for rebuilding your breast, if this is of interest to you.

Of the many choices you make during treatment, this is among the most personal. Only you know what having your breast means to you—and it may mean a lot, nothing at all or something in between.

Start by asking these common questions:

1. How important is it to me to keep my breast? Is your breast essential to your self-image and identity? Consider the role of your breast in your relationship with your partner or future partners. If you want, ask for your partner's input (but remember, this is your decision).

2. What is the risk of this cancer coming back in a distant area of the body? What were the outcomes in past clinical trials for people who had the surgery you want?

3. How do I feel about my risk for local recurrence? In some cases, lumpectomy may put you at higher risk than mastectomy for the cancer coming back in the same place. If so, what is the difference in risk?

4. How would I feel if removing the cancer takes more than two surgeries? What if only one more surgery would be needed?

5. How does the size of the cancer compare to the size of my breast? Ask how your breast is likely to look. Your doctor may even have photos. Are you pleased with the outcome, or would you rather have a mastectomy with reconstruction?

6. How could my other treatments impact my surgery choices? Ask if presurgical therapy is an option and, if so, whether you could then get a lumpectomy. Radiation could affect the choice and timing of reconstruction.

7. Can I have radiation therapy? Lumpectomy must be paired with radiation for you to get the benefit you would receive from mastectomy alone.

8. Where is the cancer in my breast? Your mammogram may show calcifications, tiny clusters of hard calcium associated with DCIS [ductal carcinoma in situ] and invasive cancers. If they are in more than one area, you may need more surgery.

9. Am I at very high risk for a future breast cancer? Possible reasons include a known BRCA [breast cancer gene] mutation or a strong family history. Are there other ways to improve your chances for living cancer-free?

10. Will removing my breast make me less worried about my risk for recurrence? Even if lumpectomy and mastectomy work equally well in cases like yours, you may simply feel better without your breast.

Lymph Node Surgery

To find out whether cancer is in the lymph nodes, a doctor first removes lymph nodes under the arm in a surgery called sentinel lymph node dissection. This surgery is done at the same time as your first breast surgery, after a biopsy shows you have breast cancer.

Removing the sentinel lymph node is standard treatment for most invasive breast cancers. If you have a non-invasive DCIS diagnosis, you and your doctor will talk about whether you need this surgery.

If cancer is found in the sentinel node, you may need an axillary lymph node dissection. This surgery removes most of the lymph nodes in the armpit and helps your doctor assign the cancer a stage. Axillary dissection increases the risk for side effects such as shoulder stiffness and lymphedema, numbness in the underarm area.

To find out whether you need axillary surgery, consider these key questions:

1. How much cancer was found in the sentinel lymph nodes? If it was a small amount, you may not need axillary surgery.

2. Were the lymph nodes in my armpit swollen at diagnosis? If so, you may need chemotherapy before surgery. The axillary lymph nodes will be removed right away, instead of starting with the sentinel nodes.

3. Do I have symptoms of inflammatory breast cancer? This cancer rarely forms a lump. Instead, the breast looks swollen, hot, pitted, or red; feels thick or heavy; and sometimes causes pain. With this diagnosis, you must have chemotherapy before surgery, and your axillary lymph nodes will be removed right away.

4. Should I get full-body treatment before surgery? If the cancer is more than three cm across, you might need chemotherapy, hormonal therapy, or targeted therapy before surgery. This is called neoadjuvant therapy.

Breast Reconstruction

Your breast may be rebuilt in a surgery called breast reconstruction. Sometimes this surgery can be done at the same time as a mastectomy in an immediate reconstruction. It is also possible to wait weeks, months, or even years. Delayed reconstruction is a good option if you need radiation therapy, which can damage rebuilt breast tissue or cause scarring around an implant.

Breasts can be rebuilt using tissue from other parts of the body, such as the stomach, thighs, or buttocks, or through an implant filled with silicone gel or saline (salt water).

If your provider forgets to talk about breast reconstruction, it is OK to bring it up. You have the right to learn more, even if you aren't ready to do anything. Deciding against reconstruction is also a valid choice.

While you may choose to ask others for opinions, this is your decision. If you do not rebuild your breast, you may get a breast form, or prosthesis, to place in your bra after surgery to maintain symmetry.

Reading Your Pathology Report

Over several days to several weeks, your pathologist will run tests on the tissues removed from the surgery on your breast and lymph nodes.

These tests look at the actions of genes that make up the cancer cells. Genes contain directions, called DNA [deoxyribonucleic acid], that tell human cells when and how to grow. The genes of cancer cells often have changes in their DNA: Extra copies, missing data, misspellings, and other problems.

Knowing the types of genetic changes helps doctors understand how the cancer is likely to behave and respond to treatments.

The results of these tests make up your final pathology report. You may get your complete report all at once or in parts; you may even get a few reports at a time. Meet with your doctors and ask them to explain each test result and what it means for your care. It is OK to ask questions during the meeting, and to contact your doctor's office later if you did not understand something.

Ten Tips for Getting Your Pathology Report

1. Practice patience. Waiting can be very trying. It is normal to feel anxious, stressed, sad, or worried.

2. Find out where the tests will be read. Some will be done at your facility, but others may need to be sent to outside labs. Early on, make sure your health insurance covers outside labs. Someone in your doctor's office can help you find out.

3. Learn when the results will arrive. Ask how long it may take and how you will be told. Call if results do not arrive on time.

4. Ask about the experience of the doctors looking at your tests. Find out whether they see many breast cancer cases. If not, consider a second opinion.

5. Inquire where, how, and how long your breast tissue will be stored. If your doctors need to run more tests, they may be able to use the samples. You can also use them for a second opinion.

6. Take someone with you or record your conversation, with your doctor's permission. A relative or friend can take notes so you can focus on the discussion.

7. When you get the report, try not to focus on any single result. Your doctors look at the findings as a whole to make your treatment plan.

8. Find out if you could benefit from a genomic test. These tests look together at several issues in the pathology report to predict how likely the cancer is to respond to certain treatments.

9. Get a copy of the full report. Your test results belong to you. Keep your report and copies of your imaging tests in a safe, secure place.

10. Exhale. Even though you have many decisions ahead, you now have vital tools to take first steps.

Parts of Your Pathology Report

Most pathology reports begin with a brief history of your medical state. They describe the anatomic site, where tissue was removed from your breast, and the size and look of the cancer, also called the gross description.

Reports vary but all have a section that names each test and gives the results. This section is important in planning treatment because it describes the cancer itself. Among the issues covered in this section of the report are:

- the size of the cancer;

- the number of lymph nodes with cancer, if any;

- whether cancer was found in one area or several areas in your breast;

- whether the surgeon removed all the cancer;

- how the cancer cells look under the microscope;

- how quickly the cancer cells grow.

At the end of the report, the pathologist will sum up what was found.

Ten Questions Answered in Your Pathology Report

Question 1: What type of cells make up the cancer?

Possible answers:

- Ductal cells: All breast cancers start in the terminal ducts, the pathways in the breast that carry milk. If the cancer cells look like ductal cells, the pathology report will say you have invasive ductal carcinoma or IDC. Noninvasive ductal cells mean you have ductal carcinoma in situ or DCIS. Cancers of the breast duct are the most common type.

- Lobular cells: The cancer cells look like lobular cells, which come from the sacs in the breast that make milk. The pathology report will say you have invasive lobular carcinoma or ILC. It could also say you have noninvasive lobular disease, called lobular carcinoma in situ or LCIS. LCIS puts you at higher-than-average risk for a future breast cancer.

- Other cancer cells: Many other types of cancer grow in the breast duct. Cribriform, medullary, mucinous, papillary, and tubular cells are subtypes of ductal cancer that are less common than ductal and lobular cancers. Cancers that involve the skin are called inflammatory breast cancer and Paget's disease.

Question 2: Did the cancer grow outside the milk ducts?

Possible answers:

- No, the cancer is noninvasive: It stayed inside the ducts or lobules of the breast, where it started. This is called in situ. It cannot travel away from the breast to the lymph nodes and other body parts.

- Yes, the cancer is invasive: It grew outside the ducts or lobules of the breast into nearby tissue. It has the potential to travel away from the breast to other areas of the body.

- Yes, the cancer is mixed: Some cancer cells stayed inside the ducts or lobules of the breast, and other cells invaded nearby tissues. Some of the cancer is invasive and some is noninvasive.

Question 3: How large is the cancer?

Possible answers: The size of the cancer after surgery, measured in centimeters across at its widest point. One inch equals about 2.5 centimeters. If the cancer is less than one centimeter (cm), the pathology report will state the size in millimeters (mm).

Doctors use size to assign the cancer a stage. Just because a cancer is small or large does not make it easy or hard to treat; it is just one piece of the puzzle.

Question 4: How do the cancer cells look and act compared to normal breast cells?

Possible answers:

- Similar to normal cells: The cancer cells are called grade 1, low grade, or well differentiated. Under the microscope, they look and act much like healthy cells.

- Unlike normal cells: The cancer cells are called grade 2, moderate grade, or moderately differentiated. They grow faster than normal breast cells.

- Not at all like normal cells: The cancer cells are called grade 3, high grade, or poorly differentiated. They look and act very different than normal breast cells. These cancer cells grow quickly.

Question 5: Are there cancer cells elsewhere in my breast?

Possible answers:

- Yes: Cancer cells were present in your breast's blood vessels and lymph channels, part of a system of tubes and tunnels that deliver blood and fluid throughout your body. Your report may call this lymphovascular invasion or LVI. It increases the chances the breast cancer may travel outside the breast or return in the future.

- No: Cancer cells were absent in the lymphovascular system, decreasing the chances they will travel away from the breast or recur (return) later.

Question 6: Did the surgeon remove all the cancer during surgery?

Possible answers:

- Yes: The test was negative (or clean) for cancer in the margins, the rim of healthy tissue removed with the cancer.

- No: The test was positive. The pathologist found cancer cells throughout the healthy tissue and to the edge of the rim of tissue.

- No: The test was close. Most of the area with cancer was removed along with a rim of healthy tissue around it, but the pathologist found some cancer cells within a few mm of the rim.

Question 7: Do I have cancer in the lymph node or nodes removed from my underarm?

Possible answers:

- No: The test was negative or clear. No cancer was found in the lymph nodes.

- Yes: The test was positive. Cancer is in the lymph nodes. The pathology report should say the number of lymph nodes with cancer and the amount of cancer in each node. Lymph nodes can hold anything from a few tiny cancer cells to large areas of cancer. A few cells may not affect your treatment.

Question 8: What is the stage of the breast cancer?

Possible answers:

- Stage 0: The cancer is noninvasive. It is ductal carcinoma in situ, confined to the ducts of the breast.

- Stage I: The breast cancer is invasive. These cancers are two cm or smaller across and are not in the lymph nodes.

- Stage II: The breast cancer is invasive. These cancers are larger than two cm across and can be as large as five cm. Usually, they are in the lymph nodes. They are put into two groups, A and B, based on size and lymph node status.

- Stage III: The breast cancer is invasive. These cancers are at least two cm across, can be larger than five cm, and may be in the lymph nodes. Sometimes the cancer is in lymph nodes near the breastbone or collarbone, or the nodes are matted (stuck) together. These cancers are put into three groups, A, B, and C, based on many factors.

- Stage IV: The breast cancer is invasive. It has grown into tissue outside the ducts or lobules of the breast and traveled to other organs, such as the bones, liver, lungs, or brain.

Note: Your doctor may change the stage if further tests show cancer in distant areas of the body.

Question 9: Do hormones fuel the growth of the cancer cells?

Possible answers:

- Yes, hormone receptor tests are positive: The cancer cells have estrogen or progesterone receptors, a type of protein that tells cancer cells to grow in the presence of these hormones. The cancer cells may test positive for one or both hormone receptors. You will see a percentage, rating, or other number that explains how sensitive the cancer is to hormones; the higher the percentage or rating, the more sensitive.

- No, hormone receptor tests are negative: Estrogen and progesterone do not fuel the growth of the cancer cells.

Question 10: Does the cancer make too much HER2 protein?

Possible answers:

- Yes: The cancer scores 3+ on the IHC or immunohistochemistry test. The cancer cells have too many copies of the HER2 [human epidermal growth factor receptor 2] gene, which directs proteins in the cancer cells to grow, divide, and travel away from the breast.

- No: The cancer scored 0 or 1+ on the IHC test. The cancer cells do not make too much HER2.

- Uncertain: The cancer scored 2+ on the IHC test. It is uncertain whether the cancer cells make too much HER2. To find out, a FISH or Florescence In Situ Hybridization test, should be done. FISH will report the cancer as positive for HER2 (yes) or negative (no). The FISH test result can also be between positive and negative (called equivocal), but this is uncommon.

Note: It is not routine to test DCIS for HER2. Treatments for HER2 positive breast cancer have only been studied in invasive disease.

Genetic Testing

A genetic test looks for gene mutations that increase the risk for developing breast and ovarian cancer. We inherit these genes, called BRCA1 and BRCA2, from our father or mother at conception. A mutation in either BRCA gene greatly increases the risk for a future breast cancer.

Between 5 and 10 percent of women with breast cancer test positive for a BRCA mutation. Because chances are low that any person has a BRCA mutation, doctors do not routinely offer this test. You might explore genetic counseling and testing if you are at higher risk for a BRCA mutation than the average person because:

- you or a family member was diagnosed with breast cancer before age 50;

- you have several family members with breast cancer on one side of your family, or who had breast cancer in both breasts;

- you have family members who had ovarian, pancreatic, or male breast cancer;

- your background is Ashkenazi (Eastern European) Jewish.

If you are interested in a genetic test, you will first meet with a genetic counselor, a healthcare provider trained to help you weigh the risks and benefits of testing and learn how the results could impact you. Your counselor will develop a pedigree, a chart of your family's medical and cancer history over time. The test itself is a simple blood test.

When health history suggests a BRCA mutation, genetic testing can be very helpful. If you have a mutation, your doctors may recommend more frequent screening, also called surveillance, watching you closely with regular and special tests such as breast MRI [magnetic resonance imaging] or pelvic ultrasound.

Chemoprevention is taking medicine to try to lower your chances of developing cancer. With prophylactic mastectomy, a healthy breast is removed to lessen the chances of a future breast cancer. Removing the ovaries in an oophorectomy surgery lowers the risk for future ovarian cancer.

The choice to have genetic testing can be complex. What you learn could impact not only your treatment but also your family and future generations, because the mutation can be passed to your children at conception. It can take several weeks to get results, and you may not want to wait to start treatment.

A plus of genetic testing is that you may do it anytime. If you prefer to wait, you can still have the test later. Even if you aren't sure, consider meeting with a genetic counselor to review your family history. You won't be able to use the results today, but you can decide later whether to take steps to reduce your risk.

Next Steps

When you first get your full pathology report, it is natural and normal to feel overwhelmed.

Remember, you do not need to absorb the report all at once. Your doctors should go through it with you, step by step, at an appointment. Consider these questions and how the answers could affect your treatment options:

- Is the breast cancer invasive, noninvasive, or mixed?

- How large is the cancer, and where is it in my breast?

- How aggressive is the cancer? Which tests suggest this?

- Did cancer cells travel away from the breast? Where?

- Did my breast surgery yield negative, close, or positive margins? How wide were the margins?

- Does the cancer grow in the presence of estrogen or progesterone?

- Does the cancer have too much HER2?

- Are any test results unclear? How can I get answers?

- Do I need more tests to find out if the cancer traveled to other parts of my body?

- Could I benefit from genomic testing or genetic testing?

If you have more questions but aren't sure where to start, call the LBBC Survivors' Helpline at 888-753-LBBC (753-5222). Volunteers can help you find the words to begin a talk with your doctor.

Section 35.2

Getting a Second Opinion after a Breast Cancer Diagnosis

Getting a second opinion after a diagnosis of breast cancer is almost always a good idea—and not just from another oncologist. Consider enlisting the expertise of another pathologist to double check the lab findings. This is important, since an accurate diagnosis is key to getting exactly the right type of treatment. Breast cancer surgery is another area where a second opinion is extremely important.

Should everyone who's diagnosed with breast cancer get a second opinion?

Generally, yes. In cases where breast cancer is in the very early stage and treatment seems straightforward, it may be safe to follow the oncologist's recommendation without getting another opinion. But when it comes to breast cancer, there are many different treatment options, and researchers are releasing new information all the time. Some doctors may be less current on the latest research than others. One way to think about it: In order to play it safe, it's almost always best to err on the side of more information and options, rather than less.

Why should I get a second opinion about a breast cancer diagnosis?

Two minds are better than one. The two doctors may agree with each other, confirming that the treatment plan is reasonable. However, if the oncologist has made a mistake—and mistakes do happen—a second opinion could make all the difference in outcome. Sometimes, for example, one doctor will say that the cancer is too advanced to operate, while another oncologist—who might be more familiar with that particular type of cancer or with the surgical procedure that would be required to remove it—will consider it operable. In other cases, bringing in a specialist leads to the discovery that it's a different kind of breast cancer altogether. The new oncologist may have more experience with a certain type of breast cancer or may interpret the test results differently or decide to run new tests, which could provide new insight. If you're trying to decide whether getting a second opinion is worth it, ask yourself whether you'd go the extra mile if a second examination discovered that the tumor is a more treatable type than the first doctor believes.

How can I avoid offending the doctor?

You may be concerned that the oncologist or surgeon will take your request for a second opinion as an expression of doubt or lack of confidence. Keep in mind that doctors receive this request very frequently. While some oncologists do resist when patients ask for a second opinion, most are supportive of the idea. No matter which way the oncologist reacts, all patients have the right to get a second opinion, and you may need to assume the role of advocate to make sure it happens. "Some doctors appreciate it when you want to bring in another expert because then the decision about treatment doesn't rest solely on their shoulders," says Bonnie Bajorek Daneker, author of *The Compassionate Caregiver's Guide to Caring for Someone With Cancer.* In cases where there's more than one treatment option to choose from, Daneker says, the doctor may welcome having another expert weigh in.

Chapter 36

Adjuvant and Neoadjuvant Therapy for Breast Cancer

What is adjuvant therapy for breast cancer?

Adjuvant therapy for breast cancer is any treatment given after primary therapy to increase the chance of long-term disease-free survival. Primary therapy is the main treatment used to reduce or eliminate the cancer. Primary therapy for breast cancer usually includes surgery—a mastectomy (removal of the breast) or a lumpectomy (surgery to remove the tumor and a small amount of normal tissue around it; a type of breast-conserving surgery). During either type of surgery, one or more nearby lymph nodes are also removed to see if cancer cells have spread to the lymphatic system. When a woman has breast-conserving surgery, primary therapy almost always includes radiation therapy.

Even in early-stage breast cancer, cells may break away from the primary tumor and spread to other parts of the body (metastasize). Therefore, doctors give adjuvant therapy to kill any cancer cells that may have spread, even if they cannot be detected by imaging or laboratory tests. Studies have shown that adjuvant therapy for breast cancer may increase the chance of long-term survival by preventing a recurrence.

Excerpted from "Adjuvant and Neoadjuvant Therapy for Breast Cancer," by the National Cancer Institute (NCI, www.cancer.gov), part of the National Institutes of Health, June 16, 2009.

What types of adjuvant therapies are used for breast cancer?

Most adjuvant therapies are systemic: They use substances that travel through the bloodstream, reaching and affecting cancer cells all over the body. Adjuvant therapy for breast cancer can include chemotherapy, hormonal therapy, the targeted drug trastuzumab (Herceptin), radiation therapy, or a combination of treatments.

Adjuvant chemotherapy uses drugs to kill cancer cells. Research has shown that adjuvant chemotherapy for early-stage breast cancer helps to prevent the cancer from returning. Usually, more than one drug is given during adjuvant chemotherapy (called combination chemotherapy).

Hormonal therapy deprives breast cancer cells of the hormone estrogen, which many breast tumors need to grow. A commonly used hormonal treatment is the drug tamoxifen, which blocks estrogen's activity in the body. Studies have shown that tamoxifen helps prevent the original cancer from returning and also helps to prevent the development of new cancers in the other breast; however, many women develop resistance to the drug over time.

Tamoxifen can be given to both premenopausal and postmenopausal women. Postmenopausal women may also receive hormonal therapy with a newer type of drug called an aromatase inhibitor (AI), either after tamoxifen therapy or instead of tamoxifen therapy. Rather than blocking estrogen's activity, as tamoxifen does, AIs prevent the body from making estrogen. Clinical trials suggest that AIs may be more effective than tamoxifen in preventing breast cancer recurrence in some women. Using AIs to block estrogen production in premenopausal women is not very effective, in part because the ovary is stimulated to make more estrogen when blood levels of estrogen fall below normal. This does not occur in postmenopausal women, whose ovaries have stopped making estrogen.

Some premenopausal women may undergo ovarian ablation or suppression, which greatly reduces the amount of estrogen produced by the body, either permanently or temporarily. Premenopausal women who have BRCA1 or BRCA2 [breast cancer susceptibility genes 1 and 2] gene mutations are at very high risk of breast cancer recurrence as well as of ovarian cancer and may decide to have their ovaries surgically removed as part of adjuvant therapy. The surgical removal of the ovaries also decreases the risk of ovarian cancer. Other premenopausal women who have a lower risk of recurrence may be prescribed drugs that temporarily suppress the function of the ovaries, in addition to tamoxifen.

Trastuzumab is a monoclonal antibody that targets cancer cells that make too much of, or overexpress, a protein called HER2 [human epidermal growth factor receptor]. When cancer cells overexpress HER2 protein, they are said to be HER2 positive. Approximately 20 percent of all breast cancers are HER2 positive. Clinical trials have shown that targeted therapy with trastuzumab in addition to chemotherapy decreases the risk of relapse for women with HER2-positive tumors.

Radiation therapy is usually given after breast-conserving surgery and may be given after a mastectomy. (When doctors give radiation therapy after breast-conserving surgery, it is usually considered part of primary therapy.) For women at high risk of recurrence, doctors may use radiation therapy after mastectomy to kill cancer cells that may be left in tissues next to the breast, such as the chest wall or nearby lymph nodes. Radiation therapy is a type of local therapy, not systemic therapy.

How is adjuvant therapy given, and for how long?

Adjuvant chemotherapy is given orally (by mouth) or by injection into a blood vessel. It is given in cycles, consisting of a treatment period followed by a recovery period. The number of cycles depends on the types of drugs used. Most patients do not have to stay in the hospital for chemotherapy—they can be treated as an outpatient or at the doctor's office. Adjuvant chemotherapy usually does not last for much more than six months.

Hormonal therapy is usually given orally, as a pill.

- Most women who undergo hormonal therapy take tamoxifen every day for five years.

- Some women may take an aromatase inhibitor every day for five years instead of tamoxifen.

- Some women may receive additional treatment with an aromatase inhibitor after five years of tamoxifen.

- Finally, some women may switch to taking an aromatase inhibitor after two or three years of tamoxifen, for a total of five or more years of hormonal therapy.

Trastuzumab is given by infusion into a blood vessel every one to three weeks for a year.

Radiation therapy given after mastectomy is divided into small doses given once a day over the course of several weeks. Radiation therapy may not be given at the same time as some types of chemotherapy or hormonal therapy.

How do doctors decide who needs adjuvant therapy?

Not all women with breast cancer need adjuvant therapy. Patients at higher risk of cancer recurrence are more likely to need adjuvant therapy. Doctors look at both prognostic and predictive factors to decide which patients might benefit from adjuvant treatments. Prognostic factors help doctors estimate how likely a tumor is to recur. Predictive factors help doctors estimate how likely cancer cells are to respond to a particular treatment.

In addition to a woman's age and menopausal status, several other prognostic factors are used to determine the risk of recurrence.

- **Stage of the cancer:** Cancer stage refers to the size of the tumor and whether it is in the breast only or has spread to nearby lymph nodes or other places in the body. Larger tumors (especially those that are more than five centimeters—about two inches—in diameter) are more likely to recur than small tumors. Breast cancer often first spreads to the lymph nodes under the arm (axillary lymph nodes). During surgery, doctors usually remove some of these underarm lymph nodes to determine whether they contain cancer cells. Cancer that has spread to these lymph nodes is more likely to recur.

- **Tumor grade:** This term refers to how closely the tumor cells resemble normal breast cells when viewed under a microscope. Tumors with cells that bear little or no resemblance to normal breast cells (called poorly differentiated tumors) are more likely to recur. Women with tumor cells that look like normal breast cells (called well-differentiated tumors) tend to have a better prognosis.

- **Proliferative capacity of the tumor:** Proliferative capacity refers to how fast the tumor cells divide, or multiply, to form more cells. Women who have tumor cells that have a low proliferative capacity (that is, the cells divide less often and grow more slowly) tend to have a better prognosis.

- **Hormone receptor status:** The cells of many breast tumors express receptors for the hormones estrogen and progesterone. Tumors with cells that do not express hormone receptors are more likely to recur. Doctors can determine whether a tumor expresses hormone receptors with laboratory tests.

- **HER2 status:** Tumors that produce too much of a protein called HER2 are more likely to recur. Doctors can determine whether a tumor produces too much HER2 with a laboratory test.

Two major predictive factors are currently used to determine whether cancer cells might respond to particular treatments:

- **Hormone receptor status:** As mentioned in the preceding text, the cells of many breast tumors express receptors for the hormones estrogen and progesterone. These hormones bind to the receptors and help the cancer cells grow. Blocking the activity of these hormones with hormonal therapy stops the growth of the cancer cells. Hormonal therapy will not help patients whose tumors do not express hormone receptors.

- **HER2 status:** Tumors that produce too much of the protein HER2 can be treated with trastuzumab, which can cut the risk of recurrence by up to about half. Women whose tumors do not produce too much HER2 do not benefit from treatment with trastuzumab.

Clinical trials are under way to see if genetic information collected from tumors can help predict which women will benefit from adjuvant chemotherapy.

Prognostic and predictive factors cannot determine exactly which patients may benefit from adjuvant therapy and which patients may benefit from primary therapy alone. Decisions about adjuvant therapy must be made on an individual basis. This complicated decision-making process is best carried out by consulting an oncologist, a doctor who specializes in cancer treatment. In addition to the factors described in the preceding text, doctors will take into account a woman's general health and her personal treatment preferences.

What is neoadjuvant therapy?

Neoadjuvant therapy is treatment given before primary therapy. A woman may receive neoadjuvant chemotherapy for breast cancer to shrink a tumor that is inoperable in its current state, so it can be surgically removed. A woman whose tumor can be removed by mastectomy may instead receive neoadjuvant therapy to shrink the tumor enough to allow breast-conserving surgery.

Neoadjuvant chemotherapy is given in the same manner as adjuvant chemotherapy. If a tumor does not respond (shrink) or continues to grow during neoadjuvant chemotherapy, the doctor may stop treatment and try another type of chemotherapy or perform surgery instead, depending on the stage of the cancer.

Clinical trials are examining whether hormonal therapy or trastuzumab is effective when given before surgery.

What are the side effects of adjuvant and neoadjuvant therapy?

Chemotherapy: The side effects of chemotherapy depend mainly on the drugs a woman receives. As with other types of treatment, side effects vary from person to person. In general, anticancer drugs affect rapidly dividing cells.

These include blood cells, which fight infection, cause the blood to clot, and carry oxygen to all parts of the body. When blood cells are affected by anticancer drugs, patients are more likely to get infections and bruise or bleed easily, and may have less energy during treatment and for some time afterward. Cells in hair follicles and cells that line the digestive tract also divide rapidly. As a result of chemotherapy, patients may lose their hair and may have other side effects, such as loss of appetite, nausea, vomiting, diarrhea, or mouth sores.

Doctors can prescribe medications to help control nausea and vomiting caused by chemotherapy. They also monitor patients for any signs of other problems and may adjust the dose or schedule of treatment if problems arise. In addition, doctors advise women who have a lowered resistance to infection because of low blood cell counts to avoid crowds and people who are sick or have colds. The side effects of chemotherapy are generally short-term. They gradually go away during the recovery part of the chemotherapy cycle or after the treatment is over. However, some chemotherapy drugs, called anthracyclines, can increase the risk of heart problems. Women who receive an anthracycline as part of their treatment should be monitored closely by their doctors for heart problems for the rest of their lives.

Hormonal therapy: In general, the side effects of tamoxifen are similar to some of the symptoms of menopause. The most common side effects are hot flashes, vaginal discharge, and nausea. Tamoxifen also increases the risk of cataract development. Not all women who take tamoxifen have these symptoms.

Most of these side effects do not require medical attention. Doctors carefully monitor women taking tamoxifen for any signs of more serious side effects. Among women who have not had a hysterectomy (surgery to remove the uterus), the risk of developing uterine cancer is increased for those taking tamoxifen. Women who take tamoxifen should talk with their doctor about having regular pelvic exams, and should be examined promptly if they have pelvic pain or any abnormal vaginal bleeding. Women taking tamoxifen, particularly those who are receiving chemotherapy along with tamoxifen, have a greater risk of developing a blood clot.

Aromatase inhibitors also cause hot flashes, vaginal dryness, and other symptoms of menopause. Women taking an aromatase inhibitor may also experience joint pain (arthralgia) or muscle pain (myalgia) during treatment.

Women taking aromatase inhibitors may have a higher risk of heart problems than those taking tamoxifen. Aromatase inhibitors also reduce bone density and increase the risk of bone fractures. Doctors should carefully monitor women taking aromatase inhibitors for any signs of heart damage or changes in bone density. A type of drug called a bisphosphonate can help reduce bone loss caused by aromatase inhibitors for patients at high risk of fractures.

Trastuzumab: Side effects from trastuzumab can include nausea, vomiting, hot flashes, and joint pain. Trastuzumab can also increase the risk of heart problems. Women receiving trastuzumab should be monitored closely by their doctors for any reduction in the heart's ability to pump blood, both during and after treatment.

Radiation therapy: Skin in the area treated by radiation may become red, dry, tender, and itchy, and the breast may feel heavy and tight. These problems usually go away over time. Women receiving radiation therapy may become very tired, especially in the later weeks of treatment.

Careful studies have shown that the risks of adjuvant therapy for breast cancer are outweighed by the benefit of treatment—that is, increasing the chance of long-term survival. However, it is important for women to share any concerns they may have about their treatment or side effects with their doctor or other health care provider.

What are doctors and scientists doing to learn more about adjuvant and neoadjuvant therapy for breast cancer?

Doctors and scientists are conducting research studies called clinical trials to learn how to treat breast cancer more effectively. In these studies, researchers compare two or more groups of patients who receive different treatments. Clinical trials allow researchers to examine the effectiveness of new treatments in comparison with standard ones, as well as to compare the side effects of the treatments.

Researchers are also investigating whether molecular information obtained from a woman's tumor can be used to decide if the woman would benefit from adjuvant therapy. Two large clinical trials sponsored by the National Cancer Institute (NCI), a part of the National Institutes of Health, are currently under way in this area of research.

The Trial Assigning Individualized Options for Treatment (TAILORx) is examining whether molecular markers that are frequently associated with risk of recurrence among women who have early-stage breast cancer can be used to assign patients to the most appropriate and effective treatment. TAILORx is using a test called Oncotype DX, which calculates the risk of recurrence based on the levels of expression of 21 genes in breast tumors, in over 10,000 women recruited at 900 sites in the United States and Canada. Based on their risk of recurrence, women will be assigned to one of three different treatment groups: Women with a high risk of recurrence will receive chemotherapy plus hormonal therapy; women with a low risk of recurrence will receive hormonal therapy alone; and women with an intermediate risk of recurrence will be randomly assigned to receive adjuvant hormonal therapy, with or without chemotherapy. Because the degree of benefit of chemotherapy for women with an intermediate risk of recurrence is unknown, TAILORx seeks to determine whether the Oncotype DX test will be helpful in future treatment planning for this group.

In the Microarray In Node-negative Disease may Avoid Chemotherapy Trial (MINDACT), investigators are studying genomic profiling compared with clinical assessment to determine the need for chemotherapy in women with node-negative breast cancer (cancer that has not spread to the axillary lymph nodes). The investigators will use both a 70-gene signature test and clinical assessment to determine the women's risk of recurrence. Women eligible to receive chemotherapy who have a high risk of recurrence according to the clinical criteria and a low risk of recurrence according to the 70-gene signature, or have a low risk of recurrence according to the clinical criteria and a high risk of recurrence according to the 70-gene signature, will be randomly assigned to receive treatment based on either the genetic or clinical criteria to determine which better predicts the need for chemotherapy.

Women with breast cancer who are interested in taking part in a clinical trial should talk with their doctor. Complete listings of current clinical trials testing adjuvant and neoadjuvant therapies for female breast cancer are available from NCI's website (www.cancer.gov).

Chapter 37

Surgical Treatments for Breast Cancer

Chapter Contents

Section 37.1

Overview of Surgeries for Early-Stage Breast Cancer

"Surgery Choices for Women with Early-Stage Cancer," by the Agency for Healthcare Research and Quality (AHRQ, www.ahrq.gov), August 2004. Reviewed by David A. Cooke, MD, FACP, April 2, 2012.

As a woman with early-stage breast cancer (DCIS or Stage I, IIA, IIB, or IIIA breast cancer) you may be able to choose which type of breast surgery to have. Often, your choice is between breast-sparing surgery (surgery that takes out the cancer and leaves most of the breast) and a mastectomy (surgery that removes the whole breast). Research shows that women with early-stage breast cancer who have breast-sparing surgery along with radiation therapy live as long as those who have a mastectomy. Most women with breast cancer will lead long, healthy lives after treatment.

Treatment for breast cancer usually begins a few weeks after diagnosis. In these weeks, you should meet with a surgeon, learn the facts about your surgery choices, and think about what is important to you. Then choose which kind of surgery to have.

Talk with Your Surgeon

Talk to a surgeon about your breast cancer surgery choices. Find out what happens during surgery, types of problems that sometimes occur, and other kinds of treatment (if any) you will need after surgery. Be sure to ask a lot of questions and learn as much as you can. You may also wish to talk with family members, friends, or others who have had breast cancer surgery.

After talking with a surgeon, you may want a second opinion. This means talking with another doctor who might tell you about other treatment options or simply give you information that can help you feel better about the choice you are making.

Don't worry about hurting your surgeon's feelings. It is common practice to get a second opinion and some insurance companies require it. Plus, it is better to get a second opinion than worry that you made the wrong choice.

Learn the Facts

Stages of Breast Cancer

Doctors talk about stages of cancer. This is a way of saying how big the tumor is and how far it has spread. If you are unsure of the stage of your cancer, ask your doctor or nurse.

Here are the stages of breast cancer discussed in this text:

- Stage 0: This means that you either have DCIS or LCIS. DCIS (ductal carcinoma in situ) is very early breast cancer that is often too small to form a lump. Your doctor may refer to DCIS as noninvasive cancer. LCIS (lobular carcinoma in situ) is not cancer but may increase the chance that you will get breast cancer. Talk with your doctor about treatment options if you are diagnosed with LCIS.

- Stage I: Your cancer is less than one inch across (two centimeters) or about the size of a quarter. The cancer is only in the breast and has not spread to lymph nodes or other parts of your body.

- Stage IIA:

  - No cancer is found in your breast, but cancer is found in the lymph nodes under your arm; or

  - your cancer is one inch (two centimeters) or smaller and has spread to the lymph nodes under your arm; or

  - your cancer is about one to two inches (two to five centimeters) but has not spread to the lymph nodes under your arm.

- Stage IIB:

  - Your cancer is about one to two inches (two to five centimeters) and has spread to the lymph nodes under your arm; or

  - your cancer is larger than two inches (five centimeters) and has not spread to the lymph nodes under your arm.

- Stage IIIA:

  - No cancer is found in the breast, but is found in lymph nodes under your arm, and the lymph nodes are attached to each other; or

311

- your cancer is two inches (five centimeters) or smaller and has spread to lymph nodes under your arm, and the lymph nodes are attached to each other; or

- your cancer is larger than two inches (five centimeters) and has spread to lymph nodes under your arm.

Find out about Your Breast Cancer Surgery Choices

Most women who have DCIS or Stage I, IIA, IIB, or IIIA breast cancer have three basic surgery choices. They are breast-sparing surgery followed by radiation therapy, mastectomy, or mastectomy with breast reconstruction surgery.

Breast-Sparing Surgery

Breast-sparing surgery means that the surgeon removes only your cancer and some normal tissue around it. This kind of surgery keeps your breast intact—looking a lot like it did before surgery. Other words for breast-sparing surgery include lumpectomy, partial mastectomy, breast-conserving surgery, or segmental mastectomy.

After breast-sparing surgery, most women also get radiation therapy. This type of treatment is very important because it could keep cancer from coming back in the same breast. Some women also need chemotherapy and hormone therapy.

Mastectomy

In a mastectomy, the surgeon removes all of your breast and nipple. Sometimes, you will also need to have radiation therapy, chemotherapy, hormone therapy, or all three types of therapy.

Here are some types of mastectomy:

- Total (simple) mastectomy: The surgeon removes all of your breast. Sometimes, the surgeon also takes out some of the lymph nodes under your arm.

- Modified radical mastectomy: The surgeon removes all of your breast, many of the lymph nodes under your arm, the lining over your chest muscles, and maybe a small chest muscle.

- Double mastectomy: The surgeon removes both your breasts at the same time, even if your cancer is in only one breast. This surgery is rare and mostly used when the surgeon feels you have a high risk for getting cancer in the breast that does not have cancer.

Breast Reconstruction Surgery

If you have a mastectomy, you can also choose to have breast reconstruction surgery. This surgery is done by a reconstructive plastic surgeon and gives you a new breast-like shape and nipple. Your surgeon
can also add a tattoo that looks like the areola (the dark area around
your nipple). Or you may not want any more surgery and prefer to
wear a prosthesis (breast-like form) in your bra. There are two types
of breast reconstruction surgery:

- Breast implants: In this kind of surgery, a reconstructive plastic surgeon puts an implant (filled with salt water or silicone
  gel) under your skin or chest muscle to build a new breast-like
  shape. While this shape looks like a breast, you will have little
  feeling in it because the nerves have been cut. Breast implants
  do not last a lifetime. If you choose to have an implant, chances
  are you will need more surgery later on to remove or replace it.
  Implants can cause problems such as breast hardness, breast
  pain, and infection. The implant may also break, move, or shift.
  These problems can happen soon after surgery or years later.

- Tissue flaps: In tissue flap surgery, a surgeon builds a new
  breast-like shape from muscle, fat, and skin taken from other
  parts of your body. This new breast-like shape should last the
  rest of your life. Women who are very thin or obese, smoke, or
  have other serious health problems often cannot have tissue
  flap surgery. Tissue flap is major surgery. Healing often takes
  longer after this surgery than if you have breast implants. You
  may have other problems, as well. For example, you might lose
  strength in the part of your body where muscle was taken to
  build a new breast. Or you may get an infection or have trouble
  healing. Tissue flap surgery is best done by a reconstructive
  plastic surgeon who has done it many times before.

Section 37.2

Mastectomy

A mastectomy is surgery to remove the entire breast. It is usually done to treat breast cancer.

Description

You will be given general anesthesia (unconscious and pain-free). The surgeon will make a cut in your breast:

For a subcutaneous mastectomy, the surgeon removes the entire breast but leaves the nipple and areola (the pigmented circle around the nipple) in place.

For a total or simple mastectomy, the surgeon cuts breast tissue free from the skin and muscle and removes it. The nipple and the areola are also removed. The surgeon may do a biopsy of lymph nodes in the underarm area to see if the cancer has spread.

For a modified radical mastectomy, the surgeon removes the entire breast along with some of the lymph nodes underneath the arm.

For a radical mastectomy, the surgeon removes the overlying skin, all of the lymph nodes underneath the arm, and the chest muscles. This surgery is rarely done.

The skin is closed with sutures (stitches).

One or two small plastic drains or tubes are usually left in your chest to remove extra fluid from where the breast tissue used to be.

A plastic surgeon may be able to reconstruct the breast (with artificial implants or tissue from your own body) during the same operation. You may also choose to have reconstruction later.

Mastectomy generally takes two to three hours.

Why the Procedure Is Performed

The most common reason for a mastectomy is breast cancer.

Woman Diagnosed with Breast Cancer

If you are diagnosed with breast cancer, talk to your doctor about your choices:

- Lumpectomy is when only the breast cancer and tissue around the cancer are removed. This is also called breast conservation therapy or partial mastectomy. Part of your breast will be left.

- Mastectomy is when all breast tissue is removed. Mastectomy is a better choice if the area of cancer is too large to remove without deforming the breast.

You and your doctor should consider:

- the size of your tumor, where in your breast it is located, whether you have more than one tumor in your breast, how much of your breast the cancer affects, and the size of your breasts; and

- your age, family history, overall health, and whether you have reached menopause.

The choice of what is best for you can be difficult. Sometimes, it is hard to know whether lumpectomy or mastectomy is best. You and the health care providers who are treating your breast cancer will decide together what is best.

Women at High Risk for Breast Cancer

Women who have a very high risk of developing breast cancer may choose to have a prophylactic mastectomy. Your doctor may do either a subcutaneous or total mastectomy to reduce your risk of breast cancer if you are at very high risk for developing breast cancer. This is called prophylactic mastectomy.

You may have a higher risk of getting breast cancer if one or more close family relatives has had breast cancer, especially at an early age. Genetic tests (such as BRCA1 or BRCA2 [breast cancer susceptibility genes 1 and 2]) may also show you have a high risk. This surgery should be done only after very careful thought and discussion with your doctor, a genetic counselor, your family, and others.

Mastectomy greatly reduces, but does not eliminate, the risk of breast cancer.

Risks

Risks for any surgery are:

- blood clots in the legs that may travel to the lungs;
- blood loss;
- breathing problems;
- infection, including in the surgical wound, lungs (pneumonia), bladder, or kidney;
- heart attack or stroke during surgery;
- reactions to medications.

Scabbing, blistering, or skin loss along the edge of the surgical cut may occur.

Risks when more invasive surgery, such as a radical mastectomy, is done are:

- Shoulder pain and stiffness. You may also feel pins and needles where the breast used to be and underneath the arm.
- Swelling of the arm (called lymphedema) on the same side as the breast that is removed. This swelling is not common, but it can be an ongoing problem.
- Damage to nerves that go to the muscles of the arm, back, and chest wall.

Before the Procedure

You may have many blood and imaging tests (such as CT [computed tomography] scans, bone scans, and chest x-ray) after your doctor finds breast cancer. Your surgeon will want to know whether your cancer has spread to the lymph nodes, liver, lungs, bones, or somewhere else.

Always tell your doctor or nurse if:

- you could be pregnant;
- you are taking any drugs or herbs you bought without a prescription.

During the week before the surgery:

- Several days before your surgery, you may be asked to stop taking aspirin, ibuprofen (Advil, Motrin), naproxen (Aleve, Naprosyn), vitamin E, clopidogrel (Plavix), warfarin (Coumadin), and any other drugs that make it hard for your blood to clot.
- Ask your doctor which drugs you should still take on the day of the surgery.

On the day of the surgery:

- Follow instructions from your doctor or nurse about eating or drinking before surgery.

- Take the drugs your doctor told you to take with a small sip of water.

- Your doctor or nurse will tell you when to arrive at the hospital.

After the Procedure

You may stay in the hospital for one to three days, depending on the type of surgery you had. If you have a simple mastectomy, you may go home on the same day. Most women go home after one to two days. You may stay longer if you have breast reconstruction.

Many women go home with drains still in their chest. The doctor then removes them later during an office visit.

You may have pain around the site of your cut after surgery.

Fluid may collect in the area of your mastectomy after all the drains are removed. This is called a seroma. It usually goes away on its own, but it may need to be drained using a needle (aspiration).

Outlook (Prognosis)

Most women recover well after mastectomy.

In addition to surgery, you may need other treatments for breast cancer. These treatments may include hormonal therapy, radiation therapy, and chemotherapy. All have their own side effects. Talk to your doctor.

Section 37.3

Lumpectomy

Breast lump removal, called lumpectomy, is surgery to remove a breast cancer or other lump in the breast, along with some surrounding tissue from the breast.

This text covers lumpectomy that is done to remove breast cancer. Other reasons to perform a lumpectomy include:

- fibroadenoma;

- other noncancerous tumors of the breast.

Description

If the breast cancer can be seen on a mammogram or ultrasound but the doctor cannot feel the cancer on a physical exam, a wire localization will be done before the surgery:

- A radiologist will use a mammogram or ultrasound to place a needle (or needles) in or near the abnormal breast area.

- This will help the surgeon know where the cancer is so that it can be removed.

Breast lump removal is usually done in an outpatient clinic. You will be given general anesthesia (you will be asleep, but pain free) or local anesthesia (awake, but sedated and pain free). The procedure takes about one hour.

The surgeon makes a small cut on your breast. The surgeon then removes the cancer with some breast tissue around it.

- The goal is to remove breast cancer, along with a rim of normal breast tissue around it. When no cancer cells are near the edges of the tissue removed, it is called a clear margin.

- Your surgeon may also remove lymph nodes in your armpit (axilla) to see if cancer has spread to the lymph nodes.

- The surgeon will close the skin with stitches. These may dissolve or need to be removed later. A drain tube may be placed to remove excess fluid.

Your doctor will send the lump to a laboratory for testing.

Why the Procedure Is Performed

Surgery to remove a breast cancer is usually the first step in treatment.

The choice of which surgery is best for you can be difficult. Sometimes, it is hard to know whether lumpectomy or mastectomy is best. You and the health care providers who are treating your breast cancer will decide together.

Lumpectomy is often preferred, because it is a smaller procedure and it has about the same chance of curing breast cancer as a mastectomy.

Mastectomy, when all breast tissue is removed, may be done if the area of cancer is too large to remove without deforming the breast.

You and your doctor should consider:

- the size of your tumor, where in your breast it is located, whether you have more than one tumor in your breast, how much of your breast the cancer affects, and the size of your breasts;

- your age, family history, whether you have reached menopause, and your overall health.

Risks

Risks for any surgery are:

- bleeding;
- infection;
- reactions to medications.

Risks for this procedure are:

- The appearance of your breast may change. After surgery, you may notice dimpling, a scar, or a difference in shape between the two breasts.
- You may also have numbness in the breast area.

The breast tissue that is removed will be looked at under a microscope after the surgery. If the cancer is too close to the edge of this tissue, you may need another procedure to remove more breast tissue.

319

Before the Procedure

Always tell your doctor or nurse:

- if you could be pregnant;
- what drugs you are taking, even drugs or herbs you bought without a prescription.

During the days before the surgery:

- You may be asked to stop taking aspirin, ibuprofen (Advil, Motrin), naproxen (Aleve, Naprosyn), clopidogrel (Plavix), warfarin (Coumadin), and any other drugs that make it hard for your blood to clot.
- Ask your doctor which drugs you should still take on the day of the surgery.
- Always try to stop smoking. Your doctor or nurse can help.

On the day of the surgery:

- Follow your doctor's instructions about eating or drinking before surgery.
- Take the drugs your doctor told you to take with a small sip of water.
- Your doctor or nurse will tell you when to arrive for the procedure.

After the Procedure

The recovery period is very short for a simple lumpectomy.

You should have little pain. If you do feel pain, you can take pain medicine, such as acetaminophen (Tylenol).

The skin should heal in about a month. You will need to take care of the surgical cut area. Change dressings as your doctor or nurse tells you to. Watch for signs of infection when you get home (such as redness, swelling, or drainage).

You may need to empty a fluid drain a few times a day for one to two weeks. Your doctor will remove the drain later.

Most women can go back to their usual activities in a week or so. Avoid heavy lifting, jogging, or activities that cause pain in the surgical area for one to two weeks.

If cancer is found, you will need to schedule follow-up treatment with your doctor.

Outlook (Prognosis)

The outcome of a lumpectomy for breast cancer depends mostly on the size of the cancer and whether it has spread to lymph nodes underneath your arm.

A lumpectomy for breast cancer is usually followed by radiation therapy and chemotherapy, hormone therapy, or both.

Women usually do not need breast reconstruction after lumpectomy.

Section 37.4

Using Lasers and Heat to Remove Cancer Tumors

This section contains text excerpted from "Lasers in Cancer Treatment," by the National Cancer Institute (NCI, www.cancer.gov), part of the National Institutes of Health, September 13, 2011, and excerpted from "Radiofrequency Thermal Ablation as Tumor Therapy," by Radiology and Imaging Sciences, part of the National Institutes of Health Clinical Center (clinicalcenter.nih.gov), March 6, 2009.

Lasers in Cancer Treatment

What is laser light?

The term "laser" stands for light amplification by stimulated emission of radiation. Ordinary light, such as that from a light bulb, has many wavelengths and spreads in all directions. Laser light, on the other hand, has a specific wavelength. It is focused in a narrow beam and creates a very high-intensity light. This powerful beam of light may be used to cut through steel or to shape diamonds. Because lasers can focus very accurately on tiny areas, they can also be used for very precise surgical work or for cutting through tissue (in place of a scalpel).

What is laser therapy, and how is it used in cancer treatment?

Laser therapy uses high-intensity light to treat cancer and other illnesses. Lasers can be used to shrink or destroy tumors or precancerous growths. Lasers are most commonly used to treat superficial cancers (cancers on the surface of the body or the lining of internal organs) such as basal cell skin cancer and the very early stages of some cancers, such as cervical, penile, vaginal, vulvar, and non-small cell lung cancer.

Lasers also may be used to relieve certain symptoms of cancer, such as bleeding or obstruction. For example, lasers can be used to shrink or destroy a tumor that is blocking a patient's trachea (windpipe) or esophagus. Lasers also can be used to remove colon polyps or tumors that are blocking the colon or stomach.

Laser therapy can be used alone, but most often it is combined with other treatments, such as surgery, chemotherapy, or radiation therapy. In addition, lasers can seal nerve endings to reduce pain after surgery and seal lymph vessels to reduce swelling and limit the spread of tumor cells.

How is laser therapy given to the patient?

Laser therapy is often given through a flexible endoscope (a thin, lighted tube used to look at tissues inside the body). The endoscope is fitted with optical fibers (thin fibers that transmit light). It is inserted through an opening in the body, such as the mouth, nose, anus, or vagina. Laser light is then precisely aimed to cut or destroy a tumor.

Laser-induced interstitial thermotherapy (LITT), or interstitial laser photocoagulation, also uses lasers to treat some cancers. LITT is similar to a cancer treatment called hyperthermia, which uses heat to shrink tumors by damaging or killing cancer cells. During LITT, an optical fiber is inserted into a tumor. Laser light at the tip of the fiber raises the temperature of the tumor cells and damages or destroys them. LITT is sometimes used to shrink tumors in the liver.

Photodynamic therapy (PDT) is another type of cancer treatment that uses lasers. In PDT, a certain drug, called a photosensitizer or photosensitizing agent, is injected into a patient and absorbed by cells all over the patient's body. After a couple of days, the agent is found mostly in cancer cells. Laser light is then used to activate the agent and destroy cancer cells. Because the photosensitizer makes the skin and eyes sensitive to light afterward, patients are advised to avoid direct sunlight and bright indoor light during that time.

What types of lasers are used in cancer treatment?

Three types of lasers are used to treat cancer: carbon dioxide (CO_2) lasers, argon lasers, and neodymium:yttrium-aluminum-garnet (Nd:YAG) lasers. Each of these can shrink or destroy tumors and can be used with endoscopes.

CO2 and argon lasers can cut the skin's surface without going into deeper layers. Thus, they can be used to remove superficial cancers, such as skin cancer. In contrast, the Nd:YAG laser is more commonly applied through an endoscope to treat internal organs, such as the uterus, esophagus, and colon.

Nd:YAG laser light can also travel through optical fibers into specific areas of the body during LITT. Argon lasers are often used to activate the drugs used in PDT.

What are the advantages of laser therapy?

Lasers are more precise than standard surgical tools (scalpels), so they do less damage to normal tissues. As a result, patients usually have less pain, bleeding, swelling, and scarring. With laser therapy, operations are usually shorter. In fact, laser therapy can often be done on an outpatient basis. It takes less time for patients to heal after laser surgery, and they are less likely to get infections. Patients should consult with their health care provider about whether laser therapy is appropriate for them.

What are the disadvantages of laser therapy?

Laser therapy also has several limitations. Surgeons must have specialized training before they can do laser therapy, and strict safety precautions must be followed. Laser therapy is expensive and requires bulky equipment. In addition, the effects of laser therapy may not last long, so doctors may have to repeat the treatment for a patient to get the full benefit.

Radiofrequency Thermal Ablation as Tumor Therapy

Recent developments in radiofrequency thermal ablation (RFA) have expanded the treatment options for certain oncology patients. Minimally invasive, image-guided therapy may now provide effective local treatment of isolated or localized neoplastic disease, and can also be used as an adjunct to conventional surgery, systemic chemotherapy, or radiation. RFA expands the medical application of heat, which for decades has been used as a cautery device to cut tissue. In the procedure, the tumors are located with ultrasound, computed tomography (CT), or magnetic resonance (MR) imaging devices. Then, essentially the patient is turned into an electrical circuit by placing grounding pads on the thighs. A small needle-electrode with an insulated shaft and an uninsulated distal tip is inserted through the skin and directly into the tumor. Ionic vibration at the needle tip leads to frictional heat. After 10 to 30 minutes of contact with the tumor, the radiofrequency energy kills a 2.5- to 5-cm sphere. The dead cells are not removed, but become scar tissue and eventually shrink. RFA continues to play a time-tested, major role in the treatment of patients with painful osteoid osteomas in the bone and heart arrhythmias. In addition, RFA has been used to treat painful trigeminal neuralgia for 25 years. Today, the mainstream applications of RFA are increasing. In particular, this minimally invasive, percutaneous technique is showing promise as a treatment option for patients with cancer.

Many times RFA can be an alternative to risky surgery, and sometimes it can change a patient from having an inoperable tumor to being a candidate for surgery. The procedure is proving useful as an adjunct to conventional treatments and as a palliative treatment. What's more, the cauterizing effect of the heated needle prevents excessive bleeding, leading to low complication rates. Although RFA may not be a magic bullet, it clearly can be a cure in some cases.

Radiofrequency thermal ablation can usually be performed as an outpatient procedure under general anesthesia or conscious sedation. Alternatively, RFA may be performed laparoscopically or during open surgery.

Under light sedation, lidocaine or bupivacaine is administered subcutaneously at the needle entry site and down to the liver capsule. A needle is placed through the skin and into the tumor with imaging guidance. Treatment sessions of percutaneous RFA are easily monitored using real-time ultrasound imaging, computed tomography, or magnetic resonance imaging. Most patients feel little pain during the procedure and go home the same day or the day after the procedure, usually with minimal to no pain or soreness, although there is a spectrum, and some patients will experience severe pain the day of the procedure.

During a 10- to 30-minute treatment session, nitrogen microbubbles gradually create a hyperechoic area on ultrasound that provides a rough estimation of the treated tissue, which is 2.5 to 5 cm per 10- to 30-minute treatment sphere. CT, MR imaging, or positron emission tomography (PET) imaging may provide more exquisite detail for follow-up verification of the treatment zone and for finding residual or recurrent neoplastic tissue. Although real-time MR imaging and CT are available, they are not in widespread use. Ultrasound is a safe, common, and easy guidance method, although it is somewhat operator dependent.

Once the needle has been properly positioned within the tumor, the tissue is heated. At temperatures exceeding 50 degrees Celsius, cells are destroyed. To treat tumors of different size and shape, the needle is available in different lengths and shapes of exposed tips.

Energy is transferred from the uninsulated distal tip of the needle to the tissue as current rather than as direct heat. The circuit is completed with grounding pads placed on the patient's thighs. As the alternating current flows to the grounding pads, it agitates ions in the surrounding tissue, resulting in frictional heat. The tissue surrounding the needle is desiccated, creating an oval or spherical lesion of coagulation necrosis, typically 2.5 to 5 cm in diameter for each 10- to 30-minute treatment. These spheres are added together in three dimensions to overlap and completely envelop the tumor. Ideally, the treated tissue will contain the entire tumor plus a variable rim of healthy tissue as a safety margin.

Failure to ablate the entire tumor with clean edges results in regrowth of the tumor. Depending on the size and configuration of new growth, the patient may or may not be suited for another treatment session. Over months to years, as the dead necrotic cells are reabsorbed and replaced by scar tissue and fibrosis, the size of the thermal lesion shrinks, although the remaining cells are ideally dead. The possibility of successful surgical resection may be augmented by decreasing the number of tumors. Due to the natural course of the disease, new or recurrent tumors may be suited for additional treatment sessions as well.

At the end of a treatment session, the active needle is slowly retracted to heat and cauterize the needle pathway. This action prevents bleeding and tumor seeding of the needle track by destroying any cell that becomes attached to the needle or dislodged in the needle tract.

Three companies (RITA Medical Systems, Radionics, and Radio-Therapeutics) market RFA systems. They currently have FDA 510-K clearance for soft tissue ablation, and have or are pursuing FDA 510-K clearance for unresectable liver tumor ablation. Although it is in its infancy as a technique, RFA is no longer a completely experimental procedure.

Patients with functional or tumorous disorders of the brain, such as Parkinson's disease, and benign or malignant lesions may be candidates for RFA, although it is experimental for brain tumors. One feasibility series on RFA for breast cancer in five patients suggests that it might play a role in select patient populations; however, this is also experimental.

What are the complications?

Although RFA is relatively safe and minimally invasive, the benefits do not come without slight risks. The reported complication rate has been estimated at nearly 2 percent, and may include bleeding, effusion, fever, and infection. The proximity to vital structures may influence the risk for collateral damage. The risks are kept to a minimum by attention to detail as well as continuous monitoring of vital signs and oxygenation and pre-procedural blood tests. Complications are usually managed nonoperatively.

The heating treatment inherent to RFA actually stops bleeding. The 14 to 17.5 gauge needles are very small; they are the same size needles used for biopsy, with the added benefits of cauterization and coagulation. The low rate of bleeding seen with RFA is likely the result of this cauterization effect, which is similar to electrocautery used to stop bleeding during surgery. This same treatment of the needle track should minimize the risk of needle-track seeding in the systems that are capable of cauterizing the track. The predictable nature of RFA allows for little collateral damage during treatments situated near vital structures. In fact, the "heat sink effect" actually preserves the vessels near a treatment area. However, with this effect, the inflow of "cool" blood at body temperature (cool relative to the cooked tissue) may impair the heating of the tumor cells closest to the vessels. The protected vessel often harbors an adjacent tumor that may regrow adjacent to large vessels.

Combining RFA therapy with chemoembolization can selectively block blood flow to a tumor, and thus may provide more effective treatment for larger tumors. Combining local radiation or local chemotherapy infusion with RFA could also be more effective than any one treatment alone. Doxorubicin has been shown in mice to enhance the effects of RFA by increasing the volume of tumor treated. Early reports of combining RFA with chemotherapy infusion and chemoembolization should lead to larger studies of such combination therapies.

Are there clinical applications for RFA?

A wide variety of clinical applications for RFA are being developed. If a target can be seen with CT, MR, or ultrasound, then a needle can be placed into it. If a needle can be placed, then the target tissue or tumor can be ablated and destroyed. If a clean margin is created, then the tumor will not recur at that site. Recent developments in RFA allow this treatment process to be done in a safe, predictable, and cheap fashion with low complication rates and minimal discomfort, on an outpatient basis. Further study is required to assess which patients will benefit from this new treatment, and most cancer patients will not be candidates due to the size or location of the tumor. Although long-term data have yet to be reported, early results suggest that RFA may prove to be an effective treatment option or adjunct for many oncology patients.

Section 37.5

Breast Reconstruction Surgery with Artificial Implants

After a mastectomy, some women choose to have cosmetic surgery to recreate their breast. This surgery can be performed during mastectomy itself or later.

The breast is usually reshaped in two stages. First a tissue expander is used. Then a saline implant is placed. Sometimes the implant can be inserted in the first stage.

Description

If you are having reconstruction at the same time as your mastectomy, your surgeon may do a skin sparing mastectomy. This means only the area around your nipple and areola is removed and more skin is left to make reconstruction easier.

If you will have breast reconstruction later, your surgeon will remove enough skin over your breast during the mastectomy to be able to close the skin flaps.

Breast reconstruction with implants is usually done in two stages. You will receive general anesthesia (asleep and pain-free).

In the first stage:

- Your surgeon will place a small tissue expander under your chest muscle and skin. The expander is a pouch made out of silicone, similar to a balloon.

- Your chest will still look flat right after this surgery.

- Starting about two to three weeks after surgery, you will see your surgeon every one or two weeks. During these visits, your surgeon will inject a small amount of saline (salt water) through your skin into the pouch through a valve.

- The pouch or tissue expander slowly enlarges the pouch in your chest to the right size for the surgeon to place an implant.

- When it reaches the right size, you will wait one to three months before the permanent breast implant is placed (the second stage).

In the second stage:

- Your surgeon will remove the tissue expander from your chest and replace it with a breast implant. This surgery takes one to two hours.

- Before this surgery, you will have talked with your surgeon about the different kinds of breast implants. Implants may be filled with either saline or a silicone gel.

You may have another minor procedure later that remakes the nipple and areola area.

Why the Procedure Is Performed

You and your doctor will decide together about whether to have breast reconstruction, and when to have it.

Having breast reconstruction does not make it harder to find a tumor if your breast cancer comes back.

Getting breast implants does not take as long as breast reconstruction (which uses your own muscle tissue). You will also have fewer scars. The size, fullness, and shape of the new breasts are more natural with reconstruction that uses muscle tissue.

Many women choose not to have breast reconstruction or implants. They may use a prosthesis (an artificial breast) in their bra that gives them a natural shape, or they may choose to use nothing at all.

Women who have had a lumpectomy rarely need to have breast reconstruction.

Risks

Risks for any surgery are:

- blood clots in the legs that may travel to the lungs;
- blood loss;
- breathing problems;
- heart attack or stroke during surgery;
- infection, including in the surgical wound, lungs (pneumonia), bladder, or kidney;
- reactions to medicines.

The risks for breast reconstruction with implants are:

- The implant in one out of every 10 women will break or leak in the first 10 years. If this happens, you will need more surgery.
- A scar may form around the implant in your breast. If the scar becomes tight, your breast may feel hard and you may have pain or discomfort. This is called capsular contracture. You will need more surgery if this happens.
- Infection soon after surgery: You would need to have the expander or the implant removed.
- Breast implants can shift. This will cause a change in the shape of your breast.
- One breast may be larger than the other (asymmetry of the breasts).
- You may have a loss of sensation around the nipple and areola.

Before the Procedure

Always tell your doctor or nurse if you are taking any drugs, supplements, or herbs you bought without a prescription.

During the week before your surgery:

- Several days before surgery, you may be asked to stop taking aspirin, ibuprofen (Advil, Motrin), vitamin E, clopidogrel (Plavix), warfarin (Coumadin), and other drugs like these.
- Ask your doctor which drugs you should still take on the day of surgery.

On the day of your surgery:

- Do not eat or drink anything after midnight the night before surgery.

• Take your drugs your doctor told you to take with a small sip of water.

• Shower the night before or the morning of surgery.

• Your doctor or nurse will tell you when to arrive at the hospital.

After the Procedure

You may be able to go home the same day as the surgery, or you may need to stay in the hospital for one or two days.

Outlook (Prognosis)

Results of this surgery are usually very good. It is nearly impossible to make a reconstructed breast look exactly the same as the remaining natural breast. You may need more "touch up" procedures to get the result you want.

Reconstruction will not restore normal sensation to the breast or the new nipple.

Having cosmetic surgery after breast cancer can improve your sense of well-being and your quality of life.

Section 37.6

Breast Reconstruction Surgery with Natural Tissue

After a mastectomy, some women choose to have cosmetic surgery to remake their breast. This type of surgery is called breast reconstruction.

During breast reconstruction therapy using natural tissue, the breast is reshaped using muscle, skin, and fat from another part of your body.

This surgery can be performed at the same time as mastectomy or later.

Description

If you are having breast reconstruction at the same time as your mastectomy, your surgeon may do a skin sparing mastectomy. This means only the area around your nipple and areola is removed, and more skin is left to make reconstruction easier.

If you will have breast reconstruction later, your surgeon will remove enough skin over your breast to be able to close the skin flaps.

The two most common methods of breast reconstruction are transverse rectus abdominous muscle flap (TRAM) and latissimus muscle flap with a breast implant. For both of these procedures, you will have general anesthesia (asleep and pain-free).

For TRAM Surgery

- Your surgeon will make a cut across your lower belly, from one hip to the other. Your scar will be hidden later by most clothing and bathing suits.

- Your surgeon will loosen skin, fat, and muscle in this area. The surgeon will then tunnel this tissue under the skin of your abdomen up to the breast area. Your surgeon will use this tissue to create your new breast. Blood vessels remain connected to the area from where the tissue is taken.

- In another method, the skin, fat, and muscle tissue are removed from your lower belly. Then the surgeon places this tissue in your breast area to create your new breast. In this method, the arteries and veins are cut and reattached to blood vessels under your arm.

- This tissue is then shaped into a new breast. Your surgeon will match the size and shape of your remaining natural breast as closely as possible.

- Your surgeon will close your belly cut with stitches.

- If you would like a new nipple and areola created, you will need a second, much smaller surgery later.

For Latissimus Muscle Flap with a Breast Implant

- Your surgeon will make a surgical cut in your upper back, on the side of your breast that was removed.

- Your surgeon will loosen skin, fat, and muscle from this area and then tunnel this tissue under your skin to the breast area. This tissue will be used to create your new breast. Blood vessels will remain connected to the area from where the tissue was taken.

- This tissue is then shaped into a new breast. Your surgeon will match the size and shape of your remaining natural breast as closely as possible.

- An implant may be placed underneath the chest wall muscles to help match the size of your other breast.

- If you would like a new nipple and areola created, you will need a second, much smaller surgery later.

When breast reconstruction is done at the same time as a mastectomy, it adds about two to four hours to the surgery. When it is done as a second surgery, it may take more than two or six hours.

Why the Procedure Is Performed

You and your doctor will decide together about whether to have breast reconstruction, and when. The decision depends on many different factors.

Having breast reconstruction does not make it harder to find a tumor if your breast cancer comes back.

The advantage of breast reconstruction with natural tissue is that the remade breast is softer and more natural than breast implants. The size, fullness, and shape of the new breast can be closely matched to your other breast.

But muscle flap procedures are more complicated than placing breast implants. You may need blood transfusions during the procedure. You will usually spend two or three more days in the hospital after this surgery compared to other reconstruction procedures. Also, your recovery time at home will probably be longer.

Many women choose not to have breast reconstruction or implants. They may use a prosthesis (an artificial breast) in their bra that gives a natural shape, or they may choose to use nothing at all.

Risks

Risks for any surgery are:

- blood clots in the legs that may travel to the lungs;
- blood loss;
- breathing problems;
- heart attack or stroke during surgery;
- infection, including in the surgical wound, lungs (pneumonia), bladder, or kidney;
- reactions to medicines.

The risks for breast reconstruction with natural tissue are:

- loss of sensation around the nipple and areola;
- noticeable scar;
- one breast is larger than the other (asymmetry of the breasts);
- skin loss or chronic wounds on the chest wall.

There is also a risk of bleeding into the area where the breast used to be. Sometimes a second operation is needed to control this bleeding.

Before the Procedure

Always tell your doctor or nurse if you are taking any drugs, supplements, or herbs you bought without a prescription.

During the week before your surgery:

- Several days before surgery, you may be asked to stop taking aspirin, ibuprofen (Advil, Motrin), vitamin E, clopidogrel (Plavix), warfarin (Coumadin), and any other drugs that make it hard for your blood to clot.

- Ask your doctor which drugs you should still take on the day of your surgery.

On the day of your surgery:

- Do not eat or drink anything after midnight the night before surgery.

- Take your drugs your doctor told you to take with a small sip of water.

- Shower the night before or the morning of surgery.

- Your doctor or nurse will tell you when to arrive at the hospital.

After the Procedure

You will stay in the hospital for two to five days.

You may still have drains in your chest when you go home. Your surgeon will remove them later during an office visit. You may have pain around your cut after surgery.

Fluid may collect under the skin of your armpit. This is called a seroma. It is fairly common. Seromas usually go away on their own, but sometimes they need to be drained.

Outlook (Prognosis)

Results of reconstruction surgery using natural tissue are usually very good. But reconstruction will not restore normal sensation on your new breast or nipple.

Recovery is usually faster when reconstruction is done after the mastectomy wound has healed.

Having breast reconstruction surgery after breast cancer can improve your sense of well-being and quality of life.

Chapter 38

Radiation Therapy for Breast Cancer

Facts about Breast Cancer

Breast cancer is the most common type of cancer in American women, according to the American Cancer Society. This year, 230,480 women and 2,140 men will learn they have breast cancer. Another 57,650 women will learn they have noninvasive (also called in situ) breast cancer. Breast cancer can often be cured. About 80 percent of all patients with breast cancer live at least 10 years after their diagnosis.

Treating Breast Cancer

Surgery

The main curative treatment for breast cancer is surgery. This is often followed by radiation therapy to decrease the risk of cancer returning in the breast, chest wall, and/or lymph nodes.

Breast conserving surgery involves surgical removal of the cancerous tissue along with a small rim of surrounding healthy breast tissue to preserve as much of the normal breast as possible. This type of surgery is called a lumpectomy or partial mastectomy and is often followed by radiation therapy.

Mastectomy is surgical removal of the entire breast. Sometimes, breast reconstruction can be performed after the mastectomy. While less common, radiation is sometimes recommended after mastectomy as well.

Often, a select number of lymph nodes near the breast are removed to determine if they contain tumor cells. This procedure is called a sentinel node biopsy. If one or more of the selected lymph nodes are involved with tumor, a more complete removal of lymph nodes may be recommended. This procedure is called an auxiliary lymph node dissection. In most cases, an examination of the lymph nodes is performed with the breast surgery of choice.

Both mastectomy and breast conserving therapy (surgery and radiation) can be equally effective approaches in curing breast cancer. Ask your surgeon and radiation oncologist about the risks and benefits of both options.

Radiation Therapy

After surgery, radiation therapy can decrease the chance of cancer returning in the breast and improve survival. Radiation therapy involves delivering focused radiation to the breast/chest wall to treat any cancer cells not detected or removed by surgery.

Radiation therapy kills cancer cells by destroying their ability to multiply. Surrounding healthy tissue is also affected by radiation and may have some damage. However, healthy normal cells are better able to heal from radiation injury, compared to cancer cells, because they have maintained the ability to repair radiation induced damage.

Medical Therapy

While surgery and radiation focus directly on treating the breast, medication is often recommended to improve cure rates or prevent a new breast cancer from developing. A medical oncologist will evaluate you and determine what medications may be most helpful in accomplishing those goals.

Chemotherapy has the ability to destroy cancer cells by different methods. Often, two or three different types of drugs may be combined to get the best outcome. The dose and schedule for treatment varies, but chemotherapy is usually delivered every two to three weeks for a few months.

Hormonal therapy can block the effects of estrogen in the body.

The normal female hormone, estrogen, has been shown in some cases to help your tumor grow. Usually taken as a daily pill, this medication may be started during or after radiation therapy is completed.

Immunotherapy can stimulate your immune system to help target cancer cells. Some cancer cells overexpress the HER2 [human epidermal growth factor receptor 2] molecule, which somehow makes these tumors more aggressive. Currently, trastuzumab has been used to target these aggressive breast cancers with HER2 molecule overexpression.

For more details about these drugs or newer medications, ask your medical oncologist what may be best for you.

External Beam Radiation Therapy after Lumpectomy

After breast conserving surgery (lumpectomy), the usual course of radiation treats only the breast, although you may need to have nearby lymph node areas treated as well. The radiation beam comes from a machine called a linear accelerator or linac. The radiation beam is painless and treatment itself lasts only a few minutes.

Treatment is delivered every day, five days a week, Monday through Friday. The full course of treatment is usually delivered over three to seven weeks.

Before beginning treatment, you will be scheduled for a planning session to map out the area your radiation oncologist wishes to treat. This procedure is called a simulation. Simulation involves having x-rays and/or a CT [computed tomography] scan. You may also receive tiny marks on your skin, like a permanent tattoo, to help the radiation therapist precisely position you for daily treatment.

Typically, radiation therapy is done with high energy x-rays, or photons, for the bulk of the treatment. When there is a reason to focus the radiation where the lump was taken out, sometimes a "boost" will be given with electrons to treat with a less penetrating, more focused beam instead of photons.

Different techniques can be used to give radiation therapy for breast cancer. Three-dimensional conformal radiotherapy (or 3D-CRT) combines multiple radiation treatment fields to deliver very precise doses of radiation to the breast and chest wall while sparing nearby normal tissue. Intensity modulated radiation therapy (IMRT) is a form of 3D-CRT that further modifies the radiation by varying the intensity of each radiation beam. Doctors are still studying IMRT for the treatment of some types of breast cancer. Talk to your radiation oncologist for more information about the details of your treatment plan.

Recent clinical trials suggest that treatment with whole breast radiation may be shortened by treating with higher daily doses to finish in less time. Ask your doctor for details about the right dose and schedule for your case.

Additional research suggests women aged 70 or older with hormone receptor positive early stage breast cancer benefit from radiation in terms of lowering their risk of getting breast cancer again in the treated breast. This local control benefit, however, has not been shown to affect their long term survival. Because the risks and benefits of radiation differ based not only upon age but other health factors and personal preferences, discuss with your doctor whether radiation is necessary.

Accelerated Partial Breast Irradiation

The present standard of care for the treatment of early-stage breast cancer is a lumpectomy followed by several weeks of whole breast radiation. However, ongoing research suggests that it may be safe to give radiation treatment to only part of the breast, which would allow the radiation to be delivered over a shorter period of time.

In clinical trials, doctors are studying if accelerated partial breast irradiation (or APBI)—where radiation is delivered to only part of the breast over four to five days—works as well as the present standard whole breast radiation. Because APBI is still being studied, it is used more selectively than whole breast radiation.

There are two different approaches to APBI:

1. Breast brachytherapy involves placing flexible plastic tubes called catheters or a balloon directly into the cavity where the lump was taken from. After simulation, the catheters or the balloon are connected to a machine called a high-dose-rate afterloader, which stores a radioactive source. With a special computer, a small, radioactive seed is guided into the catheters or balloon near where the tumor was removed. The radioactive seed is left in place for several minutes, based upon the treatment plan designed by your radiation oncologist. After the end of the five days, the catheters or balloon are removed.

2. External beam radiation with 3D-CRT can also treat part of the breast but it is more focused around the area of surgery. Treatment is delivered using the same machine (linear accelerator) and a similar technique as what is used for standard whole breast radiation.

Treatment with both approaches of APBI are typically given twice a day, five days a week. Treatment can be completed in one week. The long-term results of these techniques appear promising but are still being studied. Talk with your radiation oncologist for more information.

Radiation after Mastectomy

After a mastectomy, your doctor may suggest radiation therapy for the chest wall and often nearby lymph node areas. Whether or not radiation therapy should be used after removal of your breast depends on several factors. These factors include the number of lymph nodes involved, tumor size, and whether or not cancer cells were found near the edge of the tissue that was removed. Many patients who have a mastectomy can safely skip radiation therapy. Ask your doctor for more information.

For women undergoing reconstruction, postmastectomy radiation may affect your options for reconstruction or the cosmetic outcome. Discuss with your surgeon and radiation oncologist to learn more.

Possible Side Effects

Side effects are usually temporary and usually go away shortly after treatment ends. Below is a list of possible side effects you might notice during your treatment. However, ask your doctor what you can expect from your specific treatment.

- Skin irritation similar to a sunburn, sometimes with a peeling reaction toward the end of treatment

- Mild to moderate breast swelling

- Mild tenderness in the breast or chest wall (This will slowly get better over time.)

- Mild fatigue that generally gets better a month or two after treatment ends

Many of these side effects can be controlled with medications. Tell your doctor or nurse if you experience any discomfort so they can help you feel better.

After the short-term side effects of radiation therapy resolve, others may become noticeable months or years later.

- Breast firmness or mild shrinkage

- Change in skin tone, rarely with fine blood vessels present

- Scarring of a small part of the lung just under the breast

Generally, no side effects are noticed but rarely it may cause a dry cough or shortness of breath that is treatable.

Mild decreased range of motion [may be present].

Hand or arm swelling, called lymphedema, can occur but depends upon the extent of surgery and radiation.

Heart injury is rare with modern treatment techniques for left-sided breast cancers.

Rarely, new tumors can be caused by radiation, but in breast cancer the benefits of treatment should outweigh the risks.

Many factors affect your risk for these side effects. Please talk to your radiation oncologist to learn more about how likely these side effects may be for you.

Caring for Yourself during Treatment

- Get plenty of rest during treatment, and don't be afraid to ask for help.

- Follow your doctor's advice. Ask if you are unsure about anything. There are no stupid questions.

- Tell your doctor about any medications or vitamins you are taking to make sure they are safe to use during radiation therapy. If you're taking any antioxidants, make sure to tell your doctor.

- Eat a balanced diet and drink plenty of fluids. If food tastes funny or if you're having trouble eating, tell your doctor, nurse, or dietician. They might be able to help you change the way you eat.

- Treat the skin exposed to radiation with special care. Stay out of the sun, avoid hot or cold packs, only use lotions and ointments after checking with your doctor or nurse, and clean the area with warm water and mild soap.

- Coping with the stress of a cancer diagnosis can be tough. It may help to seek out help from support groups and friends.

Chapter 39

Chemotherapy for Breast Cancer

The goal of chemotherapy is to kill cancer cells that are growing or dividing quickly. It is a powerful tool to fight cancer and protect you from a recurrence.

Unlike surgery or radiation, chemotherapy kills all quickly dividing cells, even healthy ones, causing some of the common side effects that often go along with treatment.

Every case is unique, so whether you receive chemotherapy depends on many factors.

These include:

- the specific type of cancer cells;
- your age and whether you have gone through menopause;
- the size of the primary tumor;
- whether you have cancer in your lymph nodes;
- the details (or prognostic factors) of the breast cancer, as explained by pathology tests and, sometimes, genomic tests.

Some of the important features in deciding whether you should receive chemotherapy include the tumor's estrogen and progesterone receptor status, HER2 [human epidermal growth factor receptor 2] status, the proliferation index, and the tumor grade.

How Chemotherapy Works

Chemotherapy involves taking anticancer medicines by injection into a vein (intravenously) or in pill form. These medicines travel throughout the body, where they destroy cancer cells that may have entered the bloodstream. Even in early-stage breast cancer, tiny cancer cells can break away from the original tumor. Typically, these cells are so small that they do not show up on any tests. Chemotherapy lowers the risk of recurrence (the cancer coming back).

Two or more chemotherapy medicines are often given together. Intravenous chemotherapy is given in cycles, with a day (or days) of treatment followed by a period of off days. The exact schedule varies depending on the medicines used; most breast cancer chemotherapy regimens are given every two or three weeks. An entire course of chemotherapy for breast cancer usually takes from three to six months.

How Do I Know If I Need Chemotherapy?

Your doctor will recommend chemotherapy if the cancer has a significant risk of developing outside your breast or has traveled outside the breast already. Chemotherapy is given if you have a large tumor, cancer in the lymph nodes, or a tumor with features that make it aggressive.

Sometimes it is unclear whether you should receive chemotherapy, and your doctor may order a genomic test. Genomic tests look at groups of genes in breast cancer cells to see whether they are present, absent, or too active. These factors help to predict how likely it is that the cancer will come back after treatment.

Genomic tests are used only for certain kinds of early-stage breast cancers. Your doctor may ask for a genomic test if the tumor is small, has not traveled to the lymph nodes, has hormone receptors on it, and does not have too many HER2 receptors on it.

If the genomic tests show it is very likely the cancer will return, your doctor will recommend you have chemotherapy and hormonal therapy. If the chances are very low that the cancer will return, your doctor will recommend hormonal therapy only.

How Is Chemotherapy Given?

Chemotherapy for breast cancer can be given before or after surgery, and it may be given as a single therapy or in various combinations.

Before or After Surgery

Most chemotherapy is given as adjuvant therapy, after and in addition to surgery. Therapy usually begins about a month after surgery, once you have a chance to heal.

Your doctor also may offer you the option of neoadjuvant treatment, which means chemotherapy before surgery. The goal of neoadjuvant therapy is to shrink the cancer, making it easier to remove with surgery. Most of the time, neoadjuvant therapy is done to avoid a mastectomy. After neoadjuvant therapy, you still may need a mastectomy, or you may be able to have breast conservation therapy.

Alone or in Combination

There are many different types of chemotherapy medicines. These may be given alone, called single-agent therapy, or together, called combination therapy. Some chemotherapy medicines do a better job of fighting the cancer when they are given together.

Your doctor will determine the best chemotherapy treatment for the cancer based on the cancer's traits and your treatment goals.

What Happens at Treatment?

Chemotherapy is put directly into your bloodstream, usually through an IV (intravenously) but sometimes by mouth as pills or capsules.

Chemotherapy can irritate the small veins in your arms, so some surgeons put in a Mediport or Port-A-Cath, a small device under the skin that allows easy access to your veins. Once you complete treatment, the port is removed.

Your doctor will determine how often and how much chemotherapy you receive. Chemotherapy may be given weekly, every two weeks, every three weeks, or monthly. Some treatments, mostly pills taken by mouth, are taken daily.

Types of Chemotherapy Medicines

Chemotherapy medicines are organized into classes. Each class has a specific mechanism and attacks a cell at a certain point as the cell rests, grows, or divides.

Classes of Chemotherapy

Classes, and some common breast cancer medicines within them, include:

- antitumor antibiotics: doxorubicin (Adriamycin) and epirubicin (Ellence);

- alkylating agents: cyclophosphamide (Cytoxan);

- antitubulins: paclitaxel (Taxol), docetaxel (Taxotere), vinorelbine (Navelbine), and ixabepilone (Ixempra);

- antimetabolites: gemcitabine (Gemzar) and capecitabine (Xeloda).

Combination Chemotherapies

Chemotherapy medicines are often given in combinations.

Some common combinations given for breast cancers that have a relatively low risk for recurrence include:

- AC (Adriamycin and Cytoxan);

- TC (Taxotere and Cytoxan).

Some common combinations given for breast cancer that have a relatively high risk for recurrence include:

- CAF (Cytoxan, Adriamycin, and fluorouracil);

- TAC (Taxotere, Adriamycin, and Cytoxan);

- AT (Adriamycin and Taxotere).

Chemotherapy Side Effects

Many of us have scary images of chemotherapy, based on rumor, movie-of-the-week melodramas, and stories from friends or family members treated many years ago. We associate cancer and sickness with chemotherapy's side effects—hair loss, nausea and vomiting, weight gain or loss, fatigue and insomnia, dry mouth, dry skin, mouth sores, and even something called chemo brain, problems with memory and concentration.

Other side effects associated with chemotherapy include low blood counts and diarrhea.

The truth is that while some people have a rough time with chemotherapy, others manage quite well. Many continue to work, and others report feeling only mild discomfort. Each person has her own individual response.

If you become uncomfortable during treatment, there are many medicines and methods to help you. Let your doctors and nurses know about your concerns before you start treatment. Ask which side effects could occur with the chemotherapy you are receiving.

If your doctor prescribes a medicine to prevent nausea, do not wait to take it until you feel upset to your stomach. Take it, as prescribed, for several days after each treatment.

If you have a new side effect or a side effect gets worse, do not hesitate to discuss it with your doctor or oncology nurse. You do not have to suffer.

Chapter 40

Hormone Therapy
for Breast Cancer

Chapter Contents

Section 40.1

What Is Hormone Therapy?

Some cancers rely on the hormones estrogen and progesterone to grow and survive. These hormones occur naturally in your body. If you deprive these types of cancers of hormones, the cancer cells die.

Hormonal therapy targets the cancer cells that have estrogen and progesterone receptors. Your pathology report will say whether the breast cancer is estrogen receptor-positive, progesterone receptor-positive, or both. If the cancer uses these hormones to grow, it may respond to this type of therapy.

Types of Hormonal Therapy Medicines

Some hormonal therapies, like tamoxifen, trick the cancer cells into thinking that they are estrogen. Other medicines, called aromatase inhibitors, prevent the body from making any estrogen or progesterone at all. The names of the FDA [U.S. Food and Drug Administration] approved aromatase inhibitor medicines are:

- letrozole (Femara);

- anastrozole (Arimidex);

- exemestane (Aromasin).

If you are postmenopausal, aromatase inhibitors are the standard treatment. Aromatase inhibitors work as well as tamoxifen, but they are not for everyone. Your treatment team should discuss the options with you.

In general, both tamoxifen and aromatase inhibitors are given for five years as a daily pill. If your doctor feels you are at high risk for recurrence but you start out taking tamoxifen, you may be able to switch to an aromatase inhibitor to finish five years of treatment. Clinical trials are helping researchers determine how aromatase inhibitors work best to help you.

Aromatase inhibitors cannot be used if you still get your menstrual period. If you are premenopausal, your doctor may recommend tamoxifen or ovarian suppression. Another option is ablation, a treatment using medicine to stop your ovaries from making estrogen. You also may consider removing your ovaries in a surgery called an oophorectomy. Researchers are studying different types of hormonal therapy in premenopausal women, so you may be able to participate in a study.

Hormonal Therapy Side Effects

Tamoxifen and aromatase inhibitors have a number of side effects.

Aromatase inhibitors put you at higher risk for bone thinning, osteoporosis, bone fractures, and problems with blood cholesterol. They cause joint pain and muscle aches in about 50 percent of women who take them. Both medicines carry an increased risk of blood clots and stroke. Tamoxifen puts you at a slight increased risk of endometrial (uterine) cancer.

Before taking hormonal therapy, you should discuss any history of heart problems or other medical conditions with your doctor. Share information about any other medicines or supplements you are taking.

The most common side effects of both types of hormonal therapy are hot flashes, fatigue, difficulty sleeping, night sweats, and vaginal dryness.

Talk with your doctor about the risks, benefits, and side effects of each type of therapy to make the best treatment decision for you.

Section 40.2

Aromatase Inhibitors

This section contains text, under the heading "What Are Aromatase Inhibitors?" from "Links to NCI Materials," an undated document by the National Cancer Institute (NCI, www.cancer.gov), part of the National Institutes of Health, reviewed by David A. Cooke, MD, FACP, April 2, 2012. It also contains text from "Aromatase Inhibitors Come of Age," also from the NCI, adapted from the *NCI Cancer Bulletin*, March 7, 2007, reviewed and revised by David A. Cooke, MD, FACP, April 4, 2012.

What Are Aromatase Inhibitors?

Many breast tumors are "estrogen sensitive," meaning the hormone estrogen helps them to grow. Aromatase inhibitors (AIs) can help block the growth of these tumors by lowering the amount of estrogen in the body.

Estrogen is produced by the ovaries and other tissues of the body, using a substance called aromatase. AIs do not block estrogen production by the ovaries, but they can block other tissues from making this hormone. That's why AIs are used mostly in women who have reached menopause, when the ovaries are no longer producing estrogen.

Another drug, tamoxifen (Nolvadex), also helps to prevent the growth of estrogen-sensitive breast tumors, but it works differently from AIs. Whereas AIs reduce the amount of estrogen in the body, tamoxifen blocks a tumor's ability to use estrogen.

Currently, three AIs are approved by the U.S. Food and Drug Administration: Anastrazole (Arimidex), exemestane (Aromasin), and letrozole (Femara).

Aromatase Inhibitors Come of Age

Aromatase inhibitors (AIs), which interfere with the body's ability to produce the hormone estrogen, are rapidly changing the standard of treatment for breast cancer. Researchers have now taken up the challenge of learning how and when to best use these drugs to reduce recurrence for women with hormone-receptor-positive breast cancer.

Two approaches dominate the development of hormone-based treatments for breast cancer. One approach focuses on preventing estrogen from binding to its receptor and activating cell-signaling pathways that accelerate tumor growth. This strategy led to the development of the drug tamoxifen (Nolvadex), which belongs to a class of drug called selective estrogen-receptor modulators (SERMs).

Since its approval by the U.S. Food and Drug Administration (FDA) for the treatment of hormone-receptor-positive breast cancer in 1977, tamoxifen has become a mainstay of therapy. However, many women develop resistance to the drug over time, leading to cancer recurrence. In addition, because tamoxifen binds directly to the estrogen receptor, it can sometimes activate the signaling pathways it was designed to block.

"We knew that tamoxifen was a partial agonist—a weak estrogen," explains Dr. Angela Brodie, professor of pharmacology and experimental therapeutics at the University of Maryland, who has worked on the development of AIs for more than 35 years. "So we thought it might not be optimally effective on tumors . . . and that it could cause side effects. In fact, it does increase the risk of stroke and endometrial cancer."

A Different Mechanism

AIs take a different approach to hormone therapy—they prevent the bodies of postmenopausal women from producing estrogen rather than blocking its activity. AIs accomplish this by interfering with the enzyme aromatase, which catalyzes the final step in the synthesis of estrogen from its steroid precursors.

Two different types of AIs are in use in the clinic today. Steroidal AIs, such as exemestane (Aromasin), bind permanently to aromatase. Nonsteroidal AIs, such as anastrozole (Arimidex) and letrozole (Femara), bind reversibly to aromatase and compete with the precursors of estrogen for the enzyme.

Both steroidal and nonsteroidal AIs have been shown in large-scale clinical trials to be superior to tamoxifen in extending survival in women with metastatic disease, and in preventing recurrence when used as primary adjuvant therapy. In addition, treatment with an AI after a full course of tamoxifen continues to improve recurrence-free survival, compared with cessation of hormone therapy.

The challenge remains to determine the best schedule for up-front AI treatment. Studies have shown that five years of an AI alone are more effective at preventing recurrence than five years of tamoxifen alone, and that switching women already taking tamoxifen to an AI after two or three years prevents more recurrences than continuing tamoxifen for a full five years.

Despite the promising data on AIs in women who had already received tamoxifen, it remained unclear whether AIs are the best initial treatment for women who hadn't received prior hormone therapy The Breast International Group trial BIG 1-98 looked this question, and its results were published in 2009. BIG 1-98 looked at the outcomes of postmenopausal women treated with tamoxifen alone, letrozole alone, tamoxifen followed by letrozole, or letrozole followed by tamoxifen. All of the women the study received five years of therapy in total. The study found that women who received sequential therapy (tamoxifen followed by letrozole, or letrozole followed by tamoxifen) did no better than those who receive letrozole alone.

Based on the BIG 1-98 results, it appears that letrozole therapy is the best initial treatment for postmenopausal women with hormone-responsive breast cancer. However, individual factors still need to be considered when choosing treatments. It also remains unclear whether the BIG 1-98 results apply to all aromatase inhibitors, as letrozole was the only AI used in this study.

New Questions

Other questions remain as AIs move to a more prominent position in breast cancer treatment. AIs have side effects of their own, most importantly loss of bone density, which can be especially hazardous for women already at risk for osteoporosis. Therefore, tamoxifen may still provide a more favorable risk/benefit ratio for some subgroups of women, which need to be identified.

In addition, the role of AIs in premenopausal patients remains to be defined. While AIs alone may not have an effect in premenopausal women, because the ovaries can override the inhibition by producing a large amount of aromatase, clinical trials are now testing AIs in premenopausal women in combination with drugs such as goserelin, which suppress ovarian function.

Because AIs have also reduced the occurrence of contralateral breast cancer in several studies, researchers are now testing the compounds as chemopreventive agents. A large-scale study of exemestane published in 2011 found that three years of treatment significantly reduced the risk of breast cancer in high-risk women over a three-year period, with fairly minimal side effects. A second study looking at anastrozole is still in progress.

Although tamoxifen was approved in 1998 for the prevention of breast cancer in high-risk women, fewer women than expected have chosen to take it.

"One reason [healthy] women don't want to take tamoxifen is fear of side effects," explains Dr. Jennifer Eng-Wong, a clinical oncologist in the National Cancer Institute's Center for Cancer Research. If AIs prove to have both efficacy in preventing breast cancer occurrence and acceptable side effects, they and the new generation of SERMs such as raloxifene will provide women at high risk with additional options to help prevent the disease.

Section 40.3

Tamoxifen

Excerpted from "Tamoxifen," by the National Cancer Institute (NCI, www.cancer.gov), part of the National Institutes of Health, March 17, 2008.

What is tamoxifen?

Tamoxifen (Nolvadex) is a drug, taken orally as a tablet, which interferes with the activity of estrogen, a female hormone. Estrogen can promote the development of cancer in the breast. Tamoxifen is approved by the U.S. Food and Drug Administration (FDA) for the prevention of breast cancer and for the treatment of breast cancer, as well as other types of cancer.

Tamoxifen has been used for more than 30 years to treat breast cancer in women and men. Tamoxifen is used to treat patients with early-stage breast cancer, as well as those with metastatic breast cancer (cancer that has spread to other parts of the body). As adjuvant therapy (treatment given after the primary treatment to increase the chances of a cure), tamoxifen helps prevent the original breast cancer from returning and also helps prevent the development of new cancers in the other breast. As treatment for metastatic breast cancer, the drug slows or stops the growth of cancer cells that are present in the body.

Tamoxifen has been used for almost 10 years to reduce the risk of breast cancer in women who are at increased risk of developing breast cancer. Tamoxifen is also used to treat women with ductal carcinoma in situ (DCIS), a noninvasive condition that sometimes leads to invasive breast cancer.

How does tamoxifen work?

Estrogen can promote the growth of breast cancer cells. Some breast cancers are classified as estrogen receptor-positive (also known as hormone sensitive), which means that they have a protein to which estrogen will bind. These breast cancer cells need estrogen to grow. Tamoxifen works against the effects of estrogen on these cells. It is often called an antiestrogen or a SERM (Selective Estrogen Receptor Modulator).

Studies have shown that tamoxifen is only effective in treating estrogen receptor-positive breast cancers. Therefore, the tumor's hormone receptor status should be determined before deciding on treatment options for breast cancer.

Although tamoxifen acts against the effects of estrogen in breast tissue, it acts like estrogen in other tissue. This means that women who take tamoxifen may derive many of the beneficial effects of menopausal estrogen replacement therapy, such as a decreased risk of osteoporosis.

How long should a patient take tamoxifen for the treatment of breast cancer?

Patients with metastatic breast cancer may take tamoxifen for varying lengths of time, depending on the cancer's response to this treatment and other factors. When used as adjuvant therapy for early-stage breast cancer, tamoxifen is generally prescribed for five years. However, the ideal length of treatment with tamoxifen is not known.

Two studies have confirmed the benefit of taking adjuvant tamoxifen daily for five years. When taken for five years, tamoxifen reduces the chance of the original breast cancer coming back in the same breast or elsewhere. It also reduces the risk of developing a second primary cancer in the other breast.

Clinical trials are ongoing to determine whether hormone therapy taken for more than five years is beneficial. These studies usually include aromatase inhibitors (AIs) (another type of antiestrogen).

What are some of the more common side effects of tamoxifen?

The known, serious side effects of tamoxifen are blood clots, strokes, uterine cancer, and cataracts. Other side effects of tamoxifen are similar to the symptoms of menopause. The most common side effects are hot flashes and vaginal discharge. Some women experience irregular menstrual periods, headaches, fatigue, nausea and/or vomiting, vaginal dryness or itching, irritation of the skin around the vagina, and skin rash. As with menopause, not all women who take tamoxifen have these symptoms. Men who take tamoxifen may experience headaches, nausea and/or vomiting, skin rash, impotence, or a decrease in sexual interest.

Does tamoxifen cause blood clots or stroke?

Data from large clinical trials suggest that there is a small increase in the number of blood clots in women taking tamoxifen, particularly in women who are receiving anticancer drugs (chemotherapy) along with tamoxifen. The total number of women who have experienced this side effect is small. The risk of having a blood clot due to tamoxifen is similar to the risk of a blood clot when taking estrogen replacement therapy.

The Breast Cancer Prevention Trial (BCPT), a large research study funded by the NCI, was designed to test the usefulness of tamoxifen in preventing breast cancer in women with an increased risk of developing this disease. This study also found that women who took tamoxifen had an increased chance of developing blood clots and an increased chance of stroke.

Does tamoxifen cause cancers of the uterus?

Tamoxifen increases the risk of two types of cancer that can develop in the uterus: Endometrial cancer, which arises in the lining of the uterus, and uterine sarcoma, which arises in the muscular wall of the uterus. Like all cancers, endometrial cancer and uterine sarcoma are potentially life-threatening. Women who have had a hysterectomy (surgery to remove the uterus) and are taking tamoxifen are not at increased risk for these cancers.

Studies have found the risk of developing endometrial cancer to be about two cases per 1,000 women taking tamoxifen each year compared with one case per 1,000 women taking placebo. Most of the endometrial cancers that have occurred in women taking tamoxifen have been found in the early stages, and treatment has usually been effective. However, for some breast cancer patients who developed endometrial cancer while taking tamoxifen, the disease was life-threatening.

Studies have found the risk of developing uterine sarcoma to be slightly higher in women taking tamoxifen compared with women taking placebo. However, it was less than one case per 1,000 women per year in both groups. Research to date indicates that uterine sarcoma is more likely to be diagnosed at later stages than endometrial cancer, and may therefore be harder to control and more life-threatening than endometrial cancer.

Abnormal vaginal bleeding and lower abdominal (pelvic) pain are symptoms of cancers of the uterus. Women who are taking tamoxifen should talk with their doctor about having regular pelvic examinations and should be checked promptly if they have any abnormal vaginal bleeding or pelvic pain between scheduled exams.

Does tamoxifen cause other types of cancer?

Tamoxifen is not known to cause any types of cancer in humans other than endometrial cancer and uterine sarcoma.

Does tamoxifen cause eye problems?

As women age, they are more likely to develop cataracts (clouding of the lens inside the eye). Women taking tamoxifen appear to be at increased risk for developing cataracts. Other eye problems, such as corneal scarring or retinal changes, have been reported in a few patients.

Should women taking tamoxifen avoid pregnancy?

Yes. Doctors advise women receiving tamoxifen to avoid pregnancy because animal studies have suggested that the use of tamoxifen during pregnancy can cause harm to the fetus. Women who have questions about fertility, birth control, or pregnancy should discuss their concerns with their doctor.

Does tamoxifen cause a woman to begin menopause?

Tamoxifen does not cause a woman to begin menopause, although it can cause some symptoms that are similar to those that may occur during menopause. In most premenopausal women taking tamoxifen, the ovaries continue to act normally and produce estrogen in the same or slightly increased amounts.

Do the benefits of tamoxifen in treating breast cancer outweigh its risks?

The benefits of tamoxifen as a treatment for breast cancer are firmly established and far outweigh the potential risks. Patients who are concerned about the risks and benefits of tamoxifen or any other medications are encouraged to discuss these concerns with their doctor.

Can tamoxifen prevent breast cancer?

Research has shown that when tamoxifen is used as adjuvant therapy for early-stage breast cancer, it reduces the chance that the original breast cancer will come back in the same breast or elsewhere. It also reduces the risk of developing new cancers in the other breast. Based on these findings, the NCI funded a study to determine whether taking tamoxifen for at least five years can prevent breast cancer in women who have never been diagnosed with breast cancer but who are at increased risk of developing the disease. This study found a reduction in diagnoses of invasive breast cancer among women who took tamoxifen for five years. Women who took tamoxifen also had fewer diagnoses of noninvasive breast tumors, such as DCIS or lobular carcinoma in situ (LCIS). After seven years of follow-up, researchers found similar results. The study found that tamoxifen reduced the occurrence of estrogen receptor-positive tumors by 69 percent, but no difference in the occurrence of estrogen receptor-negative tumors was seen.

Who should take tamoxifen to reduce breast cancer risk?

The decision to take tamoxifen is an individual one. A woman and her doctor must carefully consider the benefits and risks of therapy. At this time, there is no evidence that tamoxifen has a net benefit for women who do not have an increased risk of developing breast cancer.

What is raloxifene and how does it compare to tamoxifen?

Raloxifene is a drug approved by the FDA for the prevention and treatment of osteoporosis in postmenopausal women. Raloxifene is also approved by the FDA for reducing the risk of invasive breast cancer in postmenopausal women with osteoporosis and in postmenopausal women at high risk for invasive breast cancer.

The NCI funded the Study of Tamoxifen and Raloxifene (STAR), a clinical trial comparing raloxifene (Evista) with tamoxifen in preventing breast cancer in postmenopausal women who are at an increased risk of developing the disease. The study found that raloxifene and tamoxifen are equally effective in reducing invasive breast cancer risk in postmenopausal women who are at increased risk of the disease. The study also found that women who took raloxifene had fewer uterine cancers and fewer blood clots than the women who took tamoxifen. However, raloxifene did not reduce the risk of noninvasive breast tumors such as DCIS and LCIS. Other side effects associated with raloxifene were similar to tamoxifen and included hot flashes, vaginal dryness, joint pain, and leg cramps. Studies of raloxifene to date have only examined its role in breast cancer prevention, not treatment.

What other hormone therapy may be used for early-stage breast cancer?

Aromatase inhibitors (AIs) are another adjuvant treatment option for some women with early-stage breast cancer. AIs block the action of a protein called aromatase, which helps the body produce estrogen. Most of the estrogen in a woman's body is made in the ovaries, but other tissues can also produce this hormone. AIs are usually used in women who have reached menopause, when the ovaries are no longer producing estrogen.

Although AIs and tamoxifen both help to prevent the growth of estrogen-sensitive breast tumors, they work differently in the body. Tamoxifen blocks the tumor's ability to use estrogen, and AIs reduce the amount of estrogen in the body. Anastrozole (Arimidex), exemestane (Aromasin), and letrozole (Femara) are AIs that have been approved by the FDA.

The American Society of Clinical Oncology (ASCO) recommends that postmenopausal women with hormone-sensitive breast cancer consider one of two adjuvant treatment options:

- Begin treatment with tamoxifen for two to three years or five years, and then switch to an AI for another two to three years or five years.

- Forego tamoxifen entirely and begin adjuvant treatment with an AI for five years.

ASCO concluded that AIs are appropriate as initial treatment for women who should not take tamoxifen and that patients who cannot take AIs should receive tamoxifen.

Whether an individual patient should start therapy with an AI or begin therapy with tamoxifen and then change to an AI is a subject of medical judgment and clinical research. Patients should talk with their doctors about which drug would be best for them given their particular medical situation.

Chapter 41

Targeted (Biologic) Therapies for Breast Cancer

Targeted therapies are medicines that fight cancer by finding and killing only cancer cells. They recognize a specific feature of the cancer cell, attach to it, and destroy it.

For example, if the breast cancer tests positive for HER2 [human epidermal growth factor receptor 2], you may be able to receive a targeted therapy that affects only HER2-positive cells. Other targeted treatments block the growth of blood vessels that some tumors need to grow.

Many forms of targeted therapy are being tested in clinical trials. They are given intravenously (by vein) or by mouth as a pill. Some treatments, such as trastuzumab (Herceptin), have already been approved by the U.S. Food and Drug Administration, but others are only available to participants in clinical trials.

Types of Targeted Therapy Medicines

Some targeted therapy medicines used in breast cancer treatment target HER proteins. Others target VEGF (Vascular Endothelial Growth Factor).

HER Proteins

About 25 percent of breast cancers make too much of a protein known as HER2 (human epidermal growth factor receptor), which triggers rapid cell division and growth. HER2-positive cancers tend to be more aggressive than HER2-negative cancers, but targeting the protein has opened up new treatment options.

If the cancer is HER2 positive, then its cells make too much of a receptor protein called HER2. With too many receptors, breast cancer cells pick up too many growth signals and start growing too much and too fast.

The medicine trastuzumab (Herceptin) blocks the receptors so they do not pick up as many growth signals. Trastuzumab is the standard treatment for HER2-positive breast cancers. Other therapies that target HER2 are under study.

Treatment usually is given intravenously every week or every three weeks for 52 weeks after surgery. This medicine can cause damage to the heart, so it may not be recommended if you have certain heart conditions or heart-related risks. It cannot be given with other chemotherapy medicines that can affect the heart. Your heart function will need to be monitored before and during therapy. Talk to your treatment team about any concerns you may have related to heart health.

A newer targeted therapy called lapatinib (Tykerb) blocks the effect of HER2 and a related protein, HER1, by interfering with the pathway inside the cell instead of at its surface. This medicine is FDA approved in combination with other medicines for the treatment of metastatic (stage IV) HER2 positive breast cancer.

Lapatinib appears to offer several benefits over trastuzumab: It is taken as a pill, instead of given by vein, and studies suggest it poses fewer risks to the heart. Side effects include diarrhea, redness, and tingling in the hands and feet, rash, stomach upset, vomiting, and fatigue.

VEGF (Vascular Endothelial Growth Factor)

To get the oxygen and nutrients they need to grow and spread, tumors create new blood vessels through a process called angiogenesis.

Bevacizumab (Avastin) is a medicine that targets the VEGF protein, which plays a key role in angiogenesis. It is not FDA approved for use in breast cancer, but it is approved for use against other types of cancers. It has been studied in metastatic (stage IV) breast cancer when given with paclitaxel (Taxol) in women who have not yet gotten chemotherapy. Your doctor might offer you this treatment through a clinical trial.

Bevacizumab can cause side effects such as high blood pressure and nosebleeds, and some studies suggest a slightly higher risk of stroke and other clotting and bleeding problems.

Chapter 42

Complementary and Alternative Medicine (CAM) Therapies Used in the Treatment of Breast Cancer

Chapter Contents

Section 42.1

Questions and Answers about CAM and Cancer Treatment

Excerpted from PDQ® Cancer Information Summary. National Cancer Institute; Bethesda, MD. Complementary and Alternative Medicine in Cancer Treatment (PDQ): Treatment—Patient. Updated 03/2012. Available at: www.cancer.gov. Accessed March 15, 2012.

What is complementary and alternative medicine?

Complementary and alternative medicine (CAM), as defined by the National Center for Complementary and Alternative Medicine (NCCAM), is a group of different medical and health care systems, practices, and products that are not presently considered to be part of conventional medicine. Complementary medicine is used together with conventional medicine. Alternative medicine is used in place of conventional medicine. Conventional medicine is medicine that is practiced by holders of MD (medical doctor) or DO (doctor of osteopathy) degrees and by health professionals who work with them, including physical therapists, psychologists, and registered nurses. Other terms for conventional medicine include allopathy; Western, mainstream, orthodox, and regular medicine; and biomedicine. Some conventional medical practitioners are also practitioners of CAM.

What is integrative medicine?

NCCAM defines integrative medicine as treatment that combines conventional medicine with CAM therapies that have been reported to be safe and effective after being studied in patients. In practice, many CAM therapies used along with conventional medicine have not yet been well tested.

Are complementary and alternative therapies widely used?

Yes. Many CAM approaches are used by a large percentage of people in the general public and cancer patients.

The 2007 National Health Interview Survey reported about 4 out of 10 adults used CAM therapy in the past 12 months, with the most commonly used treatments being natural products and deep breathing exercises.

One large survey of cancer survivors reported on the use of complementary therapies. The therapies used most often were prayer and spiritual practice (61%), relaxation (44%), faith and spiritual healing (42%), and nutritional supplements and vitamins (40%). CAM therapies are used by 31–84% of children with cancer, both in and outside of clinical trials. CAM therapies have been used in the management of side effects caused by cancer or cancer treatment.

How are CAM approaches evaluated?

It is important that CAM therapies be evaluated with the same long and careful research process used to evaluate conventional treatments. The National Cancer Institute (NCI) and the Office of Cancer Complementary and Alternative Medicine (OCCAM) are sponsoring a number of clinical trials (research studies) at medical centers to evaluate CAM therapies for cancer.

Conventional cancer treatments have generally been studied for safety and effectiveness through a rigorous scientific process that includes clinical trials with large numbers of patients. Less is known about the safety and effectiveness of many CAM therapies. Research of CAM therapies has been slower for a number of reasons:

• Time and funding issues

• Problems finding institutions and cancer researchers to work with on the studies

• Regulatory issues

Some CAM therapies have undergone careful evaluation. A small number of CAM therapies originally meant to be alternative treatments are finding a place in cancer treatment as complementary therapies that may help patients feel better and recover faster. One example is acupuncture. According to a panel of experts at a National Institutes of Health (NIH) Consensus Conference in November 1997, acupuncture has been found to be effective in the management of chemotherapy-associated nausea and vomiting and in controlling pain associated with surgery. In contrast, some approaches, such as the use of laetrile, have been studied and found ineffective or possibly harmful.

What should patients do when using or considering complementary and alternative therapies?

Cancer patients using or considering complementary or alternative therapy should discuss this decision with their doctor or nurse, as they would any therapeutic approach. Some complementary and alternative therapies may interfere with standard treatment or may be harmful when used with conventional treatment. It is also a good idea to become informed about the therapy, including whether the results of scientific studies support the claims that are made for it.

When considering complementary and alternative therapies, what questions should patients ask their health care providers?

- What benefits can be expected from this therapy?
- What are the risks associated with this therapy?
- Do the known benefits outweigh the risks?
- What side effects can be expected?
- Will the therapy interfere with conventional treatment?
- Is this therapy part of a clinical trial? If so, who is sponsoring the trial?
- Will the therapy be covered by health insurance?

Section 42.2

Coenzyme Q10 and Cancer

Excerpted from PDQ® Cancer Information Summary. National Cancer Institute; Bethesda, MD. Coenzyme Q10 (PDQ): Patient version. Updated 07/2011. Available at: www.cancer.gov. Accessed January 15, 2012.

What is coenzyme Q10?

Coenzyme Q10 is a compound that is made naturally in the body. The Q and the 10 in coenzyme Q10 refer to the groups of chemicals that make up the coenzyme. Coenzyme Q10 is also known by these other names:

- CoQ10
- Q10
- Vitamin Q10
- Ubiquinone
- Ubidecarenone

A coenzyme helps an enzyme do its job. An enzyme is a protein that speeds up the rate at which natural chemical reactions take place in cells of the body.

The body's cells use coenzyme Q10 to make energy needed for the cells to grow and stay healthy. The body also uses coenzyme Q10 as an antioxidant. An antioxidant is a substance that protects cells from chemicals called free radicals. Free radicals can damage DNA (deoxyribonucleic acid). Genes, which are pieces of DNA, tell the cells how to work in the body and when to grow and divide. Damage to DNA has been linked to some kinds of cancer. By protecting cells against free radicals, antioxidants help protect the body against cancer.

Coenzyme Q10 is found in most body tissues. The highest amounts are found in the heart, liver, kidneys, and pancreas. The lowest amounts are found in the lungs. The amount of coenzyme Q10 in tissues decreases as people get older.

What is the history of the discovery and use of coenzyme Q10 as a complementary or alternative treatment for cancer?

Coenzyme Q10 was first identified in 1957. Its chemical structure was determined in 1958. Interest in coenzyme Q10 as a possible treatment for cancer began in 1961, when it was found that some cancer patients had a lower than normal amount of it in their blood. Low blood levels of coenzyme Q10 have been found in patients with myeloma, lymphoma, and cancers of the breast, lung, prostate, pancreas, colon, kidney, and head and neck.

Studies suggest that coenzyme Q10 may help the immune system work better. Partly because of this, coenzyme Q10 is used as adjuvant therapy for cancer. Adjuvant therapy is treatment given following the primary treatment to increase the chances of a cure.

What is the theory behind the claim that coenzyme Q10 is useful in treating cancer?

Coenzyme Q10 may be useful in treating cancer because it boosts the immune system. Also, studies suggest that CoQ10 analogs (drugs that are similar to CoQ10) may prevent the growth of cancer cells directly. As an antioxidant, coenzyme Q10 may help prevent cancer from developing.

How is coenzyme Q10 administered?

Coenzyme Q10 is usually taken by mouth as a pill (tablet or capsule). It may also be given by injection into a vein (IV). In animal studies, coenzyme Q10 is given by injection.

Have any preclinical (laboratory or animal) studies been conducted using coenzyme Q10?

A number of preclinical studies have been done with coenzyme Q10. Research in a laboratory or using animals is done to find out if a drug, procedure, or treatment is likely to be useful in humans. These preclinical studies are done before any testing in humans is begun. Most laboratory studies of coenzyme Q10 have looked at its chemical structure and how it works in the body. The following has been reported from preclinical studies of coenzyme Q10 and cancer:

- Animal studies found that coenzyme Q10 boosts the immune system and helps the body fight certain infections and types of cancer.

- Coenzyme Q10 helped to protect the hearts of study animals that were given the anticancer drug doxorubicin, an anthracycline that can cause damage to the heart muscle.

- Laboratory and animal studies have shown that analogs of coenzyme Q10 may stop cancer cells from growing.

Have any clinical trials (research studies with people) of coenzyme Q10 been conducted?

There have been no well-designed clinical trials involving large numbers of patients to study the use of coenzyme Q10 in cancer treatment. There have been some clinical trials with small numbers of people, but the way the studies were done and the amount of information reported made it unclear if benefits were caused by the coenzyme Q10 or by something else. Most of the trials were not randomized or controlled. Randomized controlled trials give the highest level of evidence:

- In randomized trials, volunteers are assigned randomly (by chance) to one of two or more groups that compare different factors related to the treatment.

- In controlled trials, one group (called the control group) does not receive the new treatment being studied. The control group is then compared to the groups that receive the new treatment, to see if the new treatment makes a difference.

Some research studies are published in scientific journals. Most scientific journals have experts who review research reports before they are published, to make sure that the evidence and conclusions are sound. This is called peer review. Studies published in peer-reviewed scientific journals are considered better evidence. No randomized clinical trials of coenzyme Q10 as a treatment for cancer have been published in a peer-reviewed scientific journal.

The following has been reported from studies of coenzyme Q10 in people:

Randomized trial of coenzyme Q10 and doxorubicin: A randomized trial of 20 patients looked at whether coenzyme Q10 would protect the heart from the damage caused by the anthracycline drug doxorubicin. The results of this trial and others have shown that coenzyme Q10 decreases the harmful effects of doxorubicin on the heart.

Studies of coenzyme Q10 as an adjuvant therapy for breast cancer: Small studies have been done on the use of coenzyme Q10 after standard treatment in patients with breast cancer:

- In a study of coenzyme Q10 in 32 breast cancer patients, it was reported that some signs and symptoms of cancer went away in six patients. Details were given for only three of the six patients. The researchers also reported that all the patients in the study used less pain medicine, had improved quality of life, and did not lose weight during treatment.

- In a follow-up study, two patients who had breast cancer remaining after surgery were treated with high doses of coenzyme Q10 for three to four months. It was reported that after treatment with high-dose coenzyme Q10, the cancer was completely gone in both patients.

- In a third study led by the same researchers, three breast cancer patients were given high-dose coenzyme Q10 and followed for three to five years. The study reported that one patient had complete remission of cancer that had spread to the liver, another had remission of cancer that had spread to the chest wall, and the third had no breast cancer found after surgery.

It is not clear, however, if the benefits reported in these studies were caused by coenzyme Q10 therapy or something else. The studies had the following weaknesses:

- The studies were not randomized or controlled.

- The patients used other supplements in addition to coenzyme Q10.

- The patients received standard treatments before or during the coenzyme Q10 therapy.

- Details were not reported for all patients in the studies.

Anecdotal reports of coenzyme Q10: Anecdotal reports are incomplete descriptions of the medical and treatment history of one or more patients. There have been anecdotal reports that coenzyme Q10 has helped some cancer patients live longer, including patients with cancers of the pancreas, lung, colon, rectum, and prostate. The patients described in these reports, however, also received treatments other than coenzyme Q10, including chemotherapy, radiation therapy, and surgery.

Have any side effects or risks been reported from coenzyme Q10?

No serious side effects have been reported from the use of coenzyme Q10. The most common side effects include the following:

- Insomnia (being unable to fall sleep or stay asleep)
- Higher than normal levels of liver enzymes
- Rashes
- Nausea
- Pain in the upper part of the abdomen
- Dizziness
- Feeling sensitive to light
- Feeling irritable
- Headache
- Heartburn
- Feeling very tired

It is important to check with health care providers to find out if coenzyme Q10 can be safely used along with other drugs. Certain drugs, such as those that are used to lower cholesterol, blood pressure, or blood sugar levels, may decrease the effects of coenzyme Q10. Coenzyme Q10 may change way the body uses warfarin (a drug that prevents the blood from clotting) and insulin.

As noted in the preceding text, the body uses coenzyme Q10 as an antioxidant. Antioxidants protect cells from free radicals. Some conventional cancer therapies, such as anticancer drugs and radiation treatment, kill cancer cells in part by causing free radicals to form. Researchers are studying whether using coenzyme Q10 along with conventional therapies has any effect, good or bad, on the way these conventional therapies work in the body.

Is coenzyme Q10 approved by the U.S. Food and Drug Administration (FDA) for use as a cancer treatment in the United States?

Coenzyme Q10 is sold as a dietary supplement and is not approved by the FDA for use as a cancer treatment. In the United States, dietary supplements are regulated as foods, not drugs. This means that approval by the FDA is not required before coenzyme Q10 is sold, unless specific health claims are made about the supplement. Also, the way companies make coenzyme Q10 is not regulated. Different batches and brands of coenzyme Q10 supplements may be different from each other.

Section 42.3

Flaxseed and Breast Cancer

Excerpted from "Flaxseed and Breast Cancer," © 2010 American Institute for Cancer Research. Reprinted with permission. To view the complete text of this report including references, visit www.aicr.org.

The Take-Home

General Summary

- Because human studies are extremely limited, research does not provide a basis to recommend use of flaxseed for the explicit purpose of cancer protection at this time.

- For people who wish to consume flaxseed as a source of omega-3 fat or dietary fiber, studies do not support fears that flaxseed could increase incidence or recurrence of breast cancer.

- Because there are no studies regarding the effects of flaxseed in children or women who are pregnant or breastfeeding, researchers suggest caution.

Research Specifics

- Animal studies suggest that flaxseed may decrease growth of both estrogen receptor-negative and estrogen receptor-positive breast cancers.

- In animal studies, flaxseed did not interfere with tamoxifen's actions and may have enhanced effectiveness.

- However, with no results of clinical trials of flaxseed use during tamoxifen or aromatase inhibitor treatment, decisions about flaxseed use should be discussed carefully with a patient's physician.

- Flaxseed's effects vary with individual differences including diet, hormones, and genetics.

- In limited short-term human studies using 10 to 30 g flaxseed per day (corresponding to approximately 1 to 4 level tablespoons of ground flaxseed), consumption altered estrogen metabolism in ways that may protect against breast cancer.

Research Background

Most research in flaxseed and cancer has focused on flaxseed's relationship to breast cancer, though emerging research addresses its role in cancers of the prostate and colon. Research has primarily focused on the potential for flaxseed (also known as linseed) to reduce cancer risk through its lignan compounds and its alpha-linolenic acid (ALA, an omega-3 fatty acid) content, and these will be the focus of this text, although its concentrated dietary fiber and other nutritional components may also influence cancer risk. The impact of flaxseed needs to be distinguished from that of flaxseed oil, which does not naturally contain lignans.

Few human intervention trials using flaxseed are available. Compared to a control group of postmenopausal women with newly diagnosed breast cancer, those who consumed 25 g ground flaxseed per day for approximately 32 days showed decreased tumor cell proliferation, decreased HER2 (c-erbB2) [human epidermal growth factor receptor 2] expression and increased apoptosis at the time of surgery. (HER2 leads to growth factor signaling pathways that play a role in cell proliferation, differentiation, apoptosis, and metastasis.) Estrogen and progesterone levels and receptor activity did not change.

In early animal studies, flaxseed reduced tumor incidence, number, and size when fed to carcinogen-treated rats at initiation, promotion, or later stages of cancer development. More recently, diets with 5 percent or 10 percent flaxseed (comparable to 25 to 30 g of flaxseed daily in humans) inhibited the growth of both estrogen receptor (ER)-positive and ER-negative human breast cancer cells injected in mice. It also reduced metastasis of ER-negative breast tumors. These studies maintained either high estrogen levels as a model for premenopausal breast cancer or low estrogen levels as a model of postmenopausal breast cancer. Decreased cell proliferation rates, decreased angiogenesis, and increased apoptosis seem to account for the decreased tumor growth.

Lignans in Depth

Lignans occur in a number of plant foods, but flaxseed is a particularly rich source (lignans are not to be confused with lignins, a type of insoluble fiber).

Lignans, along with isoflavones and coumestans, comprise the three major classes of phytoestrogens (plant estrogens). When plant lignans

371

are consumed, intestinal bacteria convert some into two mammalian lignans, enterolactone and enterodiol. These compounds are absorbed from the digestive tract, circulate, and are excreted in the urine. In some population studies, greater serum or urinary levels of entero-lactone are associated with decreased breast cancer risk. In others, however, serum enterolactone showed no link to breast cancer risk, and one nested case-control study showed a U-shaped relationship with increased risk at very low and very high levels of serum enterolactone.

In a series of case-control studies, women with highest estimated lignan consumption showed 28 percent to 51 percent lower risk of breast cancer, though impact varied according to menopausal and estrogen receptor status, and was not seen in all such studies. A meta-analysis of seven case control and four cohort studies found no significant association of total lignan intake and overall breast cancer risk. Separating analysis by menopausal status showed no significant link to premenopausal breast cancer, but a significant 15 percent lower risk of postmenopausal breast cancer in women with highest lignan consumption.

Another case-control study published since this meta-analysis showed highest estimated lignan consumption was associated with significantly lower postmenopausal breast cancer mortality, but showed no significant association with premenopausal breast cancer mortality.

In studies such as these, it's important to note that dietary and body levels of lignans do not represent flaxseed consumption alone. In most Western diets, vegetables, grains, fruit, tea, coffee, legumes, nuts, and seeds provide much larger amounts of lignans.

Flaxseed is by far the most concentrated source of lignans, however, so including it in a diet changes lignan consumption dramatically.

The top quartile of lignan consumption in these studies is substantially lower than amounts provided by the two to four tablespoons of ground flaxseed per day typically used in human studies.

So the effects, or lack of effects, of lignan consumption in these studies does not necessarily predict the effect of flaxseed consumption because flaxseed provides different types of lignans. In addition, the omega-3 fat in flaxseed is not likely obtained from other sources of lignans.

Lignans and Estrogen

Human estrogen occurs in two major forms: estradiol (E2) and estrone (E1). Estradiol is oxidized in the liver to estrone, which can then be hydroxylated to one of several forms of widely differing estrogenic power. The two major forms are 2-hydroxyestrone (2OHE1), a relatively weak estrogen, and 16-hydroxyestrone (16OHE1), which increases cell proliferation of human breast cancer cell lines in vitro and increases uterine growth in animal studies. Research suggests that women with a low ratio of urinary 2OHE1 to 16OHE1 have an increased risk of both pre- and postmenopausal breast cancer.

Among healthy postmenopausal women, ground flaxseed in amounts from 5 to 40 g daily may or may not reduce serum estrone and estradiol, but 5 to 25 g of ground flaxseed per day has consistently shown a shift toward the weaker (2OHE1) form of estrogen. Flaxseed also showed a significant shift to the weaker estrogen (increased 2OHE1:16OHE1 ratio) in premenopausal women.

One trial that worked up to 15 g of flaxseed per day suggests that flaxseed's impact on serum estrogens may be greater among overweight and obese postmenopausal women than those of normal weight; these women generally have higher levels of circulating estrogen. The range in response to lignans may also reflect polymorphisms in genes related to hormone metabolism.

Another way lignans may alter estrogen metabolism in postmenopausal women is through decreasing estrogen levels by moderately inhibiting the aromatase enzyme responsible for the conversion of androstenedione to estrone in adipose tissue (the major source of estrogen after menopause). Some research suggests that lignans could also reduce bioavailable estrogen by increasing synthesis of sex hormone-binding globulin (SHBG), which binds androgens and estrogens, but results have not been consistent.

Lignans and Growth Factors

Lignans could influence ER-negative and ER-positive tumors by decreasing insulin-like growth factor-1 (IGF-1), epidermal growth factor receptor (EGFR), HER2, and the vascular endothelial growth factor (VEGF) which supports angiogenesis.

Most of the studies showing effects on these growth factors involve xenografts of human breast cancer in mice. However, Thompson also found decreased HER2 (c-erbB2) expression in breast tumor tissue at time of surgery compared with time of diagnosis in postmenopausal women given 25 g of flaxseed daily for about 32 days.

Flaxseed as a Source of Omega-3 Fat

Flaxseed's omega-3 fat provides both hope for potential benefits and concerns of potential risks for some people. Alpha-linolenic acid (ALA,

18:3) comprises almost half of the fat in flaxseed. Each tablespoon of ground flaxseed provides 1.6 g ALA and each tablespoon of flaxseed oil has 7.3 g ALA, about four times the content of linoleic acid (LA, 18:2), an essential omega-6 fatty acid.

Role of ALA and LA in Cancer Cell Growth

Humans can use ALA to synthesize eicosapentaenoic acid (EPA), the source of anti-inflammatory eicosanoids. Eicosanoids are signaling compounds involved in balancing and controlling inflammation and immunity. Emerging research suggests that EPA could influence cell-signaling pathways in ways that decrease cancer growth. In contrast, LA leads to production of pro-inflammatory eicosanoids, which in vitro and animal studies suggest could increase cancer cell proliferation and angiogenesis.

Conversion of ALA to EPA and DHA

When considering omega-3 fat's impact on cancer, it's important to note that effects seen with a particular amount of EPA and DHA (docosahexaenoic acid, another omega-3 fatty acid present in fish) should not be expected from an equal amount of ALA. Conversion of ALA to DHA is particularly inefficient, estimated at less than four percent in men and up to nine percent in women of reproductive age. Estimates of ALA conversion to EPA, the source of anti-inflammatory and other potentially cancer-inhibiting compounds, range from 0.3 to 8 percent in men and up to 21 percent in women of childbearing age.

Overall diet, including consumption of ALA, LA, DHA, and EPA, affects rates of conversion as well.

Despite inefficient conversion, the 5.7 to 6.8 g of ALA in the approximately 25 to 30 g daily doses of ground flaxseed generally used in studies of flaxseed and breast cancer-related biomarkers could increase circulating EPA levels significantly.

The effect on breast cancer incidence is unknown.

Animal and Human Studies and ALA

In a study of mice with xenografts of ER- human breast cancer, flaxseed oil alone decreased tumor cell proliferation and increased apoptosis, but best protection, including decreased overall metastasis, came from flaxseed or a combination of its lignans and its oil. A prospective study of ALA consumption and breast cancer risk concluded that the effect of ALA or total omega-3 fat consumption depends on interactions among antioxidants, fatty acids and other components of the diet.

A review by the Natural Standard Research Collaboration concludes that evidence is not currently adequate to support recommending alpha-linolenic acid as a way to reduce risk of breast or prostate cancer. *Food, Nutrition, Physical Activity and the Prevention of Cancer,* AICR's second expert report, notes biological plausibility of a relationship of omega-3 fat intake and reduced risk of breast and possibly other cancers, but found evidence was too limited to draw any conclusions.

Flaxseed and Special Populations

People at bleeding risk: The ALA in flaxseed is converted to EPA, which forms compounds that decrease blood clotting and this raises questions about its safety for people at risk of bleeding. EPA and DHA in amounts less than 3 g per day are unlikely to increase bleeding tendencies. Therefore, because of the inefficient conversion of ALA to EPA, flaxseed in typical amounts (two to four tablespoons of ground flaxseed or one tablespoon of flaxseed oil per day) poses little risk of bleeding in healthy people. People who take high dose EPA and DHA supplements or medications with anticoagulant effects, such as aspirin, clopidogrel (Plavix), dipyridamole (Persantine), enoxaparin (Lovenox), heparin, ticlopidine (Ticlid), and warfarin (Coumadin), should talk with their doctor before beginning daily flaxseed use and have their coagulation status monitored.

Women on adjuvant breast therapy: Tamoxifen is an adjuvant therapy for breast cancer that seems to work principally by competing with estrogen for binding to estrogen receptors.

Health professionals often question whether the lignans in flaxseeds could interfere with tamoxifen.

However, studies of mice injected with ER+ human breast cancer suggest that in both high- and low estrogen conditions (modeling pre- and postmenopausal breast cancer), flaxseed either enhanced or maintained the effectiveness of tamoxifen in decreasing tumor growth, decreasing cell proliferation, and increasing apoptosis. However, no results of clinical trials of flaxseed use during tamoxifen treatment are currently available. Research is in progress regarding flaxseed use during treatment with aromatase inhibitors.

Interactions with other medications: Flaxseed may slow or decrease absorption of oral medications or nutrients, so it should be taken one hour before or two hours after any prescription or non-prescription medicine.

In addition to the interactions with anticoagulant medications above, the potential for glucose lowering due to flaxseed combined with antidiabetes medications increases the chances of hypoglycemia.

Pregnancy, breastfeeding, children: Researchers have no conclusive data on the safety of flaxseed taken daily by children or by women who are pregnant or breastfeeding. The Natural Medicines Comprehensive Database says there is no reliable clinical evidence of safety during pregnancy or lactation. It lists flaxseed use during pregnancy as "possibly unsafe" and recommends avoidance during breastfeeding.

Questions That Need to Be Answered

What is the impact of regular long-term consumption of flaxseed on bone health?

Bone strength seems to be particularly increased by the 16OHE1 form of estrogen, so especially for cancer survivors who may be at increased risk of osteoporosis, it's important to know whether changing the 2OHE1:16OHE1 ratio decreases bone mineral density. No significant effects—positive or negative—on biomarkers of bone health or bone mineral density were observed in postmenopausal women taking 25 g daily for sixteen weeks, 40 g flaxseed daily for three months, or 40 g flaxseed daily for one year. It is however, an important issue to investigate and consider in the decision about regular use of flaxseed.

What is the impact of flaxseed on risk of other cancers?

Prostate: Limited studies have shown that flaxseed inhibits the growth and metastasis of prostate cancer in mice, and lowers tumor biomarkers or pre-surgery cell proliferation rates in men with prostate cancer, with or without a low-fat diet. Conflicting reports link ALA consumption with increased, decreased, or unchanged prostate cancer risk, and impact likely varies with the food source of ALA and overall fatty acid composition of the diet.

Colon: Laboratory studies suggest that flaxseed could protect against colon cancer through anti-inflammatory effects of its omega-3 fat, its lignans promotion of apoptosis, and perhaps through its dietary fiber content, but human studies are lacking.

Uterine: Limited data does not suggest a protective role for flaxseed against uterine cancer. In an animal study, it did not seem to decrease estrogen-stimulated uterine growth and endometrial thickness (a measure of uterine cancer) did not change in postmenopausal women who took 25 g flaxseed for 3 months. Some evidence suggests that flaxseed may, however, reduce uterine growth that can be promoted with tamoxifen use.

How do the lignan phytoestrogens in flaxseed compare and interact with lignans from sesame seeds, grains, and other foods, and with the isoflavone phytoestrogens in soybeans?

Preliminary evidence suggests that different lignans may have very different effects, and that flaxseed may interact in beneficial ways with soy.

Talking with Patients about Flaxseed

Does flaxseed lower risk for cancer?

Flaxseed may contribute to lower cancer risk, but research is too limited to recommend it for cancer protection.

Flaxseed's effects vary depending on diet, hormones, genetics, and more.

One to four tablespoons of ground flaxseed per day appears to be safe and potentially protective against breast cancer based on studies using those amounts.

I heard that flaxseed might increase risk for getting breast cancer.

Studies have not shown that flaxseed increases incidence or recurrence of breast cancer.

Is it safe to take flaxseed if I'm on tamoxifen or aromatase inhibitor treatment?

Although in animal studies flaxseed did not interfere with tamoxifen's actions, there are no clinical study results available.

Research with aromatase inhibitors is not yet available.

It is best to discuss flaxseed use with your physician.

Does flaxseed interfere with any medications or supplements?

Flaxseed may slow or decrease absorption of medications, so discuss with your doctor. (You may need to take it at different times than your prescription or nonprescription medicine.)

It is also important to talk with your doctor before taking flaxseed if you take fish oil, EPA + DHA supplements, or anticoagulant medications (aspirin or blood thinners such as clopidogrel (Plavix), heparin, and warfarin (Coumadin).

Can pregnant women and children take flaxseed?

The effects of flaxseed supplements in pregnant and breastfeeding women and children are not known, so caution is advised. Talk with your doctor.

If I decide to take flaxseed, what's the best way to get started?

- Start with one tablespoon of ground flaxseed at a time; wait a few days to get used to the increased fiber before adding more.

- Use ground flaxseed ("flaxseed meal") so you'll absorb more omega-3 fats and the cancer-fighting lignans.

- Buy flaxseed pre-ground or grind the whole seeds in a coffee grinder or food processor.

- Drink at least 64 ounces of liquids daily to help move the fiber through your digestive system.

- Add to cereal, yogurt, or salads. Include in baked muffins or quick breads as cooking does not change lignan content significantly.

- Bars and cereals with flaxseeds often contain small amounts of the omega-3 fats.

- Refrigerate in a closed container; it will stay fresh for three to four months.

What about taking flaxseed oil?

Flaxseed oil provides omega-3 fat, but no fiber or lignans (unless they have been added to the oil), so effects may be different than those of ground flaxseed.

The oil may be an attractive option if the fiber content of flaxseed causes discomfort for you, or if you are in one of the groups where research about safety of regular flaxseed is lacking (pregnant women and children).

Flaxseed oil should not be used in cooking, but you could use about one tablespoon daily to be drizzled over vegetables after cooking or used in salad dressings. It is essential to store it in the refrigerator.

Chapter 43

Treating Breast Cancer during Pregnancy

Breast cancer is sometimes detected (found) in women who are pregnant or have just given birth.

In women who are pregnant or who have just given birth, breast cancer occurs most often between the ages of 32 and 38. Breast cancer occurs about once in every 3,000 pregnancies.

Signs and Symptoms of Breast Cancer

Breast cancer may cause any of the following signs and symptoms. Check with your doctor if any of the following problems occur:

- A lump or thickening in or near the breast or in the underarm area.

- A change in the size or shape of the breast.

- A dimple or puckering in the skin of the breast.

- A nipple turned inward into the breast.

- Fluid, other than breast milk, from the nipple, especially if it's bloody

- Scaly, red, or swollen skin on the breast, nipple, or areola (the dark area of skin that is around the nipple)

Excerpted from PDQ® Cancer Information Summary. National Cancer Institute; Bethesda, MD. Breast Cancer Treatment and Pregnancy (PDQ): Patient version. Updated 07/2011. Available at: www.cancer.gov. Accessed January 18, 2012.

- Dimples in the breast that look like the skin of an orange, called peau d'orange

Other conditions that are not breast cancer may cause these same symptoms.

Detecting Breast Cancer Early in Pregnant or Nursing Women

Women who are pregnant, nursing, or have just given birth usually have tender, swollen breasts. This can make small lumps difficult to detect and may lead to delays in diagnosing breast cancer. Because of these delays, cancers are often found at a later stage in these women.

To detect breast cancer, pregnant and nursing women should examine their breasts themselves. Women should also receive clinical breast examinations during their routine prenatal and postnatal examinations.

If an abnormality is found, one or all of the following tests may be used:

- Ultrasound exam: A procedure in which high-energy sound waves (ultrasound) are bounced off internal tissues or organs and make echoes. The echoes form a picture of body tissues called a sonogram.

- Mammogram: An x-ray of the breast. A mammogram can be performed with little risk to the fetus. Mammograms in pregnant women may appear negative even though cancer is present.

- Biopsy: The removal of cells or tissues by a pathologist so they can be viewed under a microscope to check for signs of cancer.

Prognosis and Treatment

The prognosis (chance of recovery) and treatment options depend on the following:

- The stage of the cancer (whether it is in the breast only or has spread to other places in the body)

- The size of the tumor

- The type of breast cancer

- The age of the fetus

- Whether there are symptoms

- The patient's general health

Treatment options for pregnant women depend on the stage of the disease and the age of the fetus.

Three types of standard treatment are used: Surgery, radiation therapy, and chemotherapy.

Surgery

Most pregnant women with breast cancer have surgery to remove the breast. Some of the lymph nodes under the arm are usually taken out and looked at under a microscope to see if they contain cancer cells.

Types of surgery to remove the breast include:

- Simple mastectomy: A surgical procedure to remove the whole breast that contains cancer. Some of the lymph nodes under the arm may also be removed for biopsy. This procedure is also called a total mastectomy.

- Modified radical mastectomy: A surgical procedure to remove the whole breast that has cancer, many of the lymph nodes under the arm, the lining over the chest muscles, and sometimes, part of the chest wall muscles.

Breast-conserving surgery, an operation to remove the cancer but not the breast itself, includes the following:

- Lumpectomy: A surgical procedure to remove a tumor (lump) and a small amount of normal tissue around it. Most doctors also take out some of the lymph nodes under the arm.

- Partial mastectomy: A surgical procedure to remove the part of the breast that contains cancer and some normal tissue around it. Some of the lymph nodes under the arm may also be removed for biopsy. This procedure is also called a segmental mastectomy.

Even if the doctor removes all of the cancer that can be seen at the time of surgery, the patient may be given radiation therapy, chemo-therapy, or hormone therapy after surgery to try to kill any cancer cells that may be left. Treatment given after surgery, to lower the risk that the cancer will come back, is called adjuvant therapy.

Radiation Therapy

Radiation therapy is a cancer treatment that uses high-energy x-rays or other types of radiation to kill cancer cells. There are two types of radiation therapy. External radiation therapy uses a machine outside the body to send radiation toward the cancer. Internal radiation therapy uses a radioactive substance sealed in needles, seeds, wires, or catheters that are placed directly into or near the cancer. The way the radiation therapy is given depends on the type and stage of the cancer being treated.

Radiation therapy should not be given to pregnant women with early stage (stage I or II) breast cancer because it can harm the fetus. For women with late stage (stage III or IV) breast cancer, it should not be given during the first three months of pregnancy.

Chemotherapy

Chemotherapy is a cancer treatment that uses drugs to stop the growth of cancer cells, either by killing the cells or by stopping the cells from dividing. When chemotherapy is taken by mouth or injected into a vein or muscle, the drugs enter the bloodstream and can reach cancer cells throughout the body (systemic chemotherapy). When chemotherapy is placed directly into the cerebrospinal fluid, an organ, or a body cavity such as the abdomen, the drugs mainly affect cancer cells in those areas (regional chemotherapy). The way the chemotherapy is given depends on the type and stage of the cancer being treated.

Chemotherapy should not be given during the first three months of pregnancy. Chemotherapy given after this time does not usually harm the fetus but may cause early labor and low birth weight.

Other Considerations for Pregnancy and Breast Cancer

- Because ending the pregnancy is not likely to improve the mother's chance of survival, it is not usually a treatment option.

- If surgery is planned, breastfeeding should be stopped to reduce blood flow in the breasts and make them smaller. Breastfeeding should also be stopped if chemotherapy is planned. Many anticancer drugs, especially cyclophosphamide and methotrexate, may occur in high levels in breast milk and may harm the nursing baby. Women receiving chemotherapy should not breastfeed. Stopping lactation does not improve survival of the mother.

- Breast cancer cells do not seem to pass from the mother to the fetus.

- Some doctors recommend that a woman wait two years after treatment for breast cancer before trying to have a baby, so that any early return of the cancer would be detected. This may affect a woman's decision to become pregnant. The fetus does not seem to be affected if the mother has previously had breast cancer.

- The effects of treatment with high-dose chemotherapy and a bone marrow transplant, with or without radiation therapy, on later pregnancies are not known.

Chapter 44

Treating Male Breast Cancer

Breast cancer may occur in men. Men at any age may develop breast cancer, but it is usually detected (found) in men between 60 and 70 years of age. Male breast cancer makes up less than 1% of all cases of breast cancer.

The following types of breast cancer are found in men:

- Infiltrating ductal carcinoma: This is cancer that has spread beyond the cells lining ducts in the breast. Most men with breast cancer have this type of cancer.

- Ductal carcinoma in situ: A type of cancer in which abnormal cells are found in the lining of a duct; also called intraductal carcinoma.

- Inflammatory breast cancer: This is a type of cancer in which the breast looks red and swollen and feels warm.

- Paget disease of the nipple: This is a tumor that has grown from ducts beneath the nipple onto the surface of the nipple.

- Lobular carcinoma in situ (abnormal cells found in one of the lobes or sections of the breast) sometimes occurs in women and has not been seen in men.

Excerpted from PDQ® Cancer Information Summary. National Cancer Institute; Bethesda, MD. Male Breast Cancer Treatment (PDQ)—Patient version. Updated 09/2011. Available at: www.cancer.gov. Accessed January 18, 2012.

Radiation exposure, high levels of estrogen, and a family history of breast cancer can increase a man's risk of developing breast cancer.

Anything that increases your risk of getting a disease is called a risk factor. Having a risk factor does not mean that you will get cancer; not having risk factors doesn't mean that you will not get cancer. People who think they may be at risk should discuss this with their doctor. Risk factors for breast cancer in men may include the following:

- Being exposed to radiation

- Having a disease related to high levels of estrogen in the body, such as cirrhosis (liver disease) or Klinefelter syndrome (a genetic disorder)

- Having several female relatives who have had breast cancer, especially relatives who have an alteration of BRCA2 [breast cancer gene 2]

Male Breast Cancer and Inherited Gene Mutations

The genes in cells carry the hereditary information that is received from a person's parents. Hereditary breast cancer makes up approximately 5% to 10% of all breast cancer. Some altered genes related to breast cancer are more common in certain ethnic groups. Men who have an altered gene related to breast cancer have an increased risk of developing this disease.

Tests have been developed that can detect altered genes. These genetic tests are sometimes done for members of families with a high risk of cancer.

Finding Breast Cancer in Men

Men with breast cancer usually have lumps that can be felt.

Lumps and other symptoms may be caused by male breast cancer. Other conditions may cause the same symptoms. A doctor should be seen if changes in the breasts are noticed.

Tests that examine the breasts are used to detect (find) and diagnose breast cancer in men.

The following tests and procedures may be used:

- Biopsy: Biopsy is the removal of cells or tissues so they can be viewed under a microscope by a pathologist to check for signs of cancer. The following are different types of biopsies:

  - Fine-needle aspiration (FNA) biopsy: This involves the removal of tissue or fluid using a thin needle.

- Core biopsy: This involves the removal of tissue using a wide needle.

- Excisional biopsy: This involves the removal of an entire lump of tissue.

- Estrogen and progesterone receptor test: This is a test to measure the amount of estrogen and progesterone (hormones) receptors in cancer tissue. If cancer is found in the breast, tissue from the tumor is checked in the laboratory to find out whether estrogen and progesterone could affect the way cancer grows. The test results show whether hormone therapy may stop the cancer from growing.

- HER2 test: This is a test to measure the amount of HER2 [human epidermal growth factor receptor 2] in cancer tissue. HER2 is a growth factor protein that sends growth signals to cells. When cancer forms, the cells may make too much of the protein, causing more cancer cells to grow. If cancer is found in the breast, tissue from the tumor is checked in the laboratory to find out if there is too much HER2 in the cells. The test results show whether monoclonal antibody therapy may stop the cancer from growing.

Survival and Prognosis in Men with Breast Cancer

Survival for men with breast cancer is similar to that for women with breast cancer when their stage at diagnosis is the same. Breast cancer in men, however, is often diagnosed at a later stage. Cancer found at a later stage may be less likely to be cured.

The prognosis (chance of recovery) and treatment options depend on the following:

- The stage of the cancer (whether it is in the breast only or has spread to other places in the body)

- The type of breast cancer

- Estrogen-receptor and progesterone-receptor levels in the tumor tissue

- Whether the cancer is also found in the other breast

- The patient's age and general health

Stages of Male Breast Cancer

After breast cancer has been diagnosed, tests are done to find out if cancer cells have spread within the breast or to other parts of the body. This process is called staging. The information gathered from the staging process determines the stage of the disease. It is important to know the stage in order to plan treatment. Breast cancer in men is staged the same as it is in women. The spread of cancer from the breast to lymph nodes and other parts of the body appears to be similar in men and women.

The following tests and procedures may be used in the staging process:

- Chest x-ray: This is an x-ray of the organs and bones inside the chest. An x-ray is a type of energy beam that can go through the body and onto film, making a picture of areas inside the body.

- CT scan (computed tomography, or CAT scan): This is a procedure that makes a series of detailed pictures of areas inside the body, taken from different angles. The pictures are made by a computer linked to an x-ray machine. A dye may be injected into a vein or swallowed to help the organs or tissues show up more clearly. This procedure is also called computed tomography, computerized tomography, or computerized axial tomography.

- Bone scan: A procedure to check if there are rapidly dividing cells, such as cancer cells, in the bone. A very small amount of radioactive material is injected into a vein and travels through the bloodstream. The radioactive material collects in the bones and is detected by a scanner.

- PET scan (positron emission tomography scan): A procedure to find malignant tumor cells in the body. A small amount of radioactive glucose (sugar) is injected into a vein. The PET scanner rotates around the body and makes a picture of where glucose is being used in the body. Malignant tumor cells show up brighter in the picture because they are more active and take up more glucose than normal cells do.

Ways That Cancer Spreads in the Body

The three ways that cancer spreads in the body are the following:

- Through tissue: Cancer invades the surrounding normal tissue.

- Through the lymph system: Cancer invades the lymph system and travels through the lymph vessels to other places in the body.

- Through the blood: Cancer invades the veins and capillaries and travels through the blood to other places in the body.

When cancer cells break away from the primary (original) tumor and travel through the lymph or blood to other places in the body, another (secondary) tumor may form. This process is called metastasis. The secondary (metastatic) tumor is the same type of cancer as the primary tumor. For example, if breast cancer spreads to the bones, the cancer cells in the bones are actually breast cancer cells. The disease is metastatic breast cancer, not bone cancer.

Stage 0 (Carcinoma In Situ)

There are two types of breast carcinoma in situ:

- Ductal carcinoma in situ (DCIS) is a noninvasive condition in which abnormal cells are found in the lining of a breast duct. The abnormal cells have not spread outside the duct to other tissues in the breast. In some cases, DCIS may become invasive cancer and spread to other tissues, although it is not known at this time how to predict which lesions will become invasive.

- Lobular carcinoma in situ (LCIS) is a condition in which abnormal cells are found in the lobules of the breast. This condition has not been seen in men.

Stage I

In stage I, cancer has formed. Stage I is divided into stages IA and IB.

- In stage IA, the tumor is 2 cm or smaller and has not spread outside the breast.

- In stage IB, either no tumor is found in the breast, but small clusters of cancer cells (larger than 0.2 mm but not larger than 2 mm) are found in the lymph nodes; or the tumor is 2 cm or smaller and small clusters of cancer cells (larger than 0.2 mm but not larger than 2 mm) are found in the lymph nodes.

Stage II

Stage II is divided into stages IIA and IIB.

- In stage IIA no tumor is found in the breast, but cancer is found in the axillary lymph nodes (lymph nodes under the arm); or the tumor is 2 cm or smaller and has spread to the axillary lymph nodes; or the tumor is larger than 2 cm but not larger than 5 cm and has not spread to the axillary lymph nodes.

- In stage IIB, the tumor is either larger than 2 cm but not larger than 5 cm and has spread to the axillary lymph nodes; or larger than 5 cm but has not spread to the axillary lymph nodes.

Stage IIIA

In stage IIIA:

- no tumor is found in the breast. Cancer is found in axillary lymph nodes that are attached to each other or to other structures, or cancer may be found in lymph nodes near the breastbone; or

- the tumor is 2 cm or smaller. Cancer has spread to axillary lymph nodes that are attached to each other or to other structures, or cancer may have spread to lymph nodes near the breastbone; or

- the tumor is larger than 2 cm but not larger than 5 cm. Cancer has spread to axillary lymph nodes that are attached to each other or to other structures, or cancer may have spread to lymph nodes near the breastbone; or

- the tumor is larger than 5 cm. Cancer has spread to axillary lymph nodes that may be attached to each other or to other structures, or cancer may have spread to lymph nodes near the breastbone.

Stage IIIB

In stage IIIB, the tumor may be any size and cancer:

- has spread to the chest wall and/or the skin of the breast; and

- may have spread to axillary lymph nodes that may be attached to each other or to other structures, or cancer may have spread to lymph nodes near the breastbone.

Cancer that has spread to the skin of the breast is inflammatory breast cancer.

Stage IIIC

In stage IIIC, there may be no sign of cancer in the breast or the tumor may be any size and may have spread to the chest wall and/or the skin of the breast. Also, cancer:

- has spread to lymph nodes above or below the collarbone; and

- may have spread to axillary lymph nodes or to lymph nodes near the breastbone.

Cancer that has spread to the skin of the breast is inflammatory breast cancer.

Stage IIIC breast cancer is divided into operable and inoperable stage IIIC.

In operable stage IIIC, the cancer:

- is found in 10 or more axillary lymph nodes; or

- is found in lymph nodes below the collarbone; or

- is found in axillary lymph nodes and in lymph nodes near the breastbone.

In inoperable stage IIIC breast cancer, the cancer has spread to the lymph nodes above the collarbone.

Stage IV

In stage IV, the cancer has spread to other organs of the body, most often the bones, lungs, liver, or brain.

Inflammatory Male Breast Cancer

In inflammatory breast cancer, cancer has spread to the skin of the breast and the breast looks red and swollen and feels warm. The redness and warmth occur because the cancer cells block the lymph vessels in the skin. The skin of the breast may also show the dimpled appearance called peau d'orange (like the skin of an orange). There may not be any lumps in the breast that can be felt. Inflammatory breast cancer may be stage IIIB, stage IIIC, or stage IV.

Recurrent Male Breast Cancer

Recurrent breast cancer is cancer that has recurred (come back) after it has been treated. The cancer may come back in the breast, in the chest wall, or in other parts of the body.

Treatment Options

Different types of treatment are available for men with breast cancer. Some treatments are standard (the currently used treatment), and some are being tested in clinical trials. A treatment clinical trial is a research study meant to help improve current treatments or obtain information on new treatments for patients with cancer. When clinical trials show that a new treatment is better than the standard treatment, the new treatment may become the standard treatment.

For some patients, taking part in a clinical trial may be the best treatment choice. Many of today's standard treatments for cancer are based on earlier clinical trials. Patients who take part in a clinical trial may receive the standard treatment or be among the first to receive a new treatment.

Patients who take part in clinical trials also help improve the way cancer will be treated in the future. Even when clinical trials do not lead to effective new treatments, they often answer important questions and help move research forward.

Some clinical trials only include patients who have not yet received treatment. Other trials test treatments for patients whose cancer has not gotten better. There are also clinical trials that test new ways to stop cancer from recurring (coming back) or reduce the side effects of cancer treatment.

Four types of standard treatment are used to treat men with breast cancer.

Surgery

Surgery for men with breast cancer is usually a modified radical mastectomy (removal of the breast, many of the lymph nodes under the arm, the lining over the chest muscles, and sometimes part of the chest wall muscles).

Breast-conserving surgery, an operation to remove the cancer but not the breast itself, is also used for some men with breast cancer. A lumpectomy is done to remove the tumor (lump) and a small amount of normal tissue around it. Radiation therapy is given after surgery to kill any cancer cells that are left.

Chemotherapy

Chemotherapy is a cancer treatment that uses drugs to stop the growth of cancer cells, either by killing the cells or by stopping them from dividing. When chemotherapy is taken by mouth or injected into a vein or muscle, the drugs enter the bloodstream and can reach cancer cells throughout the body (systemic chemotherapy). When chemotherapy is placed directly into the cerebrospinal fluid, an organ, or a body cavity such as the abdomen, the drugs mainly affect cancer cells in those areas (regional chemotherapy). The way the chemotherapy is given depends on the type and stage of the cancer being treated.

Hormone Therapy

Hormone therapy is a cancer treatment that removes hormones or blocks their action and stops cancer cells from growing. Hormones are substances made by glands in the body and circulated in the bloodstream. Some hormones can cause certain cancers to grow. If tests show that the cancer cells have places where hormones can attach (receptors), drugs, surgery, or radiation therapy is used to reduce the production of hormones or block them from working.

Radiation Therapy

Radiation therapy is a cancer treatment that uses high-energy x-rays or other types of radiation to kill cancer cells or keep them from growing. There are two types of radiation therapy. External radiation therapy uses a machine outside the body to send radiation toward the cancer. Internal radiation therapy uses a radioactive substance sealed in needles, seeds, wires, or catheters that are placed directly into or near the cancer. The way the radiation therapy is given depends on the type and stage of the cancer being treated.

Targeted Therapy

Targeted therapy is a type of treatment that uses drugs or other substances to identify and attack specific cancer cells without harming normal cells. Monoclonal antibody therapy is a type of targeted therapy being studied in the treatment of male breast cancer.

Monoclonal antibody therapy uses antibodies made in the laboratory from a single type of immune system cell. These antibodies can identify substances on cancer cells or normal substances that may help cancer cells grow. The antibodies attach to the substances and kill the cancer cells, block their growth, or keep them from spreading. Monoclonal antibodies are given by infusion. They may be used alone or to carry drugs, toxins, or radioactive material directly to cancer cells. Monoclonal antibodies are also used in combination with chemotherapy as adjuvant therapy (treatment given after surgery to lower the risk that the cancer will come back).

Trastuzumab (Herceptin) is a monoclonal antibody that blocks the effects of the growth factor protein HER2.

Chapter 45

Treating Advanced and Recurrent Breast Cancer

Chapter Contents

Section 45.1

Treating Cancer That Has Metastasized

"Metastatic Cancer," by the National Cancer Institute (NCI, www.cancer
.gov), part of the National Institutes of Health, May 23, 2011.

What is metastatic cancer?

Metastatic cancer is cancer that has spread from the place where
it first started to another place in the body. A tumor formed by metastatic cancer cells is called a metastatic tumor or a metastasis. The
process by which cancer cells spread to other parts of the body is also
called metastasis.

Metastatic cancer has the same name and the same type of cancer
cells as the original, or primary, cancer. For example, breast cancer
that spreads to the lungs and forms a metastatic tumor is metastatic
breast cancer, not lung cancer.

Under a microscope, metastatic cancer cells generally look the same
as cells of the original cancer. Moreover, metastatic cancer cells and
cells of the original cancer usually have some molecular features in
common, such as the expression of certain proteins or the presence of
specific chromosome changes.

Although some types of metastatic cancer can be cured with current
treatments, most cannot. Nevertheless, treatments are available for all patients with metastatic cancer. In general, the primary goal of these treatments is to control the growth of the cancer or to relieve symptoms caused
by it. In some cases, metastatic cancer treatments may help prolong life.
However, most people who die of cancer die of metastatic disease.

Can any type of cancer form a metastatic tumor?

Virtually all cancers, including cancers of the blood and the lymphatic system (leukemia, multiple myeloma, and lymphoma), can form
metastatic tumors. Although rare, the metastasis of blood and lymphatic system cancers to the lungs, heart, central nervous system, and
other tissues has been reported.

Where does cancer spread?

The most common sites of cancer metastasis are the lungs, bones, and liver. Although most cancers have the ability to spread to many different parts of the body, they usually spread to one site more often than others.

Breast cancer's main sites of metastasis are the lungs, liver, and bones.

How does cancer spread?

Cancer cell metastasis usually involves the following steps:

- Local invasion: Cancer cells invade nearby normal tissue.

- Intravasation: Cancer cells invade and move through the walls of nearby lymph vessels or blood vessels.

- Circulation: Cancer cells move through the lymphatic system and the bloodstream to other parts of the body.

- Arrest and extravasation: Cancer cells arrest, or stop moving, in small blood vessels called capillaries at a distant location. They then invade the walls of the capillaries and migrate into the surrounding tissue.

- Proliferation: Cancer cells multiply at the distant location to form small tumors known as micrometastases.

- Angiogenesis: Micrometastases stimulate the growth of new blood vessels to obtain a blood supply. A blood supply is needed to obtain the oxygen and nutrients necessary for continued tumor growth.

Because cancers of the lymphatic system or the blood system are already present inside lymph vessels, lymph nodes, or blood vessels, not all of these steps are needed for their metastasis. Also, the lymphatic system drains into the blood system at two locations in the neck.

The ability of a cancer cell to metastasize successfully depends on its individual properties; the properties of the noncancerous cells, including immune system cells, present at the original location; and the properties of the cells it encounters in the lymphatic system or the bloodstream and at the final destination in another part of the body. Not all cancer cells, by themselves, have the ability to metastasize. In addition, the noncancerous cells at the original location may be able to block cancer cell metastasis. Furthermore, successfully reaching another location in the body does not guarantee that a metastatic tumor will form. Metastatic cancer cells can lie dormant (not grow) at a distant site for many years before they begin to grow again, if at all.

Does metastatic cancer have symptoms?

Some people with metastatic tumors do not have symptoms. Their metastases are found by x-rays or other tests.

When symptoms of metastatic cancer occur, the type and frequency of the symptoms will depend on the size and location of the metastasis. For example, cancer that spreads to the bones is likely to cause pain and can lead to bone fractures. Cancer that spreads to the brain can cause a variety of symptoms, including headaches, seizures, and unsteadiness. Shortness of breath may be a sign of lung metastasis. Abdominal swelling or jaundice (yellowing of the skin) can indicate that cancer has spread to the liver.

Sometimes a person's original cancer is discovered only after a metastatic tumor causes symptoms. For example, a man whose prostate cancer has spread to the bones in his pelvis may have lower back pain (caused by the cancer in his bones) before he experiences any symptoms from the original tumor in his prostate.

Can someone have a metastatic tumor without having a primary cancer?

No. A metastatic tumor is always caused by cancer cells from another part of the body.

In most cases, when a metastatic tumor is found first, the primary cancer can also be found. The search for the primary cancer may involve lab tests, x-rays, computed tomography (CT) scans, magnetic resonance imaging (MRI) scans, positron emission tomography (PET) scans, and other procedures.

However, in some patients, a metastatic tumor is diagnosed but the primary tumor cannot be found, despite extensive tests, because it either is too small or has completely regressed. The pathologist knows that the diagnosed tumor is a metastasis because the cells do not look like those of the organ or tissue in which the tumor was found. Doctors refer to the primary cancer as unknown or occult (hidden), and the patient is said to have cancer of unknown primary origin (CUP).

Because diagnostic techniques are constantly improving, the number of cases of CUP is going down.

If a person who was previously treated for cancer gets diagnosed with cancer a second time, is the new cancer a new primary cancer or metastatic cancer?

The cancer may be a new primary cancer, but, in most cases, it is metastatic cancer.

What treatments are used for metastatic cancer?

Metastatic cancer may be treated with systemic therapy (chemotherapy, biological therapy, targeted therapy, hormonal therapy), local therapy (surgery, radiation therapy), or a combination of these treatments. The choice of treatment generally depends on the type of primary cancer; the size, location, and number of metastatic tumors; the patient's age and general health; and the types of treatment the patient has had in the past. In patients with CUP, it is possible to treat the disease even though the primary cancer has not been found.

Are new treatments for metastatic cancer being developed?

Yes, researchers are studying new ways to kill or stop the growth of primary cancer cells and metastatic cancer cells, including new ways to boost the strength of immune responses against tumors. In addition, researchers are trying to find ways to disrupt individual steps in the metastatic process.

Before any new treatment can be made widely available to patients, it must be studied in clinical trials (research studies) and found to be safe and effective in treating disease. NCI and many other organizations sponsor clinical trials that take place at hospitals, universities, medical schools, and cancer centers around the country. Clinical trials are a critical step in improving cancer care. The results of previous clinical trials have led to progress not only in the treatment of cancer but also in the detection, diagnosis, and prevention of the disease. Patients interested in taking part in a clinical trial should talk with their doctor.

Section 45.2

Recurrent Breast Cancer

When and Where Do Recurrences Occur?

Breast cancer can recur at any time, but most recurrences occur in the first three to five years after initial treatment. Breast cancer can come back as a local recurrence (in the treated breast or near the mastectomy scar) or as a distant recurrence somewhere else in the body. The most common sites of recurrence include the lymph nodes, the bones, liver, or lungs.

How Do I Know There Is a Recurrence?

Women who have been treated for breast cancer should continue to practice breast self-examination, checking both the treated area and the other breast each month. A woman should report any changes to her doctor right away. Breast changes that might indicate a recurrence include:

- an area that is distinctly different from any other area on either breast;
- a lump or thickening, in or near the breast or in the underarm, that persists through the menstrual cycle;
- a change in the size, shape, or contour of the breast;
- a mass or lump, which may feel as small as a pea;
- a marble-like area under the skin;
- a change in the feel or appearance of the skin on the breast or nipple (dimpled, puckered, scaly, or inflamed [red, warm, or swollen]);
- bloody or clear fluid discharge from the nipples;
- redness of the skin on the breast or nipple.

In addition to performing monthly breast self-exams, keep your scheduled follow-up appointments with your health care provider. During these appointments, your health care provider will perform a breast exam, order lab or imaging tests as needed, and ask you about any symptoms you might have. Initially, these follow-up appointments may be scheduled every three to four months. The longer you are cancer-free, the less often you will need to see your health care provider. Continue to follow your health care provider's recommendations on screening mammograms (usually recommended once a year).

Prognostic Indicators

Prognostic indicators are characteristics of a patient and her tumor that may help a physician predict a cancer recurrence. These are some common indicators:

Lymph node involvement: Women who have lymph node involvement are more likely to have a recurrence.

Tumor size: In general, the larger the tumor, the greater the chance of recurrence.

Hormone receptors: About two-thirds of all breast cancers contain significant levels of estrogen receptors, which means the tumors are estrogen receptor positive (ER+). ER+ tumors tend to grow less aggressively and may respond favorably to treatment with hormones.

Histologic grade: This refers to how much the tumor cells resemble normal cells when viewed under the microscope. The grading scale is 1 to 4. Grade 4 tumors contain very abnormal and rapidly growing cancer cells. There is a greater chance of recurrence the higher the histologic grade.

Nuclear grade: This is the rate at which cancer cells in the tumor divide to form more cells. Cancer cells with a high nuclear grade (also called proliferative capacity) are usually more aggressive (faster growing).

Oncogene expression: An oncogene is a gene that causes or promotes cancerous changes within the cell. Tumors that contain certain oncogenes may increase a patient's chance of recurrence.

Treatment Team

Following local breast cancer treatment, the treatment team will determine the likelihood that the cancer will recur outside the breast.

401

This team usually includes a medical oncologist, a specialist trained in using medicines to treat breast cancer. The medical oncologist, who works with the surgeon, may advise the use of tamoxifen (tamoxifen citrate, Nolvadex) or possibly chemotherapy. These treatments are used in addition to, but not in place of, local breast cancer treatment with surgery and/or radiation therapy.

Treatment of Breast Cancer Recurrence

The type of treatment for local breast cancer recurrences depends on the woman's initial treatment. If she had a lumpectomy, local recurrence is usually treated with mastectomy, since radiation therapy cannot be delivered twice to the same area. If the initial treatment was mastectomy, recurrence near the mastectomy site is treated by removing the tumor whenever possible, usually followed by radiation therapy. In either case, hormone therapy and/or chemotherapy may be used after surgery and/or radiation therapy. If breast cancer is found in the other breast, it may be a new tumor unrelated to the first breast cancer. Treatment would include a lumpectomy or mastectomy and, sometimes, systemic therapy.

Women with distant recurrence involving organs such as the bones, lungs, brain, or other organs, are treated with systemic therapy using chemotherapy, hormonal therapy, or both. Radiation therapy or surgery also may be recommended to relieve certain symptoms.

Immunotherapy with trastuzumab (Herceptin) alone or with chemotherapy may be recommended for women whose cancer cells have high levels of the HER2/neu [human epidermal growth factor receptor 2/neu] protein. Immunotherapy is generally started after hormonal or chemotherapy is no longer effective.

Chapter 46

Clinical Trials

Chapter Contents

Section 46.1

What Is a Clinical Trial?

"What Is a Clinical Trial?," by the National Cancer Institute (NCI, www
.cancer.gov), part of the National Institutes of Health, April 8, 2008.

Clinical trials are research studies in which people help doctors find
ways to improve health and cancer care. Each study tries to answer
scientific questions and to find better ways to prevent, diagnose, or
treat cancer.

Why are there clinical trials?

A clinical trial is one of the final stages of a long and careful cancer
research process. Studies are done with cancer patients to find out
whether promising approaches to cancer prevention, diagnosis, and
treatment are safe and effective.

What are the different types of clinical trials?

Treatment trials test new treatments (like a new cancer drug, new
approaches to surgery or radiation therapy, new combinations of treatments, or new methods such as gene therapy).

Prevention trials test new approaches, such as medicines, vitamins,
minerals, or other supplements that doctors believe may lower the risk
of a certain type of cancer. These trials look for the best way to prevent cancer in people who have never had cancer or to prevent cancer
from coming back or a new cancer from occurring in people who have
already had cancer.

Screening trials test the best way to find cancer, especially in its
early stages.

Quality of Life trials (also called Supportive Care trials) explore
ways to improve comfort and quality of life for cancer patients.

What are the phases of clinical trials?

Most clinical research that involves the testing of a new drug
progresses in an orderly series of steps, called phases. This allows

researchers to ask and answer questions in a way that results in reliable information about the drug and protects the patients. Most clinical trials are classified into one of three phases:

- **Phase I trials:** These first studies in people evaluate how a new drug should be given (by mouth, injected into the blood, or injected into the muscle), how often, and what dose is safe. A phase I trial usually enrolls only a small number of patients, sometimes as few as a dozen.

- **Phase II trials:** A phase II trial continues to test the safety of the drug, and begins to evaluate how well the new drug works. Phase II studies usually focus on a particular type of cancer.

- **Phase III trials:** These studies test a new drug, a new combination of drugs, or a new surgical procedure in comparison to the current standard. A participant will usually be assigned to the standard group or the new group at random (called randomization). Phase III trials often enroll large numbers of people and may be conducted at many doctors' offices, clinics, and cancer centers nationwide.

In addition, after a treatment has been approved and is being marketed, the drug's maker may study it further in a phase IV trial. The purpose of phase IV trials is to evaluate the side effects, risks, and benefits of a drug over a longer period of time and in a larger number of people than in phase III clinical trials. Thousands of people are involved in a phase IV trial.

Section 46.2

How to Find a Cancer Treatment Trial

Excerpted from "How to Find a Cancer Treatment Trial: A 10-Step Guide," by the National Cancer Institute (NCI, www.cancer.gov), part of the National Institutes of Health, June 8, 2010.

Step 1: Understand Clinical Trials

Clinical trials are research studies that involve people. They are the final step in a long process that begins with laboratory research and testing in animals. Many treatments used today are the result of past clinical trials.

Step 2: Talk with Your Doctor

When thinking about clinical trials, your best starting point is your doctor or another member of your health care team.

Usually, it is a doctor who may know about a clinical trial, or search for one, that could be a good option for you and your type of cancer. He or she can provide information and answer questions while you think about joining a clinical trial.

In some cases, your doctor may not be taking part in clinical trials or may not be very familiar with them. If your doctor doesn't have information to give you about clinical trials, you may want to get a second opinion about your treatment options and about participating in a clinical trial.

Step 3: Complete a Cancer Details Checklist

If you decide to look for a clinical trial, you must know certain details about your cancer diagnosis. You will need to compare these details with the eligibility criteria of any trial that interests you. Eligibility criteria are the guidelines for who can and cannot take part in a certain clinical trial. They are also called entry criteria or enrollment criteria.

To help you know which trials you may be eligible to join, complete a Cancer Details Checklist [www.cancer.gov/clinicaltrials/learningabout/

treatment-trial-guide/page15] as much as possible. This form asks questions about your cancer and provides space to write down your answers. Keep the form with you during your search for a clinical trial.

To get the information you need for the form, ask your doctor, a nurse, or social worker at your doctor's office for help. Explain to them that you are interested in looking for a clinical trial and that you need these details before starting to look. They may be able to review your medical records and help you fill out the form. The more information you can find to complete the form, the easier it will be to find a clinical trial that might fit your situation.

Step 4: Search the U.S. National Cancer Institute's List of Cancer Clinical Trials

Many websites have lists of cancer clinical trials that are taking place in the United States. Some trials are sponsored by non-profit organizations, including the U.S. federal government, and others are sponsored by for-profit groups, such as drug companies. In addition, there are hospitals and academic medical centers that sponsor trials conducted by their own researchers. Unfortunately, because of the many types of sponsors, no single list of clinical trials is complete.

The National Cancer Institute (NCI), which is part of the U.S. federal government, has one of the most complete lists of cancer clinical trials available. This list can be searched on NCI's website at www.cancer .gov/clinicaltrials/search.

Step 5: Search Other Lists of Cancer Clinical Trials

In addition to NCI's list of cancer clinical trials, you may want to check a few other trial lists. Why? Because some may include a few trials not found in NCI's list and you may prefer the way you can search those lists.

Other places to look for lists of cancer clinical trials are included in the following text.

Websites of Research Organizations that Conduct Cancer Clinical Trials

Many cancer centers across the United States, including NCI-designated Cancer Centers, sponsor or take part in cancer clinical trials. The websites of these centers usually have a list of the clinical trials taking place at their location. Some of the trials included in these lists, mainly phase I clinical trials (also called phase 1 trials), may not be in NCI's list.

Keep in mind that the amount of information about clinical trials on these websites can vary considerably. You may have to contact a cancer center's clinical trials office to get more information about the trials that interest you. See a list of NCI-designated Cancer Centers at cancercenters.cancer.gov/cancer_centers/cancer-centers -list.html.

Another place to look is the TrialCheck® Website [www.cancer trialshelp.org/cancer-trial-search]. This website is managed by an organization called the Coalition of Cancer Cooperative Groups (CCCG). The CCCG includes groups of doctors and other health professionals who conduct many of the large cancer clinical trials sponsored by NCI. The TrialCheck website has a clinical trials questionnaire that helps you search for trials based on your cancer type and the treatment(s) you have already received. Most of the clinical trials listed on the TrialCheck website are the same as those found in NCI's clinical trials list.

Drug and Biotechnology Company Websites

Drug and biotechnology companies also sponsor cancer clinical trials. Many of these trials are included in NCI's list of cancer clinical trials, but some are not.

How to search for company-sponsored trials: Search the U.S. websites of drug and biotechnology companies. Many companies provide lists of the clinical trials that they sponsor on their websites. Sometimes, a company's website may refer you to the website of another organization that helps the company find patients for its trials. The other organization may be paid fees for this service.

The website of the Pharmaceutical Research and Manufacturers of America (PhRMA) includes a list of its member companies at [www .phrma.org], many of which sponsor cancer clinical trials. PhRMA is a trade organization that represents drug and biotechnology companies in the United States.

Search the Clinical Trials Portal of the International Federation of Pharmaceutical Manufacturers & Associations (IFPMA) [clinicaltrials .ifpma.org/clinicaltrials/no_cache/en/myportal/index.htm]. The IFPMA web portal includes trials found in NCI's list of cancer clinical trials, as well as some other trials. You can search for clinical trials based on cancer type or other medical condition, drug name, and geographic location (for example, the United States).

Clinical Trial Listing Services

Other organizations provide lists of clinical trials as a major part of their business. These organizations generally do not sponsor or take part in clinical trials. Some of them may receive fees from drug or biotechnology company sponsors of trials for listing their trials or helping them find patients for their trials.

Keep the following points in mind:

- The trial lists provided by these organizations often rely heavily on trial lists that are available at no cost from the U.S. federal government (NCI and ClinicalTrials.gov).

- The trial lists provided by these organizations may have a few more trials than NCI's list, or they may have fewer trials.

- Unlike the NCI website (and ClinicalTrials.gov), the websites of these organizations may not be updated regularly.

- Unlike the NCI website (and ClinicalTrials.gov), the websites of these organizations may require you to register to search for clinical trials or obtain trial contact information for trials that interest you.

Links to the websites of several clinical trial listing services are given below. Visiting the links will help you learn more about the websites, what the organizations that manage the sites have to offer, and their clinical trial lists.

- Acurian.com
- BreastCancerTrials.org
- Cancer411.org
- CenterWatch.com
- ClinicalTrialsSearch.org
- eCancerTrials.com
- EmergingMed.com

Cancer Advocacy Group Websites

Cancer advocacy groups work on behalf of people diagnosed with cancer and their loved ones. They provide education, support, financial assistance, and advocacy to help patients and families who are dealing with cancer, its treatment, and survivorship. These organizations recognize that clinical trials are important to improving cancer care. They work to educate and empower people to find information and obtain access to appropriate treatment.

Advocacy groups work hard to know about the latest advances in cancer research. They will sometimes have information about certain government-sponsored clinical trials, as well as some trials sponsored by cancer centers or drug and biotechnology companies.

How to search for trials through a cancer advocacy group: Search the websites of advocacy groups for specific types of cancer. Many of these websites have lists of clinical trials or refer you to the websites of organizations that match patients to trials. The CancerActionNow.org website, managed by the non-profit Marti Nelson Cancer Foundation, provides a partial list of cancer advocacy groups [http://www.cancer actionnow.org/living/cancerresources.php#disease]. Or, you can contact an advocacy group directly for assistance in finding clinical trials.

Step 6: Make a List of Potential Clinical Trials

At this point, you should have completed a Cancer Details Checklist, found one or more trials of interest to you, and printed out or saved a summary for each trial.

Key questions to ask about each trial:

- Trial objective: What is the main purpose of the trial? Is it to cure your cancer? To slow its growth or spread? To lessen the severity of cancer symptoms or the side effects of treatment? To determine whether a new treatment is safe and well tolerated? Read this information carefully to learn whether the trial's main objective matches your goals for treatment.

- Eligibility criteria: Do the details of your cancer diagnosis and your current overall state of health match the trial's entry criteria? This may tell you whether or not you can qualify for the trial. If you're not sure, keep the trial on your list for now.

- Trial location: Is the location of the trial manageable for you? Some trials take place at more than one location. Look carefully at how often you will need to receive treatment during the course of the trial. Decide how far and how often you are willing to travel. You will also need to ask whether the sponsoring organization will pay for some or all of your travel costs.

- Study length: How long will the trial run? Not all clinical trial summaries provide this information. If they do, consider the time involved and whether it will work for you and your family.

After considering these questions, if you are still interested in one or more of the clinical trials you have found, then you are ready for Step 7.

Step 7: Contact the Clinical Trial Team

There are many ways to contact the clinical trial team.

Contact the trial team directly. The clinical trial summary should include the phone number of a person or an office that you can contact for more information. You do not need to talk to the lead researcher (called the "protocol chair" or "principal investigator") at this time, even if his or her name is given along with the telephone number. Instead, call the number and ask to speak with the "trial coordinator," the "referral coordinator," or the "protocol assistant." This person can answer questions from patients and their doctors. It is also this person's job to decide whether you are likely to be eligible to join the trial. (A final decision will probably not be made until you have had a visit with a doctor who is taking part in the trial.)

Ask your doctor or another health care team member to contact the trial team for you. Because the clinical trial coordinator will ask questions about your cancer diagnosis and your current general health, you may want to ask your doctor or someone else on your health care team to contact the clinical trial team for you.

The trial team may contact you. If you have used the website of a clinical trial listing service and found a trial that interests you, you may have provided your name, phone number, and e-mail address so the clinical trial team can contact you directly.

You will need to refer to your Cancer Details Checklist during this conversation, so keep it handy.

Step 8: Ask Questions about the Trial

Whether you or someone from your health care team calls the clinical trial team, this is the time to get answers to questions that will help you decide whether or not to take part in this particular clinical trial.

It will be helpful if you can talk about your cancer and your current general health in a manner that is brief and to the point. Before you make the call, you may want to rehearse how you will present key information about your cancer diagnosis and general health with a family member or a friend. This will make you more comfortable when you are talking with the clinical trial team member, and it will help you answer his or her questions more smoothly. Remember to keep your Cancer Details Checklist (from Step 3) handy to help you answer some of the questions that may be asked.

Questions to ask the trial coordinator:

- Is the trial still open? On occasion, clinical trial listings will be out of date and will include trials that are no longer accepting new participants.

- Am I eligible for this trial? The trial team member will ask you many, if not all, of the questions listed on your Cancer Diagnosis Checklist (Step 3). This is the time to confirm that you are a candidate for this trial. However, a final decision will likely not be made until you have had your first visit with a doctor who is taking part in the clinical trial (Step 10).

- Why do researchers think the new treatment might be effective? Results from previous research have indicated that the new treatment may be effective in people with your type of cancer. Ask about the previous research studies. Results from studies in humans are stronger than results from laboratory or animal studies.

- What are the potential risks and benefits associated with the treatments I may receive in this trial? Every treatment has risks, whether you receive the treatment as part of a clinical trial or from your doctor outside of a clinical trial. Be sure you understand the possible risks and side effects of each treatment you may receive as a participant in this trial. Also, ask for a detailed description of how the treatments you may receive could benefit you.

- Who will watch over my care and safety? Primary responsibility for the care and safety of people taking part in a cancer clinical trial rests with the clinical trial team. Also, clinical trials are governed by safety and ethical regulations set by the federal government and the organization sponsoring and carrying out the trial. One of these groups is called the Institutional Review Board (IRB). The trial team will be able to give you more information.

- Can I get a copy of the trial's protocol document? A trial's protocol document is an action plan for the trial. It includes the reason(s) for doing the trial, the number of people that will be included, the eligibility criteria for participation, the treatments that will be given, the medical tests that will be done and how often, and what information will be collected. These documents are usually written in highly technical language and are often confidential. In some cases, however, the trial team may be allowed to release the protocol document to you.

- Can I get a copy of the informed consent document? Yes. The U.S. Food and Drug Administration (FDA) and the Office for Human Research Protections (OHRP) require that potential participants in a clinical trial receive detailed, understandable information about the trial. This process is known as "informed consent," and it must be in writing. It may be helpful to see a copy of this document before you make your final decision about joining the trial.

- Is there a chance that I will receive a placebo? Placebos (sham or inactive treatments) are rarely used alone in cancer treatment trials. When they are used, they are most often given along with a standard (usual) treatment. In such cases, a trial will compare a standard treatment plus a new treatment with the same standard treatment plus a placebo. If a placebo is used alone, it's because no standard treatment exists. In this case, a trial will compare the effects of a new treatment with the effects of a placebo. Be sure you understand the treatments that are being used in any trial you are thinking of joining.

- Is the trial randomized? In a randomized clinical trial, participants are assigned by chance to different treatment groups or "arms" of the trial. Neither you nor your doctor can choose which arm you are in. All participants in an arm receive the same treatment. At the end of the trial, the results from the different treatment arms are compared. In a randomized trial, you may or may not receive the new treatment that is being tested.

- What is the dose and schedule of the treatments given in each arm of the trial? Dose refers to the amount of treatment given, and schedule refers to when and how often treatment is given. You will want to think about this information when you are discussing your treatment options with your health care team. Is the treatment schedule manageable for you?

- What costs will I or my health insurance plan have to pay? In many cases, the research costs are paid by the organization sponsoring the trial. Research costs include the treatments being studied and any tests performed purely for research purposes. However, you or your insurance plan would be responsible for paying "routine patient care costs." These are the costs of medical care (for example, doctor visits, hospital stays, x-rays) that you would receive whether or not you were taking part in a clinical trial. Some insurance plans don't cover these costs once you join a trial.

- If I have to travel, who will pay for my travel and lodging? Clinical trials rarely cover travel and lodging expenses. Usually, you will be responsible for these costs. However, you should still ask this question.

- Will participation in this trial require more time (hours/days) than standard care? Will participation require a hospital stay? Understanding how much time is involved and whether a hospital stay is required, compared to the usual treatment for your type of cancer, may influence your decision. This information will also be important if you decide to take part in the trial because it will help you in making plans.

- How will participating in this trial affect my everyday life? A diagnosis of cancer can disrupt the routine of your everyday life. Many people seek to keep their routine intact as they deal with their cancer and its treatment. This information will be useful in making plans and in determining whether you need any additional help at home.

Step 9: Discuss Your Options with Your Doctor

To make a final decision, you will want to know the potential risks and benefits of all treatment options available to you. Through the research that you have done, you likely have a good idea about the possible risks and benefits of the treatment(s) in clinical trials that interest you. If you have any remaining questions or concerns, you should discuss them with your doctor. You should also ask your doctor about the risks and benefits of standard, or usual, treatment for your type of cancer. Then, you and your doctor can compare the risks and benefits of standard treatment with those of treatment in a clinical trial. You may decide that joining a trial is your best option, or you may decide not to join a trial. It's your choice.

Step 10: Schedule an Appointment

If you decide to join a clinical trial for which you are eligible, schedule a visit with the trial team (most likely, the same person you spoke with in Step 8).

Part Six

Managing Side Effects and Complications of Breast Cancer Treatment

Chapter 47

Side Effects and Complications of Breast Cancer Treatment

Living with Metastatic Breast Cancer

As new treatments help people live longer with advanced breast cancer, symptoms of the disease and side effects of treatment have become a growing area of concern. More than ever before, you and your healthcare providers are looking for new ways to balance treatment for the disease with your general well-being, doing whatever possible to keep the cancer under control while maintaining the best possible quality of life.

Treatment for advanced breast cancer can cause all kinds of side effects. And the disease itself may cause symptoms that also require treatment. Sometimes it's hard to tell what's causing discomfort, because it could be a symptom of the disease or a side effect of treatment. Whatever the cause, it is extremely important to tell your healthcare team about any discomfort or new symptom you may have. Together you can figure out if it's the cancer, treatment, or both, and find ways to help you feel better.

The purpose of this text is to help you when you have symptoms of advanced breast cancer or side effects of treatment, and also to prepare you, so you know what to expect with different treatments.

Being prepared can decrease worry and give you ways to cope right away, so you don't have to wait until a symptom or side effect becomes difficult to manage. In some cases, you may even be able to prevent a side effect from happening, if you know about it ahead of time.

In this text you will find medical information and advice from women who have been living with advanced breast cancer for as long as 10 years and who have had a wide variety of treatments and side effects. What worked for them might not always work for you. But we hope their advice gives you as many options as possible in dealing with your own symptoms and treatment side effects.

Tips to Keep in Mind When You're Dealing with Symptoms and Side Effects

- Be prepared. Knowing about possible side effects ahead of time can help you prepare mentally as well as physically for what might happen with each treatment. Keep in mind that your team is required to tell you about all possible side effects, but just because side effects could happen does not mean that they will.

- Know your options. Discuss and understand the different options you have for treatment and why your doctor chose or recommended a certain option. Ask in advance what signs and side effects you should monitor and what interventions are used to prevent and treat them.

- Focus on your quality of life. With advanced breast cancer, the goal of treatment is to extend survival with the best possible quality of life, so getting help with symptoms and side effects is key.

- Keep a log. Record any side effects you have along with medicines you take to treat them. Include how long and severe the side effects are and to what extent the recommended treatment impacts them. Jot down questions that may come up, so you can remember and review them at your next office visit.

- Speak up! Always tell healthcare providers what's bothering you and ask for help if anything interferes with your daily life, whether or not you think you know what is causing the discomfort.

- Speak to others. Many women find it very helpful to talk to others who are going through the same types of treatments and having similar symptoms/side effects. You may want to try the LBBC Helpline at 888-753-LBBC (753-5222), with a personalized matching service that connects you to women in similar circumstances.

- Find what works for you. Treatments, as well as the cancer, affect each woman differently. Listen to what others have to say, then take the time to see how your body responds to each treatment and find remedies for symptoms and side effects that work best for you.

The Top Three Symptoms/Side Effects: Pain, Fatigue, and Depression

The women who helped us prepare this text said pain, fatigue, and depression, or emotional issues, are the three things that bothered them most.

In this portion of text, we will discuss these concerns in depth. Many also said three things helped most to combat these symptoms/side effects: Exercise, complementary therapies, and emotional counseling or support.

Exercise

Moving your body is one of the best ways to improve your physical, as well as your psychological, well-being. The tricky part is finding the right kind of movement or exercise for you. With metastatic breast cancer, you might not be able to work out as strenuously as you used to, but you can usually find a routine that provides a good level of activity, even if it is a brief walk or stretch. Always talk with your doctor before starting any exercise routine.

Remember to listen to your body: If the exercise is painful, or if it's too stressful, slow down. And if something is not working for you anymore, find a new routine.

When you're going through treatment for advanced breast cancer, your needs and activity levels are constantly changing. It helps to keep a flexible attitude about what exercise might be right at different times in your treatment: What is right today might not be right tomorrow.

Complementary Therapies

There are many complementary therapies that may be helpful. They include acupuncture, meditation, music, relaxation, massage, yoga, and more. These types of treatments can help improve overall physical and emotional well-being while also addressing specific areas of pain, discomfort, or stress.

Note: It's extremely important to talk to your doctor about any complementary option you want to try. In most cases, these treatments do not interfere with conventional medical treatment (and vice versa). But sometimes you need to take special precautions, and your doctor can advise you. Some breast cancer medicines may be less effective when used with certain complementary treatments, like herbs and supplements. We know little about how effective most complementary therapies are, but many resources exist to guide you and your doctors in making decisions about them.

Psychological and Emotional Support

This type of support is essential, but "support" might mean something different for you than for someone else you know. There are many ways of getting support: From family and friends, professional therapists and counselors, religious guides, support groups, and more. As with exercise, different types of support work for different people, and your needs will probably change as you go through different phases of treatment.

Dealing with Pain

Pain can make you feel miserable, and if left untreated, can have a big impact on your quality of life. Thankfully, there are many effective ways to manage pain. Don't hesitate to ask about them.

Pain in metastatic breast cancer can have many different causes. It may be caused by the cancer itself in bones and other areas of metastasis.

Enlarged lymph nodes can press on nerves and cause pain. Chemotherapy, radiation, hormonal treatments, and targeted therapies may cause skin, joint, bone, or muscle pain.

Pain Medicine

There are many different types of pain medicine, and they work differently for different people.

In general, you might find it helpful to have two types on hand: Long-acting and short-acting.

Long-acting pain medicine stays in the body for a long time and helps with chronic (ongoing) pain.

You take it on a regular schedule. Short-acting pain medicine can start relieving pain within 30 minutes or so, and you take it as needed. It helps with breakthrough pain, or extra-strong pain that can break through the long-acting pain medicine.

If your healthcare team has a hard time finding pain medicine that works for you, pain specialists and specialized pain clinics can help. Ask your doctor for a referral if pain is a problem for you.

Getting Effective Pain Treatment

- Never ignore the pain. Always tell your healthcare team if you feel any pain or discomfort, whether you think you know the cause or not.

- Keep a record of the type of pain and its intensity. Do not hesitate to explore complementary options (like acupuncture or massage) as well.

- Seeking effective pain relief does not mean you are weak or a whiner. It's essential for maintaining your best possible quality of life.

- Keep trying until you find pain relief that works. Many treatments, medical and complementary, relieve pain and work differently for different people. Don't settle for a treatment that's not working for you.

- Do not worry about getting addicted to pain medicine. When you get medicine for pain associated with metastatic breast cancer, it is not addictive. This is because your body needs the medicine to help reduce the pain. Addiction happens when you crave the treatment without having the symptoms. You can and should get as much treatment as you need to relieve the pain every time.

- Give yourself time to get used to the side effects of pain medicine. Side effects may include grogginess or nausea (with opioid pain medicines like morphine and oxycodone). Often, these side effects improve with time, so you and your doctors can fine-tune the dose and schedule to best control the pain and allow you to continue your usual routine.

- Stool softeners or laxatives are almost always given along with opioids to prevent constipation.

Dealing with Fatigue

Cancer-related fatigue is unlike any other kind of tiredness. It can be caused by the disease itself or by the effects of ongoing treatment on the body. Many people describe it as feeling drained and tired all

421

the time, so that even sleep does not relieve the feeling of constant drowsiness, muddleheadedness, and need for rest.

The most important first step is to recognize that the fatigue is real, that it will not go away on its own, and that there are many different ways to deal with it—you need to find the way that works for you.

Medical Treatments for Fatigue

Treating anemia: One specific cause of fatigue can be anemia, or low red blood cell counts. This may be caused by chemotherapy treatments that affect how many blood cells are made in your body.

There are some treatments that can increase red blood cell counts, called growth factors. However, recent research suggests they can be harmful to people in some situations, and new guidelines have been issued for their use. For this reason, if you have serious or persistent anemia, your doctor is likely to recommend blood transfusions instead.

If you have anemia, talk to your doctor about treatment options that might be appropriate for you.

Medicine for fatigue: Sometimes medicines can help with fatigue. These include methylphenidate (brand name: Ritalin) and modafinil (brand name: Provigil). Talk to your doctor about whether these might be right for you.

Managing Fatigue Day-to-Day

The women who helped us with this text say fatigue is something you learn to live with and work around. Here are some tips they keep in mind:

- Listen to your body and pay attention to its needs: If you're feeling tired, take a break. Don't push yourself to do more than feels comfortable.

- Exercise is one of the best ways to combat fatigue. Try to get a little bit of exercise as often as you can. Even a short walk once a day can help increase your overall energy.

- Be flexible: If you can't finish everything you planned for today, let it go until you feel more energetic.

- Pay attention to the time of day when you feel most energetic, and try to plan activities—including as much exercise as you feel comfortable doing—for that time.

- Get help with chores and anything else that drains your energy. Your loved ones will be thankful for the opportunity to help, and you'll be thankful for the chance to focus on what matters most to you.

- Get treatment for depression, if it's an issue for you. Depression can make fatigue even worse, and there are very effective treatments for it.

Dealing with Depression/Anxiety/Emotional Issues

Nearly everyone diagnosed with metastatic cancer experiences depression, anxiety, or other emotional issues. This is normal for anyone facing a serious illness, and there are effective remedies, both medical and psychological. If you had depression earlier in your life, you are more likely to have it again with your diagnosis of advanced cancer.

Don't let depression go untreated. Feeling bad emotionally can make it difficult for you to cope with physical symptoms and treatment and can seriously affect your quality of life.

Remember: Accepting that you are depressed or anxious and asking for help are not signs of weakness.

In fact, you may find that it requires a great deal of strength to ask for help. Once you ask, you may actually feel empowered and relieved.

Signs of Depression and Anxiety

Some common signs of depression are:

- uncontrollable crying;
- overwhelming sadness;
- losing interest in what used to make you happy;
- not looking forward to anything;
- trouble sleeping or sleeping all the time;
- not wanting to eat at all or wanting to eat all the time.

If you have any of these signs for more than two weeks, you may be suffering from depression. Even if you have none of these but think you might be depressed, talk to your healthcare team and ask for help.

Medical Treatments for Depression

Medicines called antidepressants can be very effective in making you feel better. Each one works a little differently and could cause different side effects.

It may take a few weeks before they start working.

Don't give up. Keep trying until you find the medicine that makes you feel better.

Note: Some studies suggest that the antidepressants fluoxetine (brand name: Prozac), paroxetine (brand name: Paxil), bupropion (brand name: Wellbutrin), and duloxetine (brand name: Cymbalta) lessen the effectiveness of tamoxifen. Talk to your doctor about which antidepressants are safe for you to try.

Counseling and Support Groups

Sometimes talking to someone who is not a friend or a relative can be a big help in relieving sadness.

It can be easier to talk to a professional counselor or therapist because you don't have to worry about how your feelings might affect the counselor. You can be completely honest about what's bothering you.

There are so many different types of counselors: Social workers, therapists, psychologists, psychiatrists, religious counselors, and more. As with everything else, it is important to find someone who makes you feel better. If one therapist or counselor is not giving you the support you feel you need, look for someone else.

There are also many types of support groups that can be a huge help in dealing with both emotional and physical issues. LBBC volunteers say it's important to find a group specifically for people with metastatic cancer. Groups with people who have early-stage cancer seem to be less helpful. Still, remember that not everyone finds help in a group.

If you are one of those people, there is no reason to feel guilty. There are many other sources of support that may work better for you.

Ask your doctor or nurse about groups in your area that might be right for you. You may also want to look for online support groups or other virtual support communities, or try the toll-free LBBC Helpline at 888-753-LBBC (753-5222), with a personalized matching service that connects you to women in similar circumstances.

Even if you do not use counseling or a support group, research has shown that staying connected to friends and family and keeping up with your social activities and networks can make a big difference for your quality of life.

Specific Treatment Side Effects

In this portion of text you will learn about side effects that are specific to certain advanced breast cancer treatments. Remember that not everyone gets every side effect. And you do not have to read about all of them at once. It can help, however, to know what might happen with a treatment you're going to get, so you can try to prepare ahead of time.

Dealing with Side Effects of Radiation

In advanced breast cancer, radiation is sometimes used to try to reduce the size or slow the growth of a tumor that is causing pain or that might cause pain in the future.

The main side effects of radiation are fatigue and skin burns. There is no single remedy for skin burns, but there are different ointments and creams you may want to try. Talk to your radiation oncologist about what might work best for you.

Depending on what area of your body receives radiation, you may have other side effects, like diarrhea or irritation of the bladder. In general, your radiation oncologist will treat as small an area as possible to best manage the symptoms and risks.

Before you start treatment, ask your doctor what benefits and side effects you should expect in the area to be treated. This information will help you make informed decisions and prepare, just as you would with any other cancer treatment.

Dealing with Side Effects of Chemotherapy

There are so many different types of chemotherapy for metastatic breast cancer, with so many different possible side effects, that it's difficult to cover them all.

The good news is that there are effective treatments that help prevent or lessen some of the most distressing side effects of chemotherapy, especially nausea and vomiting.

The more difficult part of chemotherapy is that everyone's body responds to it differently, so it's hard to know what side effects you might have.

How you respond to a particular type of chemotherapy also depends on what types and amounts of different treatments you have already had or other health conditions you have.

Chemotherapy affects many systems in your body and can make you feel tired and run-down. After a few cycles, you should know how your body responds to a particular type of chemotherapy. This makes it possible to plan the best time of day to get the treatment. You also can plan ahead for side effects and prepare so you can prevent or minimize them.

Hair loss: Not all treatments or types of chemotherapy cause hair loss. Ask your doctor or nurse if the type you are getting is likely to have this side effect. If it is, you can do some things to prepare:

• Cut your hair short before treatment starts. When the hair falls out, it will be less of a shock.

• If you want to cover your head, go ahead of time to find wigs, hats, scarves, or other head coverings that are comfortable for you. You may want to leave your head uncovered during the warm seasons because head coverings can make you feel hot.

With metastatic breast cancer, you may get several different types of treatment and may lose your hair more than once. Some hormonal therapies also can cause hair loss or thinning, although the loss is usually not as dramatic as with chemotherapy. After you lose your hair a few times, it might not grow back as thick as it used to be. You may prefer to continue using a head covering, if your hair grows back less fully.

Scalp pain and itching sometimes happen with chemotherapy-caused hair loss. They usually improve over time.

Also be aware that you might lose hair from other areas of your body: Eyelashes, eyebrows, armpits, and pubic hair can all be affected by chemotherapy.

Nausea and vomiting: Not all types of chemotherapy cause nausea and vomiting. Ask your doctor or nurse ahead of time whether the type you are getting is likely to have these side effects. If so, there are effective treatments you can take to prevent or lessen them.

In many cases, you can take treatments before you get the chemotherapy, or while you're getting it, to prevent or lessen nausea and vomiting. Ask which anti-nausea medicines your doctor recommends. If one doesn't work, ask for another.

Diet and lifestyle changes also can help you with nausea and vomiting. These include the following:

• Eating more, smaller meals: Eating a lot all at once can make nausea worse. It helps to eat small meals, or snacks, through the day, rather than sitting down for a three-course lunch or dinner.

• Eating at the time or times of day when you feel best: If nausea tends to strike in the mornings, eat less or nothing, and wait until later. If you know you tend to get more nauseated at dinnertime, try to eat more in the earlier hours of the day.

- Avoiding spicy and high-fat foods: Bland choices like rice, plain pasta, bananas, and crackers can be easier on your stomach. Gingersnaps can be soothing.

Other digestive system side effects: These side effects are typically caused by chemotherapy but also can be caused by radiation to certain areas of the body in or near the digestive system.

Taste loss or taste changes are side effects you may not hear about, but they can be unpleasant while they last. The important thing to remember is that taste may come back if/when you switch to a different treatment.

Gas is another side effect you might not hear about, but it can be embarrassing and make it difficult to be in company. It usually lasts for a limited time right after treatment. Try to eat foods less likely to cause gas right before and after you get treatment.

Diarrhea also tends to last for a limited time after treatment. Imodium and other over-the-counter remedies usually help. Ask your doctor or nurse for other medicines if these are not helpful.

Mouth sores can be very unpleasant and can affect your mouth, throat, and nose. Try sucking on ice chips during treatment. Keeping the area cold might prevent the chemotherapy from settling in and causing side effects. Avoid hot foods for a while after treatment to reduce the chance of sores developing.

Side effects in your hands and feet (nail side effects): Chemotherapy can cause fingernails and toenails to become discolored, painful, cracked, and even fall off. You could try keeping your hands and feet in bags of ice during treatment to prevent the chemotherapy from settling in the fingers and toes.

You might need to look for roomier shoes if your toenails become painful. If you go to a dermatologist, make sure to explain that you are getting chemotherapy. The nail changes can look like fungus, and you do not want to get an antifungal treatment if you don't need it.

Hand-and-foot syndrome is similar to the nail side effects, but it happens to the skin of the hands or feet, which can become dry, blistered, cracked, and painful. You can try keeping your hands and feet "on ice" during treatment. If that doesn't work, moisturizing your hands and feet and keeping your hands in gloves and feet in socks at night can help.

Neuropathy is pain, tingling, and numbness, usually in the hands and feet. It's not the same as hand-and-foot syndrome, and it does not go away when chemotherapy is over, so it's crucial to tell your healthcare provider right away if you feel it. If neuropathy gets too severe, your doctor might decide to cut back on the chemotherapy dose or try a different treatment. There are a few treatments available to relieve some of the discomfort.

Neutropenia: Most chemotherapy treatments cause low blood counts, or neutropenia. This means you have lower than the normal amounts of red blood cells, white blood cells and platelets in your body. This can lead to:

- anemia, if your red blood counts are low;
- increased risk of infection, if your white blood cell counts are low;
- increased risk of bleeding, if your platelet levels are low.

Medicines called growth factors can help increase blood counts. Filgrastim (brand name: Neupogen) and pegfilgrastim (brand name: Neulasta) can help with white blood cell counts. Sometimes these medicines are not enough to get your white blood cell counts back up. If white blood counts stay very low between chemotherapy cycles, your doctor might adjust your treatment schedule.

Some growth factors can help increase red blood cell counts. But research shows they may be harmful to people with certain types of cancer, including breast cancer. New guidelines for these medicines limit how and when they are used. If you have anemia, which means your red blood cell counts are low, and it doesn't get better, your doctor is more likely to recommend blood transfusions than growth factors. Nowadays, transfusions are much safer than they were in the past, and they can make a big difference with severe anemia.

Chemo brain: For a long time women who took chemotherapy complained about changes in memory, concentration, and other cognitive functions. And for a long time, people thought this was mainly the result of fatigue, depression, or other symptoms of cancer.

Now research shows that these cognitive changes, known as chemo brain, may indeed be related to the chemotherapy, as well as the other causes.

Still, very little is known about how often chemo brain occurs, whether it gets better and how to best measure it. So if you're feeling fuzzy in the head and think it's from the chemotherapy or other treatments, you're not crazy. Breast cancer treatments, as well as the cancer itself, could be causing these side effects.

These issues could also be caused, or made worse, by fatigue and depression, so it is extremely important to address them.

You also may be able to find ways to help your mind stay focused and to help you remember important things.

Dealing with Side Effects of Hormonal and Targeted Therapies

Hormonal treatments affect the amount and activity of the hormones estrogen and progesterone in your body. These hormones can stimulate some types of breast cancer to grow, so lowering their impact can help slow the growth of the cancer.

With lower hormone levels, you also may have side effects that are similar to the discomforts of menopause, a time when the level of hormones in your body naturally decreases.

Sometimes, if you go through breast cancer treatment and menopause at the same time, it can be hard to know the cause of the symptoms. Many remedies work for symptoms caused both by menopause and by hormonal treatments.

Effects of hormonal treatment on younger women: If you are premenopausal and your hormonal treatment includes taking out or shutting down your ovaries, you will have menopausal symptoms. Some things to remember:

- Knowing ahead of time can help you prepare and take steps right away to lessen unpleasant side effects.

- If you are concerned about fertility (having children), you should talk to your healthcare team ahead of time about your options.

The good news is that remedies exist for many of the symptoms of menopause and side effects of hormonal treatments.

Many of the symptoms lessen over time, as your body adjusts to new, lower levels of hormones.

Hot flashes: Hot flashes are a common and unpleasant symptom of menopause and a side effect of hormonal treatment.

Not everyone has this side effect, but if you do, it can make you hot and sweaty, disrupt your sleep, and generally hurt your quality of life.

Thankfully, there are medicines that can help with hot flashes. These include:

- Antidepressants (for example: venlafaxine [brand name: Effexor]): For hot flashes you take lower doses of these medicines than you would for treating depression. It takes a while for these treatments to work against hot flashes, so be patient. It's reasonable to wait about a month to see if they are working. If by then they don't seem to lower the frequency or intensity of your hot flashes, ask for something else. Note: Research suggests that some antidepressants, including fluoxetine (brand name: Prozac), duloxetine (brand name: Cymbalta), bupropion (brand name: Wellbutrin), and paroxetine (brand name: Paxil) lower the effectiveness of tamoxifen. Talk to your doctor about which anti-depressant you might try to help with your hot flashes.

- Gabapentin (brand name: Neurontin), an antiseizure medicine: Studies suggest gabapentin can be effective in treating hot flash-es. As with antidepressants, gabapentin takes a while to work, so wait before switching to something else.

- Megestrol acetate (brand name: Megace) at low doses can be very effective in treating hot flashes, but it can also increase your appetite and lead to weight gain. This medicine is proges-terone, a hormone, so talk to your doctor about whether it might be an option for you.

- Clonidine, a blood pressure medicine, can decrease the sweating and rapid heart rate which sometimes come with hot flashes. But it can also make you feel tired and without energy. Cloni-dine may not be an option if you have low blood pressure.

Follow these lifestyle dos and don'ts. Do:

- Wear layers of cotton clothes that you can easily take on and off.

- Find a moderate exercise routine that works for you.

- Try relaxation, acupuncture, or other complementary methods that can help with overall well-being and sometimes specifically with hot flashes.

Don't:

- Take hot showers or baths.

- Eat spicy foods.

- Drink alcohol.

- Drink caffeine.

- Smoke.

Vaginal dryness/discomfort: This symptom of menopause or side effect of hormonal treatment can be hard to deal with because your doctor may not mention it, and you may find it embarrassing to talk about.

It's important to try to get past the embarrassment if vaginal dryness is bothering you, or if it makes sex unpleasant or painful. Over-the-counter lubricants and vaginal moisturizers can help. Prescription vaginal estrogens also can be very effective. However, this type of treatment involves hormones that can affect breast cancer growth, so talk to your doctor about whether it may be right for you.

Loss of libido: Overall loss of libido, or sexual drive, can be the real problem with hormonal treatments (and breast cancer treatments in general), rather than the more specific symptoms of hot flashes or vaginal dryness.

Loss of libido can result from so many different things, including the hormonal changes caused by hormonal therapy, but also the general physical discomfort caused by multiple treatments, as well as psychological factors. As several women we talked to put it: "When you're going through all these difficult treatments for advanced breast cancer, who has the time, energy, or desire to have sex?"

But if you're in an intimate relationship with a partner, loss of libido can become a serious issue that you want to address. You can try creating a romantic atmosphere, experimenting with different types of physical intimacy, and so on, but many women say this type of advice misses the point.

What you and your partner really need are patience and open communication, both in and out of the bedroom, so you can:

- acknowledge each other's fears about physical intimacy;
- reassure your partner that she or he will not hurt you by initiating physical intimacy;
- let your partner know you may not want to initiate intimacy, but that it's OK if she or he does;
- discuss what makes you feel good physically and what feels uncomfortable or painful.

It also can help to know that you are not alone. There are other women who are going through similar experiences.

Bone loss/bone pain: Bone loss and bone pain can be caused by hormonal treatment and also by metastases to the bone.

Menopause also contributes to bone loss. While you're on hormonal treatment, or if you have metastases in your bones, you will have different types of bone scans to monitor for bone loss and fractures, and to see how well treatments you get might be working.

431

Some of these treatments may include:

- Medicines called bisphosphonates: These help with some bone problems. They can reduce pain and lower the risk of fractures. Research suggests that they can even help slow the growth of cancer that has spread to the bones. Two of these medicines are pamidronate (brand name: Aredia) and zoledronic acid (brand name: Zometa). A serious but rare side effect of these medicines is osteonecrosis of the jaw, which means that the jawbone becomes brittle and can splinter and break. Because this is a rare side effect that takes a while to develop, you and your doctors may not be looking out for it. Although it does not happen often, when it does, it can be very upsetting, and you may realize what it is too late to lessen the damage. Although the chances that you will have this side effect are small, try to get any dental work you need before starting this type of treatment. And if you start to feel jaw pain, tell your doctor about it right away, before it becomes a serious problem. Rarely, bisphosphonates can cause side effects in the kidneys, so your doctor may order regular blood tests to monitor them. Depending on the test results, your doctor may adjust the dose of the medicine.

- Kyphoplasty: In this procedure a cement-like substance is injected into the bones to strengthen them from the inside. If your bones are very weak and at high risk for fractures, kyphoplasty might be an option to consider.

- Exercise and weight loss: Although it's hard to exercise when you're in pain, the right amount and type of exercise can ease painful bones as well as other body aches and pains. Losing weight helps lower the load that weak bones have to bear. The most important thing to remember is to listen to your body and find the right type and level of exercise for you.

Muscle and joint pain: Sometimes you may feel pain in your muscles or joints and think that you twisted or hurt something while exercising. In fact, these aches and pains can be caused by various breast cancer treatments, especially hormonal therapy and some targeted therapies.

Be sure to mention any pain or discomfort you're feeling to your healthcare team so you can figure out what is causing it and how to relieve it. There may be exercises that can help stop the pain. If pain really bothers you, medicine also can help.

Other side effects: Even though targeted, or biological, therapies generally have fewer side effects than chemotherapy, you may still have some side effects.

In rare cases trastuzumab (brand name: Herceptin), which is used in HER2 [human epidermal growth factor receptor 2] positive breast cancer, can weaken the heart. This can put you at risk for congestive heart failure, a weakening of the heart that leads to fluid build-up. Your doctor will monitor your heart before and during treatment. If your heart suffers any damage, your doctor might stop the treatment. This heart damage usually is not permanent—once you stop treatment, it goes away—but it can sometimes persist. Trastuzumab also can cause runny nose, watery eyes, and mild diarrhea.

Lapatinib (brand name: Tykerb), another treatment for metastatic HER2 positive breast cancer, can cause diarrhea, which is treated with over-the-counter or prescription diarrhea medicines. It can also cause a skin rash. If the rash is more than mild, your doctor can give you antibiotics or steroids to put on the skin.

Chapter 48

Fatigue after Cancer Treatment

Fatigue occurs in 14% to 96% of people with cancer, especially those receiving treatment for their cancer. Fatigue is complex, and has biological, psychological, and behavioral causes. Fatigue is difficult to describe and people with cancer may express it in different ways, such as saying they feel tired, weak, exhausted, weary, worn-out, heavy, or slow. Health professionals may use terms such as asthenia, fatigue, lassitude, prostration, exercise intolerance, lack of energy, and weakness to describe fatigue.

Fatigue can be described as a condition that causes distress and decreased ability to function due to a lack of energy. Specific symptoms may be physical, psychological, or emotional. To be treated effectively, fatigue related to cancer and cancer treatment needs to be distinguished from other kinds of fatigue.

Fatigue may be acute or chronic. Acute fatigue is normal tiredness with occasional symptoms that begin quickly and last for a short time. Rest may alleviate fatigue and allow a return to a normal level of functioning in a healthy individual. Chronic fatigue syndrome describes prolonged debilitating fatigue that may persist or relapse, and is not related to cancer. Fatigue related to cancer is called chronic because it lasts over a period of time and is not completely relieved by sleep and rest. Chronic fatigue diagnosed in patients with cancer may be called "cancer fatigue," "cancer-related fatigue," or "cancer treatment-related fatigue." Although

Excerpted from PDQ® Cancer Information Summary. National Cancer Institute; Bethesda, MD. Fatigue (PDQ): Patient version. Updated 11/2011. Available at: www.cancer.gov. Accessed February 7, 2012.

many treatment- and disease-related factors may cause fatigue, the exact process of fatigue in people with cancer is not known.

Fatigue can become a very important issue in the life of a person with cancer. It may affect how the person feels about him- or herself, his or her daily activities, family care, and relationships with others, and whether he or she continues with cancer treatment. Patients receiving some cancer treatments may miss work or school, withdraw from friends, need more sleep, and, in some cases, may not be able to think clearly or perform any physical activities because of fatigue. Finances can become difficult if people with fatigue need to take disability leave or stop working completely. Job loss may result in the loss of health insurance or the inability to get medical care. Understanding fatigue and its causes is important in determining effective treatment and in helping people with cancer cope with fatigue. Tests that measure the level of fatigue have been developed.

How long fatigue lasts and how much fatigue the patient feels depends on the type and schedule of cancer treatment. For example, patients treated with cycles of chemotherapy usually have the most fatigue in the days following treatment, then less fatigue until the next treatment. Patients treated with external-beam radiation therapy usually have more fatigue as their treatment continues. It is likely that most patients beginning cancer treatment already feel fatigued following diagnostic tests, surgery, and the emotional distress of coping with a cancer diagnosis.

Causes

Most of the causes of fatigue in patients with cancer are poorly understood, and patients are likely to be coping with many possible causes of fatigue at the same time. Fatigue commonly is an indicator of disease progression and is frequently one of the first symptoms of cancer in both children and adults. For example, parents of a child diagnosed with acute lymphocytic leukemia or non-Hodgkin lymphoma frequently seek medical care because of the child's extreme fatigue. Tumors can cause fatigue directly or indirectly by spreading to the bone marrow, causing anemia, and by forming toxic substances in the body that interfere with normal cell functions. People who are having problems breathing, another symptom of some cancers, may also experience fatigue.

Fatigue can occur for many reasons. The extreme stress that people with cancer experience over a long period of time can cause them to use more energy, leading to fatigue. However, there may be other reasons that patients with cancer suffer from fatigue. The central nervous system (the brain and spinal cord) may be affected by the cancer or the cancer therapy (especially biological therapy) and cause fatigue. Medication to treat pain, depression, vomiting, seizures, and other problems related to cancer may also cause fatigue. Tumor necrosis factor (TNF), a protein made mainly by white blood cells, can cause necrosis (death) of some types of tumor cells and may be given to a patient as a cancer treatment. TNF may cause the loss of protein stores in muscles, making the body work harder to perform normal functions and causing fatigue. There are many chemical, physical, and behavioral factors that are thought to cause fatigue.

Factors Related to Fatigue

It is not always possible to determine the factors that cause fatigue in patients with cancer. Possible factors include the following:

- Cancer treatment
- Anemia
- Medications
- Weight loss and loss of appetite
- Changes in metabolism
- Hormone levels that are too low or too high
- Emotional distress
- Decline in physical condition
- Trouble sleeping
- Inactivity
- Trouble breathing
- Loss of strength and muscle coordination
- Pain and other symptoms
- High levels of inflammation-causing cytokines
- Poor nutrition
- Dehydration
- Infection
- Heart trouble
- Having other medical conditions in addition to cancer

Fatigue is a common symptom following radiation therapy or chemotherapy. Fatigue may also be a side effect of biologic response modifier therapy, a type of treatment to boost or restore the ability of the immune system to fight cancer, infections, and other diseases. It may be caused by anemia, or the collection of toxic substances produced by cells. In the case of radiation, it may be caused by the increased energy needed to repair damaged skin tissue.

Several factors have been linked with fatigue caused by chemotherapy. Some people may respond to the diagnosis and treatment of cancer with mood changes and disrupted sleep patterns. Nausea, vomiting, chronic pain, and weight loss can also cause fatigue.

Studies have reported that patients have the most severe fatigue around mid-way through all the cycles of chemotherapy. Fatigue decreases after chemotherapy is finished, but patients often don't feel back to normal even 30 days after the last treatment.

Fatigue during cancer treatment may be increased by the following factors:

• Pain

• Depression

• Anxiety

• Anemia (Some types of chemotherapy keep the bone marrow from making enough new red blood cells, causing anemia—too few red blood cells to carry oxygen to the body).

• Lack of sleep caused by certain anticancer drugs

Many patients undergoing radiation therapy report fatigue that keeps them from being as active as they want to be. After radiation therapy begins, fatigue usually increases until mid-way through the course of treatments and then stays about the same until treatments end. Fatigue usually lessens after the therapy is completed, but some fatigue may last for months or years following treatment. Patients who are older, have advanced disease, or receive combination therapy (for example, chemotherapy plus radiation therapy) are at a higher risk for developing long-term fatigue.

In men with prostate cancer, fatigue was increased by having the following symptoms before radiation therapy started:

• Poor sleep

• Depression

• Anxiety

438

- Pain

In women with breast cancer, fatigue was increased by the following:

- Working while undergoing radiation therapy
- Having children at home
- Depression
- Anxiety
- Poor sleep
- Younger age
- Being underweight
- Having advanced cancer or other medical conditions

Biological therapy frequently causes fatigue. In this setting, fatigue is one of a group of side effects known as flu-like syndrome. This syndrome also includes fever, chills, muscle pain, headache, and a sense of generally not feeling well. Some patients may also experience problems with their ability to think clearly. The type of biological therapy used may determine the type and pattern of fatigue experienced.

Many people with cancer undergo surgery for diagnosis or treatment. Fatigue is a problem following surgery, but fatigue from surgery improves with time. It can be made worse, however, when combined with the fatigue caused by other cancer treatments.

Anemia

Anemia may be a major factor in cancer-related fatigue and quality of life in people with cancer. Anemia may be caused by the cancer, cancer treatment, or may be related to other medical causes.

Nutrition Factors

Fatigue often occurs when the body needs more energy than the amount being supplied from the patient's diet. In people with cancer, three major factors may be involved, including a change in the body's ability to process food normally, an increased need by the body for energy (due to tumor growth, infection, fever, or problems with breathing), and a decrease in the amount of food eaten (due to lack of appetite, nausea, vomiting, diarrhea, or bowel obstruction).

Psychological Factors

The moods, beliefs, attitudes, and reactions to stress of people with cancer can also contribute to the development of fatigue. Anxiety and depression are the most common psychological disorders that cause fatigue.

Depression may be a disabling illness that affects approximately 15% to 25% of people who have cancer. When patients experience depression (loss of interest, difficulty concentrating, mental and physical tiredness, and feelings of hopelessness), the fatigue from physical causes can become worse and last longer than usual, even after the physical causes are gone. Anxiety and fear associated with a cancer diagnosis, as well as its impact on a person's physical, mental, social, and financial well-being are sources of emotional stress. Distress from being diagnosed with cancer may be all that is needed to trigger fatigue. Some patients report having more fatigue after cancer treatments than others do. Studies have found that patients who worry about or expect fatigue before, during, or after treatment may be more likely to report having fatigue.

Mental Ability Factors

Decreased attention span and difficulty understanding and thinking are often associated with fatigue. Attention problems are common during and after cancer treatment. Attention may be restored by activities that encourage rest. Sleep is also necessary for relieving attention problems but it is not always enough.

Sleep Disorders and Inactivity

Disrupted sleep, poor sleep habits, less sleep at night, sleeping a lot during the day, or no activity during the day may contribute to cancer-related fatigue. Patients who are less active during the daytime and awaken frequently during the night report higher levels of cancer-related fatigue.

Poor sleep affects people in different ways. For example, the time of day that fatigue is worse may be different. Some patients who have trouble sleeping may feel more fatigue in the morning. Others may have periods of severe fatigue in both the morning and the evening.

Even in patients who have poor sleep, correcting sleep problems does not always decrease fatigue. A lack of sleep may not be what is causing the fatigue.

Medications

Medications other than those used in chemotherapy may also contribute to fatigue. Opioids used in treating cancer-related pain often cause drowsiness, the extent of which may vary depending on the individual. Taking opioids over time may lower the amount of sex hormones made in the testes in men and the ovaries in women. This can lead to fatigue as well as sexual dysfunction and depression. Other types of medications such as tricyclic antidepressants and antihistamines may also produce the side effect of drowsiness. Taking several medications may compound fatigue symptoms.

Assessment

To determine the cause and best treatment for fatigue, the person's fatigue pattern must be determined, and all of the factors causing the fatigue must be identified. The doctor will look for causes of fatigue that can be treated. The following factors must be included:

1. Fatigue pattern, including how and when it started, how long it has lasted, and its severity, plus any factors that make fatigue worse or better

2. Type and degree of disease and of treatment-related symptoms and/or side effects

3. Treatment history

4. Current medications

5. Sleep and/or rest patterns and relaxation habits

6. Eating habits and appetite or weight changes

7. Effects of fatigue on activities of daily living and lifestyle

8. Psychological profile, including an evaluation for depression

9. Complete physical examination that includes evaluation of walking patterns, posture, and joint movements

10. How well the patient is able to follow the recommended treatment

11. Job performance

12. Financial resources

13. Other factors (for example, anemia, breathing problems, decreased muscle strength)

Underlying factors that contribute to fatigue should be evaluated and treated when possible. Contributing factors include anemia, depression, anxiety, pain, dehydration, nutritional deficiencies, sedating medications, and therapies that may have poorly tolerated side effects. Patients should tell their doctors when they are experiencing fatigue and ask for information about fatigue related to underlying causes and treatment side effects.

Anemia Evaluation

There are different kinds of anemia. A medical history, a physical examination, and blood tests may be used to determine the kind and extent of anemia that a person may have. In people with cancer there may be several causes.

Treatment

Most of the treatments for fatigue in cancer patients are for treating symptoms and providing emotional support because the causes of fatigue that are specifically related to cancer have not been determined. Some of these symptom-related treatments may include adjusting the dosages of pain medications, administering red blood cell transfusions or blood cell growth factors, diet supplementation with iron and vitamins, and antidepressants or psychostimulants.

Psychostimulant Drugs

Fatigue in patients who have depression may be treated with antidepressant or psychostimulant drugs. Psychostimulants may help some patients have more energy and a better mood, and may help them think and concentrate. The use of psychostimulants for treating fatigue is still under study. The doctor may prescribe low doses of a psychostimulant to be used for a short time in advanced cancer patients with severe fatigue.

Psychostimulants have side effects, especially with long-term use. Different psychostimulants have different side effects. Patients who have heart problems or are taking anticancer drugs that affect the heart may have serious side effects from psychostimulants. These drugs have boxed warnings on the label about their risks. It is important to talk with a doctor about the effects these drugs may have and use them only under a doctor's care. Some of the possible side effects include the following:

- Trouble sleeping

- Euphoria (feelings of extreme happiness)

- Headache

- Nausea

- Anxiety

- Mood changes

- Loss of appetite

- Nightmares

- Paranoia (feelings of fear and distrust of other people)

- Serious heart problems

Treatment for Anemia

Treatment for fatigue that is related to anemia may include red blood cell transfusions. Transfusions are an effective treatment for anemia; however possible side effects include infection, immediate transfusion reaction, graft-versus-host disease, and changes in immunity.

The use of drugs that cause the bone marrow to make more red blood cells may be considered for treating anemia-related fatigue in patients undergoing chemotherapy. Epoetin alfa and darbepoetin alfa are two of these drugs. This type of drug may shorten survival time, increase the risk of serious heart problems, and cause some tumors to grow faster. Patients should discuss the risks and benefits of these drugs with their doctors.

Exercise

Moderate activity for three to five hours a week may help cancer-related fatigue. Choosing a type of exercise that will be enjoyed makes an exercise plan more likely to be followed. The health care team can help with planning the best time and place for exercise and how often to exercise. Patients may need to start with light activity for short periods of time and build up to more exercise little by little. Studies have shown that exercise can be safely done during and after active cancer treatment.

People with cancer who exercise may have more physical energy, improved appetite, improved ability to function, improved quality of life, improved outlook, improved sense of well-being, enhanced sense of commitment, and improved ability to meet the challenges of cancer and cancer treatment. Findings from a study of breast cancer survivors suggest that patients may be able to lessen fatigue and pain and function better in daily activities if they take part in moderate to vigorous recreational sports after cancer treatment.

Exercise may also help patients with advanced cancer, even those in hospice care. More benefit may result when family members are involved with the patient in the physical therapy program.

Mind and body exercises such as qigong, tai chi, and yoga may also help relieve fatigue. These exercises combine activities like movement, stretching, balance, and controlled breathing with mental exercise such as meditation.

Cognitive Behavior Therapy

Cognitive behavior therapy (CBT) is a method used by therapists to treat a variety of psychological disorders. CBT aims to change a patient's awareness (the cognitive) in order to change the way he acts (the behavior). CBT sessions may be helpful in decreasing a patient's fatigue following cancer treatment by focusing on factors such as the following:

- Stress from coping with the experience of having cancer

- Fear that the cancer may come back

- Abnormal attitudes about fatigue

- Irregular sleep or activity patterns

- Lack of social support

Activity and Rest

Any changes in daily routine require the body to use more energy. People with cancer should set priorities and keep a reasonable schedule. Health professionals can help patients by providing information about support services to help with daily activities and responsibilities. An activity and rest program can be developed with a health care professional to make the most of a patient's energy. Practicing sleep habits such as not lying down at times other than for sleep, taking short naps no longer than one hour, and limiting distracting noise (TV, radio) during sleep may improve sleep and allow more activity during the day.

444

Patient Education

Treating chronic fatigue in patients with cancer means accepting the condition and learning how to cope with it. People with cancer may find that fatigue becomes a chronic disability. Although fatigue is frequently an expected, temporary side effect of treatment, other factors may cause it to continue. Learning the facts about cancer-related fatigue may help patients cope with it better and improve their quality of life. For example, some patients in active treatment worry that fatigue is a sign that the treatment is not working. They may feel that reporting fatigue is complaining. Anxiety over this can make fatigue even worse. Knowing that fatigue is a normal side effect that should be reported and treated may make it easier to manage.

Since fatigue is the most common symptom in people receiving outpatient chemotherapy, patients should learn ways to manage the fatigue. Patients should be taught the following:

- The difference between fatigue and depression
- Possible medical causes of fatigue (not enough fluids, electrolyte imbalance, breathing problems, anemia)
- To observe their rest and activity patterns during the day and over time
- To engage in attention-restoring activities (walking, gardening, bird watching)
- To recognize fatigue that is a side effect of certain therapies
- To participate in exercise programs that are realistic
- To identify activities which cause fatigue and develop ways to avoid or modify those activities
- To identify environmental or activity changes that may help decrease fatigue
- The importance of eating enough food and drinking enough fluids
- Physical therapy to help with nerve or muscle weakness
- Respiratory therapy to help with breathing problems
- To schedule important daily activities during times of less fatigue, and cancel unimportant activities that cause stress
- To avoid or change a situation that causes stress
- To observe whether treatments being used to help fatigue are working

Chapter 49

Infection after Breast Cancer Treatment

Infection Risks

A major factor in breast cancer survival is avoiding infection. Unfortunately, the most common breast cancer treatments actually increase the risk of developing a life-threatening infection. Lumpectomies, mastectomies, and radiation provide easy access points. Furthermore, chemotherapy provides the perfect environment for infections to thrive. Taking certain precautions can reduce these risks while helping to maintain the quality of life for those with breast cancer.

Chemotherapy

Chemotherapy works by destroying rapidly multiplying cells, and this targets fast-dividing cancer cells. Unfortunately, cancer cells are not the only fast-dividing cells in the human body. Some normal cell types also divide quickly, including cells in the skin, the gastrointestinal tract, and the white blood cells called neutrophils. Chemotherapy also hurts these normal cells, and numbers of protective neutrophils can drop very low. Without adequate white blood cells, the body is vulnerable to infections that it otherwise would be able to fight off. Even typically mild illnesses, such as the flu, can become life-threatening if the body is unable to mount an effective response due to low white blood cell counts.

"Guarding against Infection," by Valarie Juntunen. © 2010 Omnigraphics, Inc. All rights reserved.

Neutropenia is the condition where the number of neutrophils sinks to dangerously low levels. Due to the risk of a life-threatening infection, chemotherapy treatments may need to be decreased or stopped until the neutrophil levels increase. This can decrease the effectiveness of chemotherapy. Additionally, neutropenia may require extended hospitalizations with intravenous (IV) antibiotic treatment and isolation precautions.

During chemotherapy treatments your physician will carefully monitor your white blood cell count. There are various tests and calculations that can be used to measure the number of white blood cells but the most commonly monitored during chemotherapy treatment is the absolute neutrophil count (ANC). According to the American Cancer Society, neutropenic levels start when the ANC falls below 1,000 with severe neutropenia occurring at levels below 500.

Permanent venous access points, such as central lines, may be used to make chemotherapy easier but they can also be a conduit for infection. Keep these areas dry. Wrap the access point with plastic wrap prior to showering. Discuss dressing changes around these access points with your physician or nurse.

Surgery

Any opening in the skin is a portal for infection, including surgical lumpectomies or mastectomies. The larger the incision or the more involved the surgery, the greater the risk for infection. Surgical teams take special precautions to minimize the risk of infection but it is important that follow-up care be performed exactly as recommended by the physician.

Avoid changing the bandage until directed to do so by the physician. If you notice, prior to the first scheduled dressing change, that bleeding or drainage has soaked the bandage, reinforce it with a clean, dry bandage and contact the physician. Any necessary dressing changes should be done as scheduled. Always wash your hands thoroughly prior to initiating any dressing change and avoid any unnecessary touching of the incision.

In some cases, mastectomy patients have a drain in place to help remove excess fluids from the area. This drain is another potential portal for infection. Make sure your hands are washed prior to emptying the drain and that the drainage spout does not come into contact with another surface.

Watch for any sign of infection, especially at the incision or drain site. Signs of infection include redness, swelling, excessive drainage, and fever. Remember that depending on other treatments, the risk for infection continues long past the date when the dressing is removed. If at any time you notice excessive warmth or tenderness at the site, contact your physician.

Mastectomies often require the removal of associated lymph nodes. This drastically increases the risk for infection on the affected side. The lymphatic system works with the immune system to reduce the risk of serious infection by providing a conduit for white blood cell-rich lymph fluid.

An infection on the side of the body where the lymph nodes have been removed can also cause lymphedema (swelling from excess lymph fluids). As the body responds to the infection, more lymph fluid is produced and with the disrupted pathway, the lymph fluids begin to back up, resulting in severe swelling which, in turn, decreases the ability to fight off the infection.

Radiation

Unlike chemotherapy, radiation destroys susceptible cells at a local level only. Often radiation is used after a mastectomy where the lymph nodes have been removed as well. The addition of radiation can cause increased lymphedema. It also can cause localized tissue damage that increases the risk for infection. Radiation may even lower overall white blood counts by a small margin.

Infection Prevention

In most cases, there will come a time during your treatment that you will want to return to your normal activities, like work or social engagements. Your physician will inform you if you need to remain isolated due to dangerously low neutrophil levels, but once cleared to do so you can safely return to your life, with just a few added precautions.

Hygiene

Infection control during cancer treatment requires some lifestyle modifications and skills. Proper hand washing with warm water and soap is particularly important. Always wash your hands after using the restroom, before and after eating, after touching a pet or animal, and upon entering your home. Remember to use antibacterial hand soap and to rinse your hands thoroughly. Let your hands air dry or use disposable paper towel. Keep liquid hand sanitizer or antibacterial hand wipes with you for those times where a sink is unavailable.

In addition to proper hand washing, it is important that you pay attention to your toileting. Bladder infections can be particularly dangerous. Shower instead of soaking in a bathtub. Drink plenty of water. Urinate frequently to reduce the length of time that urine can house infecting bacteria in the bladder. Women should always wipe from front to back to avoid contaminating the urethra, the opening to the urinary tract, with bacteria from the intestines that is present in all feces.

Due to the bacteria in fecal matter, the rectum is another potential source for infection. Notify your physician if you have hemorrhoids and avoid straining to have bowel movements. Avoid using suppositories and enemas. Consult your physician about using a stool softener if constipation is an issue. Consider using personal cleansing wipes or soap and water to clean after using the restroom.

Oral hygiene is also critically important. Chemotherapy can cause damage to the gums, lips, and other tissues in the mouth and since the mouth holds many types of bacteria, any mouth sores are prone to infection. Use a mirror and flashlight to check your mouth for any open sores. Keep your mouth moisturized with saliva-producing mouthwash or gum. Avoid mouthwashes that contain alcohol. Brush your teeth with a soft toothbrush three times daily. Replace your toothbrush each month and keep it clean and dry in between uses. Avoid using floss if you develop any mouth irritation from chemotherapy. Consult your dentist throughout chemotherapy treatment and seek immediate dental treatment if you notice any open sores, cavities, or loose teeth.

Consult your physician about any piercings or tattoos you may have. Often it is advisable to remove jewelry from piercings for the duration of chemotherapy treatment. Monitor these sites for warmth, swelling, and drainage.

Environment

People are the number-one source of infection for other people. Avoid people that have recently been ill, have recently had a vaccination, and anyone that currently has symptoms such as a rash, coughing, or sneezing. Keep your distance from any children not immediately related to you and emphasize the need for immediate family members to maintain hand hygiene and to avoid coming in close contact with you if they have had a recent vaccination or illness.

Try to avoid crowds. Whenever crowds are unavoidable, try to attend outdoor venues like outdoor markets, cafés, or concerts. Indoor air recirculates and increases the chance of virus or bacterial transmission. Also consider going shopping or attending events when they will be less crowded, like late at night or mid-morning on a weekday. In any environment, keep a four-foot space between you and strangers. Also consider wearing a mask if your neutrophil count is on the lower side or if you expect that you may come into contact with individuals who are ill or are likely to carry illnesses, like at the doctor's office.

Certain places should be avoided throughout chemotherapy treatments. These include pet stores, day care centers, elementary schools, crowded theaters, indoor concerts or bars, crowded restaurants, swimming pools, and hot tubs. Remember that areas that are damp are particularly prone to facilitating infections. Traveling can also be particularly problematic. Travel by private vehicle whenever possible. Avoid public transportation unless as a last resort and wear a face mask.

Other places may require advanced planning prior to attending. At church or school, choose a seat at the back or front of the building where you can space yourself away from others. Schedule your arrival so that you arrive separately from crowds, either earlier or later and plan on leaving later than most others.

At work, it is important that you be honest with coworkers. Prepare them by explaining the disruption to the immune system and the need for assistance in reducing your risk of infection. If possible, work outside or in a private office. Place liquid hand sanitizer by the door and request anyone entering your office or work space to use it. Keep a face mask handy for anyone who has recently been ill or wear one yourself if your neutrophil levels are particularly low. Use antimicrobial wipes to wipe off telephones, door handles, and computer mice.

Food Preparation

Proper food preparation is a must because intestinal infections may cause or worsen diarrhea and vomiting. Keep the kitchen area, utensils, and sinks clean but avoid using sponges that can just move bacteria around. Thaw meat in the refrigerator and heat all meat to recommended temperatures, using a meat thermometer for confirmation. Avoid raw foods whenever possible. Make sure all produce is properly cleaned. Do not use wooden cutting boards and keep raw meat and blood away from fresh foods. Immediately refrigerate all leftovers and discard any that may be contaminated or that have been in the refrigerator for longer than 48 hours. Do not share dishes or utensils with others. All drinking water should be filtered. Avoid raw herbs or produce that cannot be thoroughly cleaned prior to consuming. Consult your physician prior to ingesting any foods with active bacterial cultures, such as yogurts.

451

Whenever possible prepare your own food but if you must eat outside your home, avoid fast food or buffet dining. Order simple foods and request that all food be cooked well done. Avoid casseroles or salads that require many components. Always eat hot food and return any food that is not served hot. Request bottled drinks rather than tap or poured drinks.

Besides avoiding infections through food, nutrition can help boost the immune system and prevent infections from other sources. Increasing water intake can help prevent bladder and intestinal infections. High-fiber diets can help reduce constipation, thereby reducing the risk of infections from anal tearing. High protein and high calorie foods, like meats and peanut butter, are needed to heal any tissue damage caused by surgical interventions or radiation treatments. Nutrients such as vitamin C, found in citrus fruits and peppers, have been shown to boost wound healing, improve gum and mouth health, and make the most of immune responses. Consider consulting a nutritionist for nutritional guidance during chemotherapy.

Reproductive Tract

Women should use sanitary napkins rather than tampons and should avoid douching. Monitor for any increase in vaginal discharge. Report any changes in amount, consistency, and odor to your physician. Do not treat yeast infections with over-the-counter products unless advised to do so by your physician. Vaginal contraceptive inserts and gels should be used with caution to avoid pinching or tearing of the sensitive tissues. Always wash your hands before using any vaginal products.

Intercourse should be avoided during periods of severe neutropenia. Consult your physician before engaging in any sexual activity. Anal and oral sex should be avoided throughout chemotherapy and any sexual activity should be gentle. Using personal water-soluble lubrication gel may be necessary to reduce the risk of damage due to dry penetration.

Medication

Depending on the type, dosage, and duration of your chemotherapy, your physician may prescribe medications to prevent severe neutropenia. These medications increase white blood cell production by stimulating the body's natural production and are called hematopoietic growth factors or HGF. HGF medications include filgrastim (Neupogen), pegfilgrastim (Neulasta), and sargramostim (Leukine). Typically, these medications are administered via injections into the stomach, thigh, or upper arm. As with all medication, these can cause side effects and should only be prescribed when the benefits outweigh these risks.

Antibiotics may be prescribed to treat any potential infection. Generally speaking, broad spectrum, or antibiotics that treat a variety of infections, are started as soon as possible after a possible infection is diagnosed. Some common broad spectrum antibiotics include ceftazidime (Fortaz), ciprofloxacin (Cipro), and amoxicillin/clavulanate (Augmentin). These antibiotics may be given orally or through intravenous access.

Signs of Infection

If at any time during your treatment you suspect you might have developed an infection, contact your physician immediately. Some signs of infection include fever, rash, drainage, bad breath, increased diarrhea, increased vomiting, chills, cough, sneezing, increased nasal discharge, sinus drainage, ear pain, tooth pain, slow healing wounds, increased fatigue, or swelling from an unknown cause.

Mastectomy Arm Care to Prevent Infection

In order to help reduce the risk of infection, the affected arm must be protected.

1. Tell any future healthcare providers that you have had a mastectomy and on what side. If at all possible, they should avoid using that side for procedures, especially needlesticks.

2. Wear gloves when doing any potentially injury producing activities such as gardening or home repair work. Use thimbles when sewing and pay close attention when using saws, knives, or scissors.

3. Protect against hangnails, scratches, or other potential portals for infection by keeping the nails trimmed and smooth. Wash hands and soak nail area in antibacterial soap prior to doing nail care. Use nail clippers with a safety guard or a nail file. Apply lotion as needed to keep the cuticle and nail bed healthy.

4. Protect the affected side or sides from environmental injuries. Use insect repellent and sunscreen regularly.

5. Treat any injury to the skin immediately. Wash with soap and warm water. Then apply an antibiotic, first-aid ointment to the area and cover with a bandage. Monitor the site for signs of infection and report any redness, warmth, or excessive discharge to your physician immediately.

Chapter 50

Lymphedema

Lymphedema occurs when the lymph system is damaged or blocked. Fluid builds up in soft body tissues and causes swelling. It is a common problem that may be caused by cancer and cancer treatment. Lymphedema usually affects an arm or leg, but it can also affect other parts of the body. Lymphedema can cause long-term physical, psychological, and social problems for patients.

The lymph system is a network of lymph vessels, tissues, and organs that carry lymph throughout the body.

The parts of the lymph system that play a direct part in lymphedema include the following:

- Lymph: A clear fluid that contains lymphocytes (white blood cells) that fight infection and the growth of tumors. Lymph also contains plasma, the watery part of the blood that carries the blood cells.

- Lymph vessels: A network of thin tubes that helps lymph flow through the body and returns it to the bloodstream.

- Lymph nodes: Small, bean-shaped structures that filter lymph and store white blood cells that help fight infection and disease. Lymph nodes are located along the network of lymph vessels found throughout the body. Clusters of lymph nodes are found in the underarm, pelvis, neck, abdomen, and groin.

Excerpted from PDQ® Cancer Information Summary. National Cancer Institute; Bethesda, MD. Lymphedema (PDQ)—Patient version. Updated 08/2011. Available at: www.cancer.gov. Accessed January 27, 2012.

The spleen, thymus, tonsils, and bone marrow are also part of the lymph system but do not play a direct part in lymphedema.

Lymphedema occurs when lymph is not able to flow through the body the way that it should.

When the lymph system is working as it should, lymph flows through the body and is returned to the bloodstream.

- Fluid and plasma leak out of the capillaries (smallest blood vessels) and flow around body tissues so the cells can take up nutrients and oxygen.

- Some of this fluid goes back into the bloodstream. The rest of the fluid enters the lymph system through tiny lymph vessels. These lymph vessels pick up the lymph and move it toward the heart. The lymph is slowly moved through larger and larger lymph vessels and passes through lymph nodes where waste is filtered from the lymph.

- The lymph keeps moving through the lymph system and collects near the neck, then flows into one of two large ducts:
  - The right lymph duct collects lymph from the right arm and the right side of the head and chest.
  - The left lymph duct collects lymph from both legs, the left arm, and the left side of the head and chest.

- These large ducts empty into veins under the collarbones, which carry the lymph to the heart, where it is returned to the bloodstream.

When part of the lymph system is damaged or blocked, fluid cannot drain from nearby body tissues. Fluid builds up in the tissues and causes swelling.

Types of Lymphedema

There are two types of lymphedema. Lymphedema may be either primary or secondary:

- Primary lymphedema is caused by the abnormal development of the lymph system. Symptoms may occur at birth or later in life.

- Secondary lymphedema is caused by damage to the lymph system. The lymph system may be damaged or blocked by infection, injury, cancer, removal of lymph nodes, radiation to the affected area, or scar tissue from radiation therapy or surgery.

This text is about secondary lymphedema in adults that is caused by cancer or cancer treatment.

Signs of Lymphedema

Possible signs of lymphedema include swelling of the arms or legs. Other conditions may cause the same symptoms. A doctor should be consulted if any of the following problems occur:

- Swelling of an arm or leg, which may include fingers and toes
- A full or heavy feeling in an arm or leg
- A tight feeling in the skin
- Trouble moving a joint in the arm or leg
- Thickening of the skin, with or without skin changes such as blisters or warts
- A feeling of tightness when wearing clothing, shoes, bracelets, watches, or rings
- Itching of the legs or toes
- A burning feeling in the legs
- Trouble sleeping
- Loss of hair

Daily activities and the ability to work or enjoy hobbies may be affected by lymphedema.

These symptoms may occur very slowly over time or more quickly if there is an infection or injury to the arm or leg.

Cancer and Lymphedema

Cancer and its treatment are risk factors for lymphedema.

Lymphedema can occur after any cancer or treatment that affects the flow of lymph through the lymph nodes, such as removal of lymph nodes. It may develop within days or many years after treatment. Most lymphedema develops within three years of surgery. Risk factors for lymphedema include the following:

- Removal and/or radiation of lymph nodes in the underarm, groin, pelvis, or neck (The risk of lymphedema increases with the number of lymph nodes affected. There is less risk with the removal of only the sentinel lymph node—the first lymph node to receive lymphatic drainage from a tumor.)

457

- Being overweight or obese

- Slow healing of the skin after surgery

- A tumor that affects or blocks the left lymph duct or lymph nodes or vessels in the neck, chest, underarm, pelvis, or abdomen

- Scar tissue in the lymph ducts under the collarbones, caused by surgery or radiation therapy

Lymphedema often occurs in breast cancer patients who had all or part of their breast removed and axillary (underarm) lymph nodes removed. Lymphedema in the legs may occur after surgery for uterine cancer, prostate cancer, lymphoma, or melanoma. It may also occur with vulvar cancer or ovarian cancer.

Tests for Lymphedema

Tests that examine the lymph system are used to diagnose lymphedema.

It is important to make sure there are no other causes of swelling, such as infection or blood clots. The following tests and procedures may be used to diagnose lymphedema:

- Physical exam and history: An exam of the body to check general signs of health, including checking for signs of disease, such as lumps or anything else that seems unusual. A history of the patient's health habits and past illnesses and treatments will also be taken.

- Lymphoscintigraphy: A procedure used to make pictures (called scintigrams) of the lymph system to check for blockages or anything else that seems unusual. A radioactive substance is injected under the skin, between the first and second fingers or toes of each hand or foot. The substance is taken up by the lymph vessels and detected by a scanner. The scanner makes images of the flow of the substance through the lymph system on a computer screen.

- MRI (magnetic resonance imaging): A procedure that uses a magnet, radio waves, and a computer to make a series of detailed pictures of areas inside the body. This procedure is also called nuclear magnetic resonance imaging (NMRI).

The swollen arm or leg is usually measured and compared to the other arm or leg. Measurements are taken over time to see how well treatment is working.

A grading system is also used to diagnose and describe lymphedema. Grades 1, 2, 3, and 4 are based on size of the affected limb and how severe the signs and symptoms are.

Stages of Lymphedema

Stages may be used to describe lymphedema.

- Stage I: The limb (arm or leg) is swollen and feels heavy. Pressing on the swollen area leaves a pit (dent). This stage of lymphedema may go away without treatment.

- Stage II: The limb is swollen and feels spongy. A condition called tissue fibrosis may develop and cause the limb to feel hard. Pressing on the swollen area does not leave a pit.

- Stage III: This is the most advanced stage. The swollen limb may be very large. Stage III lymphedema rarely occurs in breast cancer patients. Stage III is also called lymphostatic elephantiasis.

Managing Lymphedema

Taking preventive steps may keep lymphedema from developing. Health care providers can teach patients how to prevent and take care of lymphedema at home. If lymphedema has developed, these steps may keep it from getting worse.

Preventive steps include the following:

- Tell your doctor right away if you have any of the symptoms of lymphedema. The chance of improving the condition is better if treatment begins early. Untreated lymphedema can lead to problems that cannot be reversed.

- Keep skin and nails clean and cared for, to prevent infection. Bacteria can enter the body through a cut, scratch, insect bite, or other skin injury. Fluid that is trapped in body tissues by lymphedema makes it easy for bacteria to grow and cause infection. Look for signs of infection, such as redness, pain, swelling, heat, fever, or red streaks below the surface of the skin. Call your doctor right away if any of these signs appear. To prevent infection, do the following:

  - Use cream or lotion to keep the skin moist.

  - Treat small cuts or breaks in the skin with an antibacterial ointment.

  - Avoid needle sticks of any type into the limb (arm or leg) with lymphedema. This includes shots or blood tests.

- Use a thimble for sewing.
- Avoid testing bath or cooking water using the limb with lymphedema. There may be less feeling (touch, temperature, pain) in the affected arm or leg, and skin might burn in water that is too hot.
- Wear gloves when gardening and cooking.
- Wear sunscreen and shoes when outdoors.
- Cut toenails straight across. See a podiatrist (foot doctor) as needed to prevent ingrown nails and infections.
- Keep feet clean and dry and wear cotton socks.

- Avoid blocking the flow of fluids through the body. It is important to keep body fluids moving, especially through an affected limb or in areas where lymphedema may develop.
  - Do not cross legs while sitting.
  - Change sitting position at least every 30 minutes.
  - Wear only loose jewelry and clothes without tight bands or elastic.
  - Do not carry handbags on the arm with lymphedema.
  - Do not use a blood pressure cuff on the arm with lymphedema.
  - Do not use elastic bandages or stockings with tight bands.

- Keep blood from pooling in the affected limb.
  - Keep the limb with lymphedema raised higher than the heart when possible.
  - Do not swing the limb quickly in circles or let the limb hang down. This makes blood and fluid collect in the lower part of the arm or leg.
  - Do not apply heat to the limb.

Exercise does not increase the chance that lymphedema will develop in patients who are at risk for lymphedema. In the past, these patients were advised to avoid exercising the affected limb. Studies have now shown that slow, carefully controlled exercise is safe and may even help keep lymphedema from developing. Studies have also shown that, in breast-cancer survivors, upper-body exercise does not increase the risk that lymphedema will develop.

Chapter 51

Pain after Cancer Treatment

Overview

Cancer pain can be managed effectively in most patients with cancer or with a history of cancer. Although cancer pain cannot always be relieved completely, therapy can lessen pain in most patients. Pain management improves the patient's quality of life throughout all stages of the disease.

Flexibility is important in managing cancer pain. As patients vary in diagnosis, stage of disease, responses to pain and treatments, and personal likes and dislikes, management of cancer pain must be individualized. Patients, their families, and their health care providers must work together closely to manage a patient's pain effectively.

Assessment

To treat pain, it must be measured. The patient and the doctor should measure pain levels at regular intervals after starting cancer treatment. Checks should be done at each clinic visit, at each new report of pain, and after starting any type of treatment for pain. The cause of the pain must be identified and treated promptly.

PDQ® Cancer Information Summary. National Cancer Institute; Bethesda, MD. Pain (PDQ): Patient version. Updated 12/2011. Available at: www.cancer.gov. Accessed March 4, 2012.

Patient Self-Report

To help the health care provider determine the type and extent of the pain, cancer patients can describe the location and intensity of their pain, any aggravating or relieving factors, and their goals for pain control. The family/caregiver may be asked to report for a patient who has a communication problem involving speech, language, or a thinking impairment. The health care provider should help the patient describe the following:

- Pain: The patient describes the pain, when it started, how long it lasts, and whether it is worse during certain times of the day or night.

- Location: The patient shows exactly where the pain is on his or her body or on a drawing of a body and where the pain goes if it travels.

- Pattern: The patient describes if there have been changes in where the pain is, when the pain occurs, and how long it lasts, or if there is new pain.

- Intensity or severity: The patient keeps a diary of the degree or severity of pain.

- Aggravating and relieving factors: The patient identifies factors that increase or decrease the pain. The patient also identifies symptoms that are most troublesome, since they are not always the most serious or severe.

- Personal response to pain: Feelings of fear, confusion, or hopelessness about cancer, its prognosis, and the causes of pain can affect how a patient responds to and describes the pain. For example, a patient who thinks pain is caused by cancer spreading may report more severe pain or more disability from the pain.

- Behavioral response to pain: The health care provider and/or caregivers note behaviors that may suggest pain in patients who have communication problems.

- Goals for pain control: With the health care provider, the patient decides how much pain he or she can tolerate and how much improvement he or she may achieve. The patient uses a daily pain diary to increase awareness of pain, gain a sense of control of the pain, and receive guidance from health care providers on ways to manage the pain.

Physical Exam

The assessment will include an exam of the body to check general signs of health or anything that seems unusual, and to look for signs that the cancer has grown or spread. A history of the patient's health habits and past illnesses and treatments will also be taken. A neurological exam will be done. This is a series of questions and tests to check the brain, spinal cord, and nerve function. The exam checks the patient's mental status, ability to move and walk normally, and how well the muscles, senses, and reflexes work. The patient's psychological and spiritual well-being are evaluated. A personal and family history of substance abuse is taken. All of this information is taken as a whole to diagnose and treat the pain effectively.

Assessment of the Outcomes of Pain Management

The results of pain management should be measured by monitoring for a decrease in the severity of pain and improvement in thinking ability, emotional well-being, and social functioning. The results of taking pain medication should also be monitored. Drug addiction is rare in cancer patients. Developing a higher tolerance for a drug and becoming physically dependent on the drug for pain relief does not mean that the patient is addicted. Patients should take pain medication as prescribed by the doctor. Patients who have a history of drug abuse may tolerate higher doses of medication to control pain.

Management with Drugs

Basic Principles of Cancer Pain Management

The World Health Organization developed a three-step approach for pain management based on the severity of the pain:

- For mild to moderate pain, the doctor may prescribe a Step 1 pain medication such as aspirin, acetaminophen, or a nonsteroidal anti-inflammatory drug (NSAID). Patients should be monitored for side effects, especially those caused by NSAIDs, such as kidney, heart and blood vessel, or stomach and intestinal problems.

- When pain lasts or increases, the doctor may change the prescription to a Step 2 or Step 3 pain medication. Most patients with cancer-related pain will need a Step 2 or Step 3 medication. The doctor may skip Step 1 medications if the patient initially has moderate to severe pain.

463

- At each step, the doctor may prescribe additional drugs or treatments (for example, radiation therapy).

- The patient should take doses regularly, "by mouth, by the clock" (at scheduled times), to maintain a constant level of the drug in the body; this will help prevent recurrence of pain. If the patient is unable to swallow, the drugs are given by other routes (for example, by infusion or injection).

- The doctor may prescribe additional doses of drug that can be taken as needed for pain that occurs between scheduled doses of drug.

- The doctor will adjust the pain medication regimen for each patient's individual circumstances and physical condition.

Acetaminophen and NSAIDs

NSAIDs are effective for relief of mild pain. They may be given with opioids for the relief of moderate to severe pain. Acetaminophen also relieves pain, although it does not have the anti-inflammatory effect that aspirin and NSAIDs do. Patients, especially older patients, who are taking acetaminophen or NSAIDs should be closely monitored for side effects. Aspirin should not be given to children to treat pain.

Opioids

Opioids are very effective for the relief of moderate to severe pain. Many patients with cancer pain, however, become tolerant to opioids during long-term therapy. Therefore, increasing doses may be needed to continue to relieve pain. A patient's tolerance of an opioid or physical dependence on it is not the same as addiction (psychological dependence). Mistaken concerns about addiction can result in undertreating pain.

There are several types of opioids. Morphine is the most commonly used opioid in cancer pain management. Other commonly used opioids include hydromorphone, oxycodone, oxymorphone, methadone, fentanyl, meperidine (Demerol), tapentadol, and tramadol. The availability of several different opioids allows the doctor flexibility in prescribing a medication regimen that will meet individual patient needs.

Most patients with cancer pain will need to receive pain medication on a fixed schedule to manage the pain and prevent it from getting worse. The doctor will prescribe a dose of the opioid medication that can be taken as needed along with the regular fixed-schedule opioid to control pain that occurs between the scheduled doses. The amount of time between doses depends on which opioid the doctor prescribes.

The correct dose is the amount of opioid that controls pain with the fewest side effects. The goal is to achieve a good balance between pain relief and side effects by gradually adjusting the dose. If opioid tolerance does occur, it can be overcome by increasing the dose or changing to another opioid, especially if higher doses are needed.

Occasionally, doses may need to be decreased or stopped. This may occur when patients become pain free because of cancer treatments such as nerve blocks or radiation therapy. The doctor may also decrease the dose when the patient experiences opioid-related sedation along with good pain control, or when kidney failure develops or worsens.

Medications for pain may be given in several ways. When the patient has a working stomach and intestines, the preferred method is by mouth, since medications given orally are convenient and usually inexpensive. When patients cannot take medications by mouth, other less invasive methods may be used, such as rectally, through medication patches placed on the skin, or in the form of a nasal spray. Intravenous methods are used only when simpler, less demanding, and less costly methods are inappropriate, ineffective, or unacceptable to the patient. Patient-controlled analgesia (PCA) pumps may be used to determine the opioid dose when starting opioid therapy. Once the pain is controlled, the doctor may prescribe regular opioid doses based on the amount the patient required when using the PCA pump. Intraspinal administration of opioids combined with a local anesthetic may be helpful for some patients who have uncontrollable pain.

Patients should be watched closely for side effects of opioids. The most common side effects of opioids include nausea, sleepiness, and constipation. The doctor should discuss the side effects with patients before starting opioid treatment. Sleepiness and nausea are usually experienced when opioid treatment is started and tend to improve within a few days. Other side effects of opioid treatment include vomiting, difficulty in thinking clearly, problems with breathing, gradual overdose, and problems with sexual function. Chronic nausea and vomiting in patients receiving long-term opioid treatment may be caused by constipation.

Opioids slow down the muscle contractions and movement in the stomach and intestines resulting in hard stools. The key to effective prevention of constipation is to be sure the patient receives plenty of fluids to keep the stool soft. Unless there are problems such as a blocked bowel or diarrhea, patients will usually be given a regimen to follow to prevent constipation and information on how to manage bowel health while taking opioids.

Patients should talk to their doctor about side effects that become too bothersome or severe. Because there are differences between individual patients in the degree to which opioids may cause side effects, severe or continuing problems should be reported to the doctor. The doctor may decrease the dose of the opioid, switch to a different opioid, or switch the way the opioid is given (for example intravenous or injection rather than by mouth) to attempt to decrease the side effects.

Drugs Used with Pain Medications

Other drugs may be given at the same time as the pain medication. This is done to increase the effectiveness of the pain medication, treat symptoms, and relieve specific types of pain. These drugs include antidepressants, anticonvulsants, local anesthetics, corticosteroids, bisphosphonates, and stimulants. A monoclonal antibody called denosumab is used to prevent broken bones and other bone problems caused by solid tumors that have metastasized (spread) to bone. There are great differences in how patients respond to these drugs. Side effects are common and should be reported to the doctor.

The use of bisphosphonates may cause severe and sometimes disabling pain in the bones, joints, and/or muscles. This pain may develop after these drugs are used for days, months, or years, as compared with the fever, chills, and discomfort that may occur when intravenous bisphosphonates are first given. If severe muscle or bone pain develops, bisphosphonate therapy may need to be stopped.

The use of bisphosphonates is also linked to the risk of bisphosphonate-associated osteonecrosis (BON).

Physical, Integrative, Behavioral, and Psychosocial Interventions

Noninvasive physical, integrative, thinking and behavioral, and psychological methods can be used along with drugs and other treatments to manage pain during all phases of cancer treatment. These interventions may help with pain control both directly and indirectly, by making patients feel they have more control over events. The effectiveness of the pain interventions depends on the patient's participation in treatment and his or her ability to tell the health care provider which methods work best to relieve pain.

Physical Interventions

Weakness, muscle wasting, and muscle/bone pain may be treated with heat (a hot pack or heating pad); cold (flexible ice packs); exercise (to strengthen weak muscles, loosen stiff joints, help restore coordination and balance, and strengthen the heart); changing the position of the patient; restricting the movement of painful areas or broken bones; or controlled low-voltage electrical stimulation.

Integrative Interventions

Integrative interventions include massage therapy and acupuncture.

Massage therapy has been studied as part of supportive care in managing cancer-related pain. Massage may help improve relaxation and benefit mood. Preclinical and clinical trials show that massage therapy may help to do the following:

- Stimulate the release of endorphins (substances that relieve pain and give a feeling of well-being)
- Increase the flow of blood and lymphatic fluid
- Strengthen the effects of pain medications
- Decrease inflammation and edema
- Lower pain caused by muscle spasms and tension

Physical methods to help relieve pain have direct effects on tissues of the body and should be used with caution in patients with cancer. Studies suggest that massage therapy may be safe in patients with cancer with the following precautions:

- Avoid massaging any open wounds, bruises, or areas with skin breakdown.
- Avoid massaging directly over the tumor site.
- Avoid massaging areas with deep vein thrombosis (blood clot in a vein). Symptoms may include pain, swelling, warmth, and redness in the affected area.
- Avoid massaging soft tissue when the skin is sensitive following radiation therapy.

Acupuncture is an integrative intervention that applies needles, heat, pressure, and other treatments to one or more places on the skin called acupuncture points. Acupuncture may be used to manage pain, including cancer-related pain.

Thinking, Behavioral, and Psychosocial Interventions

Thinking, behavioral, and psychosocial interventions are also important in treating pain. These interventions help give patients a sense of control and help them develop coping skills to deal with the disease and its symptoms. Beginning these interventions early in the course of the disease is useful so that patients can learn and practice the skills while they have enough strength and energy. Several methods should be tried, and one or more should be used regularly.

- Relaxation and imagery: Simple relaxation techniques may be used for episodes of brief pain (for example, during cancer treatment procedures). Brief, simple techniques are suitable for periods when the patient's ability to concentrate is limited by severe pain, high anxiety, or fatigue.

- Hypnosis: Hypnotic techniques may be used to encourage relaxation and may be combined with other thinking/behavior methods. Hypnosis is effective in relieving pain in people who are able to concentrate and use imagery and who are willing to practice the technique.

- Redirecting thinking: Focusing attention on triggers other than pain or negative emotions that come with pain may involve distractions that are internal (for example, counting, praying, or saying things like "I can cope") or external (for example, music, television, talking, listening to someone read, or looking at something specific). Patients can also learn to monitor and evaluate negative thoughts and replace them with more positive thoughts and images.

- Patient education: Health care providers can give patients and their families information and instructions about pain and pain management and assure them that most pain can be controlled effectively. Health care providers should also discuss the major barriers that interfere with effective pain management.

- Psychological support: Short-term psychological therapy helps some patients. Patients who develop clinical depression or adjustment disorder may see a psychiatrist for diagnosis.

- Support groups and religious counseling: Support groups help many patients. Religious counseling may also help by providing spiritual care and social support.

Relaxation Exercises to Try

[Note: These exercises are adapted and reprinted with permission from McCaffery M, Beebe A: *Pain: Clinical Manual for Nursing Practice.* St. Louis, Mo: CV Mosby: 1989.]

Try this slow, rhythmic breathing exercise for relaxation:

1. Breathe in slowly and deeply, keeping your stomach and shoulders relaxed.

2. As you breathe out slowly, feel yourself beginning to relax; feel the tension leaving your body.

3. Breathe in and out slowly and regularly at a comfortable rate. Let the breath come all the way down to your stomach, as it completely relaxes.

4. To help you focus on your breathing and to breathe slowly and rhythmically: Breathe in as you say silently to yourself, "in, two, three" or each time you breathe out, say silently to yourself a word such as "peace" or "relax."

5. Do steps 1 through 4 only once or repeat steps 3 and 4 for up to 20 minutes.

6. End with a slow deep breath. As you breathe out say to yourself, "I feel alert and relaxed."

Here are some simple touch, massage, or warmth exercises:

- Brief touch or massage, such as hand holding or briefly touching or rubbing a person's shoulders can aid in relaxation.

- Try soaking feet in a basin of warm water or wrapping the feet in a warm, wet towel.

- Massage (3 to 10 minutes) the whole body or just the back, feet, or hands. If the patient is modest or cannot move or turn easily in bed, consider massage of the hands and feet.

- Use a warm lubricant. A small bowl of hand lotion may be warmed in the microwave oven or a bottle of lotion may be warmed in a sink of hot water for about 10 minutes.

- Massage for relaxation is usually done with smooth, long, slow strokes. Try several degrees of pressure along with different types of massage, such as kneading and stroking, to determine which is preferred.

Especially for the elderly person, a back rub that effectively produces relaxation may consist of no more than three minutes of slow, rhythmic stroking (about 60 strokes per minute) on both sides of the spine, from the crown of the head to the lower back. Continuous hand contact is maintained by starting one hand down the back as the other hand stops at the lower back and is raised. Set aside a regular time for the massage. This gives the patient something pleasant to anticipate.

Something may have happened to you a while ago that brought you peace or comfort. You may be able to draw on that experience to bring you peace or comfort now. Think about these questions:

- Can you remember any situation, even when you were a child, when you felt calm, peaceful, secure, hopeful, or comfortable?

- Have you ever daydreamed about something peaceful? What were you thinking?

- Do you get a dreamy feeling when you listen to music? Do you have any favorite music?

- Do you have any favorite poetry that you find uplifting or reassuring?

- Have you ever been active religiously? Do you have favorite readings, hymns, or prayers? Even if you haven't heard or thought of them for many years, childhood religious experiences may still be very soothing.

Additional points: Some of the things that may comfort you, such as your favorite music or a prayer, can probably be recorded for you. Then you can listen to the tape whenever you wish. Or, if your memory is strong, you may simply close your eyes and recall the events or words.

Active listening to recorded music may help you relax:

1. Obtain a cassette player or tape recorder and earphones or a headset. Choose a cassette of music you like. (Most people prefer fast, lively music, but some select relaxing music. Other options are comedy routines, sporting events, old radio shows, or stories.)

2. Mark time to the music; for example, tap out the rhythm with your finger or nod your head. This helps you concentrate on the music rather than on your discomfort.

3. Keep your eyes open and focus on a fixed spot or object. If you wish to close your eyes, picture something about the music.

4. Listen to the music at a comfortable volume. If the discomfort increases, try increasing the volume; decrease the volume when the discomfort decreases.

5. If this is not effective enough, try adding or changing one or more of the following: Massage your body in rhythm to the

music; try other music; or mark time to the music in more than one manner, such as tapping your foot and finger at the same time.

Many patients have found this technique to be helpful. It tends to be very popular, probably because the equipment is usually readily available and is a part of daily life. Other advantages are that it is easy to learn and not physically or mentally demanding. If you are very tired, you may simply listen to the music and omit marking time or focusing on a spot.

Radiation Therapy to Relieve Pain

Radiation therapy may be used for pain relief rather than as treatment for primary cancer in patients with cancer that has spread to the bone. Radiation may be given as local therapy directly to the tumor or to larger areas of the body. Local or whole-body radiation therapy may make pain medication and other noninvasive therapies work better by directly affecting the cause of the pain (for example, by shrinking tumor size). Radiation therapy may help patients with bone pain from cancer to move more freely with less pain.

Pain flare is an increase in pain after radiation therapy that develops before pain is relieved. Pain flare is being studied in patients receiving radiation therapy for cancer that has spread to the bone.

External Beam Radiation Therapy

External-beam radiation therapy (EBRT) is a type of radiation therapy that uses a machine to aim high-energy x-rays at the cancer from outside the body. EBRT relieves pain from cancer that has spread to the bone in many patients. Radiation therapy may be given in a single dose or divided into several smaller doses given over a period of time. Single dose schedules and multiple dose schedules of EBRT are both effective for pain relief but single dose therapy is more likely to need to be repeated. Single dose EBRT for pain relief has not been found to cause more long-term harm than multiple dose EBRT. The decision whether to have single or multiple dose EBRT may also depend on how convenient the treatments are and how much they cost.

Stereotactic Body Radiation Therapy

Stereotactic body radiation therapy (SBRT) is a type of external radiation therapy that uses special equipment to position a patient and precisely deliver radiation to tumors in the body (except the brain). This type of radiation therapy helps spare normal tissue. SBRT may be used to treat cancer that has spread to the bone, especially spinal tumors. SBRT may also be used to treat areas that have already received radiation.

Bisphosphonates with Radiation Therapy

The use of radiation therapy given together with bisphosphonates is being studied in patients with cancer that has spread to the bone. More studies are needed to find out if giving bisphosphonates with radiation therapy relieves pain better than radiation therapy alone.

Radiopharmaceuticals

Radiopharmaceuticals are drugs that contain a radioactive substance that may be used to diagnose or treat disease, including cancer. Radiopharmaceuticals may also be used to relieve pain from cancer that has spread to the bone. A single dose of a radioactive agent injected into a vein may relieve pain when cancer has spread to several areas of bone and/or when there are too many areas to treat with EBRT. Small areas of cancer may respond to radiopharmaceuticals while large areas usually do not. A second treatment may be helpful in patients whose pain does not respond to a single treatment. One study showed that more than two doses of a radioactive substance called samarium 153 may be safe and effective in patients who responded to their first dose. Radiopharmaceuticals have not been shown to prevent the need for EBRT in relieving pain from cancer that has spread to the bone.

Radiofrequency Ablation

Radiofrequency ablation uses a needle electrode to heat tumors and destroy them. An imaging method is used to insert the electrode through the skin and guide the needle to the right location. This procedure may relieve pain in patients who have cancer that has spread to the bone. More study is needed to learn about possible risks and benefits.

Invasive Interventions to Relieve Pain

Less invasive methods should be used for relieving pain before trying invasive treatment. Some patients, however, may need invasive therapy.

Nerve Blocks

A nerve block is the injection of either a local anesthetic or a drug that inactivates nerves to control otherwise uncontrollable pain. Nerve blocks can be used to determine the source of pain, to treat painful conditions that respond to nerve blocks, to predict how the pain will respond to long-term treatments, and to prevent pain following procedures.

Neurologic Interventions

Surgery can be performed to implant devices that deliver drugs or electrically stimulate the nerves. In rare cases, surgery may be done to destroy a nerve or nerves that are part of the pain pathway.

Management of Procedural Pain

Many diagnostic and treatment procedures are painful. Pain related to procedures may be treated before it occurs. Local anesthetics and short-acting opioids can be used to manage procedure-related pain, if enough time is allowed for the drug to work. Antianxiety drugs and sedatives may be used to reduce anxiety or to sedate the patient. Treatments such as imagery or relaxation are useful in managing procedure-related pain and anxiety.

Patients usually tolerate procedures better when they know what to expect. Having a relative or friend stay with the patient during the procedure may help reduce anxiety.

Patients and family members should receive written instructions for managing the pain at home. They should receive information regarding whom to contact for questions related to pain management.

Treating Older Patients

Older patients are at risk for under-treatment of pain because their sensitivity to pain may be underestimated, they may be expected to tolerate pain well, and misconceptions may exist about their ability to benefit from opioids. Issues in assessing and treating cancer pain in older patients include the following:

- Multiple chronic diseases and sources of pain: Age and complicated medication regimens put older patients at increased risk for interactions between drugs and between drugs and the chronic diseases.

- Visual, hearing, movement, and thinking impairments may require simpler tests and more frequent monitoring to determine the extent of pain in the older patient.

- Nonsteroidal anti-inflammatory drug (NSAID) side effects, such as stomach and kidney toxicity, thinking problems, constipation, and headaches, are more likely to occur in older patients.

- Opioid effectiveness: Older patients may be more sensitive to the pain-relieving and central nervous system effects of opioids resulting in longer periods of pain relief.

- Patient-controlled analgesia must be used cautiously in older patients, since drugs are slower to leave the body and older patients are more sensitive to the side effects.

- Other methods of administration, such as rectal administration, may not be useful in older patients since they may be physically unable to insert the medication.

- Pain control after surgery requires frequent direct contact with health care providers to monitor pain management.

- Reassessment of pain management and required changes should be made whenever the older patient moves (for example, from hospital to home or nursing home).

Chapter 52

Sexuality and Fertility Issues in People with Cancer

Sexuality is a complex characteristic that involves the physical, psychological, interpersonal, and behavioral aspects of a person. Recognizing that normal sexual functioning covers a wide range is important. Ultimately, sexuality is defined by each patient and his/her partner according to sex, age, personal attitudes, and religious and cultural values.

Many types of cancer and cancer therapies can cause sexual dysfunction. Research shows that approximately one-half of women who have been treated for breast and gynecologic cancers experience long-term sexual dysfunction. Men who have been treated for prostate cancer report problems with erectile dysfunction that varies depending on the type of treatment. Less is known about how other types of cancer, especially other solid tumors, affect sexuality.

An individual's sexual response can be affected in many ways. The causes of sexual dysfunction are often both physical and psychological. The most common sexual problems for people who have cancer are loss of desire for sexual activity in both men and women, problems achieving and maintaining an erection in men, and pain with intercourse in women. Men may also experience inability to ejaculate, ejaculation going backward into the bladder, or the inability to reach orgasm. Women may experience a change in genital sensations due to pain, loss of sensation and numbness, or decreased ability to reach orgasm.

PDQ® Cancer Information Summary. National Cancer Institute; Bethesda, MD. Sexuality and Reproductive Issues (PDQ): Patient version. Updated 08/2011. Available at: www.cancer.gov. Accessed January 14, 2012.

Unlike many other physical side effects of cancer treatment, sexual problems may not resolve within the first year or two of disease-free survival. These problems may even increase over time and can interfere with the return to a normal life. Patients recovering from cancer should discuss their concerns about sexual problems with a health care professional.

Factors Affecting Sexual Function in People with Cancer

Both physical and psychological factors contribute to the development of sexual dysfunction. Physical factors include loss of function due to the effects of cancer therapies, fatigue, and pain. Surgery, chemotherapy, and radiation therapy may have a direct physical impact on sexual function. Other factors that may contribute to sexual dysfunction include pain medications, depression, feelings of guilt from misbeliefs about the origin of the cancer, changes in body image after surgery, and stresses due to personal relationships. Getting older is often associated with a decrease in sexual desire and performance, however, sex may be important to the older person's quality of life and the loss of sexual function can be distressing.

Surgery-Related Factors

Surgery can directly affect sexual function. Factors that help predict a patient's sexual function after surgery include age, sexual and bladder function before surgery, tumor location and size, and how much tissue was removed during surgery. Surgeries that affect sexual function include breast cancer, colorectal cancer, prostate cancer, and other pelvic tumors.

Sexual function after breast cancer surgery has been the subject of much research. Surgery to save or reconstruct the breast appears to have little effect on sexual function compared with surgery to remove the whole breast. Women who have surgery to save the breast are more likely to continue to enjoy breast caressing, but there is no difference in areas such as how often women have sex, the ease of reaching orgasm, or overall sexual satisfaction. Having a mastectomy, however, has been linked to a loss of interest in sex. Chemotherapy has been linked to problems with sexual function.

Women who have surgery to remove the uterus, ovaries, bladder, or other organs in the abdomen or pelvis may experience pain and loss of sexual function depending on the amount of tissue/organ removed. With counseling and other medical treatments, these patients may regain normal sensation in the vagina and genital areas and be able to have pain-free intercourse and reach orgasm.

Chemotherapy-Related Factors

Chemotherapy is associated with a loss of desire and decreased frequency of intercourse for both men and women. The common side effects of chemotherapy such as nausea, vomiting, diarrhea, constipation, mucositis, weight loss or gain, and loss of hair can affect an individual's sexual self-image and make him or her feel unattractive.

For women, chemotherapy may cause vaginal dryness, pain with intercourse, and decreased ability to reach orgasm. In older women, chemotherapy may increase the risk of ovarian cancer. Chemotherapy may also cause a sudden loss of estrogen production from the ovaries. The loss of estrogen can cause shrinking, thinning, and loss of elasticity of the vagina, vaginal dryness, hot flashes, urinary tract infections, mood swings, fatigue, and irritability. Young women who have breast cancer and have had surgeries such as removal of one or both ovaries, may experience symptoms related to loss of estrogen. These women experience high rates of sexual problems since there is a concern that estrogen replacement therapy, which may decrease these symptoms, could cause the breast cancer to return. For women with other types of cancer, however, estrogen replacement therapy can usually resolve many sexual problems. Also, women who have graft-versus-host disease (a reaction of donated bone marrow or peripheral stem cells against a person's tissue) following bone marrow transplantation may develop scar tissue and narrowing of the vagina that can interfere with intercourse.

For men, sexual problems such as loss of desire and erectile dysfunction are more common after a bone marrow transplant because of graft-versus-host disease or nerve damage. Occasionally chemotherapy may interfere with testosterone production in the testicles. Testosterone replacement may be necessary to regain sexual function.

Radiation Therapy-Related Factors

Like chemotherapy, radiation therapy can cause side effects such as fatigue, nausea and vomiting, diarrhea, and other symptoms that can decrease feelings of sexuality. In women, radiation therapy to the pelvis can cause changes in the lining of the vagina. These changes eventually cause a narrowing of the vagina and formation of scar tissue that results in pain with intercourse, infertility, and other long term sexual problems. Women should discuss concerns about these side effects with their doctor and ask about the use of a vaginal dilator.

For men, radiation therapy can cause problems with getting and keeping an erection. The exact cause of sexual problems after radiation therapy is unknown. Possible causes are nerve injury, a blockage of blood supply to the penis, or decreased levels of testosterone. Sexual changes occur very slowly over a period of six months to one year after radiation therapy. Men who had problems with erectile dysfunction before getting cancer have a greater risk of developing sexual problems after cancer diagnosis and treatment. Other risk factors that can contribute to a greater risk of sexual problems in men are cigarette smoking, history of heart disease, high blood pressure, and diabetes.

Hormone Therapy-Related Factors

Women older than 45 years who are treated with adjuvant tamoxifen therapy may have slightly more hot flashes, night sweats, and vaginal discharge. Studies show that patients who take tamoxifen do not have less sexual activity, but may have slightly less sexual desire and more problems reaching orgasm.

In a large study of women with breast cancer who were treated with adjuvant hormone therapy, patients who took exemestane, a type of aromatase inhibitor, had fewer hot flashes and less vaginal discharge than those who took tamoxifen. However, patients who took exemestane had more vaginal dryness, bone pain, and sleep disorders than patients who took tamoxifen.

Psychological Factors

Patients recovering from cancer often have anxiety or guilt that previous sexual activities may have caused their cancer. Some patients believe that sexual activity may cause the cancer to return or pass the cancer to their partner. Discussing their feelings and concerns with a health care professional is important for patients. Misbeliefs can be corrected and patients can be reassured that cancer is not passed on through sexual contact.

Loss of sexual desire and a decrease in sexual pleasure are common symptoms of depression. Depression is more common in patients with cancer than in the general healthy population. It is important that patients discuss their feelings with their doctor. Getting treatment for depression may be helpful in relieving sexual problems.

Cancer treatments may cause physical changes that affect how an individual sees his or her physical appearance. This view can make a man or woman feel sexually unattractive. It is important that patients discuss these feelings and concerns with a health care professional. Patients can learn how to deal effectively with these problems.

The stress of being diagnosed with cancer and undergoing treatment for cancer can make existing problems in relationships even worse. The sexual relationship can also be affected. Patients who do not have a committed relationship may stop dating because they fear being rejected by a potential new partner who learns about their history of cancer. One of the most important factors in adjusting after cancer treatment is the patient's feeling about his or her sexuality before being diagnosed with cancer. If patients had positive feelings about sexuality, they may be more likely to resume sexual activity after treatment for cancer.

Assessment of Sexual Function in People with Cancer

Sexual function is an important factor that adds to quality of life. Patients should discuss their problems and concerns about sexual function with their doctor. Some doctors may not have the appropriate training to discuss sexual problems. Patients should ask for other information resources or for a referral to a health care professional who is comfortable with discussing sexuality issues.

General Factors Affecting Sexual Functioning

When a possible sexual problem is identified, the health care professional will do a detailed interview either with the patient alone or with the patient and his or her partner. The patient may be asked any of the following questions about his or her current and past sexual functioning:

- How often do you feel a spontaneous desire to have sex?

- Do you enjoy sex?

- Do you have enough energy for sexual activity?

- Do you become sexually aroused (for men, are you able to get and keep an erection, or for women, does your vagina expand and become lubricated)?

- Are you able to reach orgasm during sex? What types of stimulation can trigger an orgasm (for example, self-touch, use of a vibrator, shower massage, partner caressing, oral stimulation, or intercourse)?

- Do you have any pain during sex? Where do you feel the pain? What does the pain feel like? What kinds of sexual activity trigger the pain? Does this cause pain every time? How long does the pain last?

- When did your sexual problems begin? Was it around the same time that you were diagnosed with cancer or received treatment for cancer?

- Are you taking any medications? Did you start taking any new medications or did the doctor change the dose of any medications around the time that these sexual problems began?

- What was your sexual functioning like before you were diagnosed with cancer? Did you have any sexual problems before you were diagnosed with cancer?

Psychosocial Aspects of Sexuality

Patients may also be asked about the significance of sexuality and relationships whether or not they have a partner. Patients who have a partner may be asked about the length and stability of the relationship before being diagnosed with cancer. They may also be asked about their partner's response to the diagnosis of cancer and if they have any concerns about how their partner may be affected by their treatment. It is important that patients and their partners discuss their sexual problems and concerns and fears about their relationship with a health care professional with whom they feel comfortable.

Medical Aspects of Sexuality

Patients may be asked about current and past medical history since many medical illnesses can affect sexual function. Lifestyle risk factors such as smoking and high alcohol intake can also affect sexual function as well as prescribed and over-the-counter medications. Patients may be asked to fill out questionnaires to help identify sexual problems and may undergo a variety of physical examinations, blood tests, ultrasound studies, measurement of nighttime erections, and hormone tests.

Effects of Medicines on Sexual Function

The side effects of medicines can add to the sexual side effects of surgery, radiation therapy, and chemotherapy. Cancer patients may receive drug therapy that can affect nerves, blood vessels, and hormones that control normal sexual function. Mental alertness and moods may also be affected. These side effects may occur in cancer patients who take opioids for pain and drugs to treat depression, for example.

Treatment of Sexual Problems in People with Cancer

Many patients are fearful or anxious about their first sexual experience after cancer treatment. Fear and anxiety can cause patients to avoid intimacy, touch, and sexual activity. The partner may also feel fearful or anxious about initiating any activity that might be thought of as pressuring to be intimate or that might cause physical discomfort. Patients and their partners should discuss concerns with their doctor or other qualified health professional. Honest communication of feelings, concerns, and preferences is important.

In general, a wide variety of treatment modalities are available for patients with sexual dysfunction after cancer. Patients can learn to adapt to changes in sexual function through reading books, pamphlets, and internet resources or listening to and watching videos. Health professionals who specialize in sexual dysfunction can provide patients with these resources as well as information on national organizations that may provide support. Some patients may need medical intervention such as hormone replacement, medications, medical devices, or surgery. Patients who have more serious problems may need sexual counseling on an individual basis, with his or her partner, or in a group. Further testing and research is needed to compare the effectiveness of various treatment programs that combine medical and psychological approaches for people who have had cancer.

Fertility Issues

Radiation therapy and chemotherapy treatments may cause temporary or permanent infertility. These side effects are related to a number of factors including the patient's sex, age at time of treatment, the specific type and dose of radiation therapy and/or chemotherapy, the use of single therapy or many therapies, and length of time since treatment.

When cancer or its treatment may cause infertility or sexual dysfunction, every effort should be made to inform and educate the patient about this possibility.

Chemotherapy

For patients receiving chemotherapy, age is an important factor and recovery improves the longer the patient is off chemotherapy. Chemotherapy drugs that have been shown to affect fertility include busulfan, melphalan, cyclophosphamide, cisplatin, chlorambucil, mustine, carmustine, lomustine, vinblastine, cytarabine, and procarbazine.

In women older than 40 years, adjuvant endocrine therapy increases the risk that chemotherapy will cause permanent loss of menstrual periods.

Radiation

For men and women receiving radiation therapy to the abdomen or pelvis, the amount of radiation directly to the testes or ovaries is an important factor. In women older than 40 years, infertility may occur at lower doses of radiation. Fertility may be preserved by the use of modern radiation therapy techniques and the use of lead shields to protect the testes. Women may undergo surgery to protect the ovaries by moving them out of the field of radiation.

Procreative Alternatives

Patients who are concerned about the effects of cancer treatment on their ability to have children should discuss this with their doctor before treatment. The doctor can recommend a counselor or fertility specialist who can discuss available options and help patients and their partners through the decision-making process. Options may include freezing sperm, eggs, or ovarian tissue before cancer treatment.

Chapter 53

Dealing with Hair Loss Related to Breast Cancer Treatment

Hair loss is one side effect of breast cancer treatment that many women with breast cancer fear. After all, you can wear loose clothing to disguise the effects of breast surgery, but the loss of your hair is very public.

Hair loss may threaten your sense of self, your sexuality, and your privacy. Without hair, you see yourself differently in the mirror, and you present yourself differently to the world. Losing your hair may cause strong emotions, such as anger, depression, and feelings of intense vulnerability. These reactions are completely normal.

The How, When, and If of Hair Loss

Hair loss occurs because chemotherapy or radiation therapy attacks all rapidly dividing cells without discrimination. Thus, healthy, rapidly growing cells, like the hair follicles, may experience collateral damage—hair loss, also known as alopecia.

Some types of chemotherapy cause hair loss and some do not. With some types of chemotherapy, your hair strands may simply get more brittle and less dense on the scalp.

Hair loss usually begins 7–21 days after treatment starts. Some individuals lose hair only from the head, while others may lose eyebrows, eyelashes, underarm, leg, and pubic hair. Luckily, hair follicles recover quickly once chemotherapy ends, so if you do lose your hair, it will likely grow back.

"Coping with Hair Loss," by Jane Neff Rollins. © 2010 Omnigraphics, Inc. All rights reserved.

The amount of hair that falls out, if any, depends on what drugs you receive, how much, how often, and the way that your body reacts to the drug. Drugs that are particularly likely to cause hair thinning or hair loss include Adriamycin, anastrazole, Cytoxan, doxorubicin, 5 fluorouracil, methotrexate, paclitaxel, docetaxel, and tamoxifen. Whole brain radiation for metastatic cancer that has spread to the brain is also associated with the risk of hair loss.

Cooling the scalp may also reduce or prevent hair from falling out during treatment. This option is effective only with certain chemotherapy drugs and for certain types of cancers. In some treatment facilities, it may involve wearing a cold cap during treatment and for up to two hours afterwards. Others use a machine that circulates a coolant through a cap to cool the scalp. These procedures can be very uncomfortable and may give you a headache. Your doctor or chemotherapy nurse will be able to tell you if scalp cooling is appropriate for you.

Physical Impact of Hair Loss

For most women, hair loss is temporary. When hair grows back, the new growth may have a different color, texture, or curl—but hair will likely grow back eventually.

The speed at which you recover a full head of hair (and eyelashes, eyebrows, and pubic hair, if you lost them, too) differs from person to person and depends on the treatment you receive.

Some patients' hair starts to grow back during treatment or within two to three weeks after it ends. With others, it may take three to six months after completing treatment. The hair on the top of your head grows faster than your eyelashes or eyebrows.

Emotional Impact of Hair Loss

Women's hair is a cultural symbol of femininity and a source of self-esteem. Hair loss makes your illness public. Some woman may worry about other people pitying them, about changes in their relationships with family and friends, or about losing their jobs. During the process of diagnosis and treatment you may feel sadness, fear, anxiety, and anger. Your self-esteem, body image and sense of well-being may decline, and you may even feel alienated from yourself, as if you were actually a different person. You may avoid socializing if you feel that your hair loss may make others uncomfortable. All of these feelings are common and normal.

No matter how well prepared you may think you are for the possibility of hair loss, when you first see clumps of hair on your pillow, it will likely still be upsetting and depressing. Be honest, and talk through your feelings about losing your hair with family and friends.

If you have children who will be influenced by your loss of hair, you are not alone. One of every four women with cancer has children still living at home. Children may suspect that something is wrong even before you tell them that you have cancer. Children may find a parent's hair loss especially stressful. Many experts recommend that you tell your kids that you might lose your hair, but also reassure your children that your hair will grow back. Children may feel better if you invite them to help you pick out wigs or hats. If your kids are preteens or teens, you might rank pretty high on the cool scale if you opt to go bald and bold. On the other hand, it may be best to wear a head covering if children seem scared or uncomfortable, no matter how old they are.

There's no ignoring the obvious: Losing your hair can make you feel less attractive, especially if you're already feeling negatively about having breast surgery. You will need some new skills to cope with changes to your mane.

Before Starting Treatment

Before you start chemotherapy, your doctor or nurse educator should discuss the possibility of hair loss with you. If they don't, take the initiative and ask your doctor or nurse if the chemotherapy, hormones, or radiation treatment you'll be getting are likely to cause your hair to fall out. If the answer is yes, then planning in advance for the possibility may give you a sense of control in a situation that feels uncontrollable.

Some people cut their hair once they start chemotherapy to prepare for the loss of their hair. It's less traumatic to lose short clumps of hair than long ones. It's also easier to fit a wig when you have less hair. If you start with a short style, you'll feel like yourself more quickly, since you won't have to wait as long for your hair to grow back. Once hair does begin to fall out, many former patients recommend shaving your head to eliminate finding hair clumps on your pillow for an extended period.

Another way to prepare is to try on hats or wigs (or both) to figure out in advance what style you will feel most comfortable wearing.

Cut a swatch of your hair from the top of your head where it is lightest, and take pictures of yourself with your current hair color and style. This will help you choose a wig that closely matches your original appearance. Of course, if you want to go wild and choose a ravishing red or blonde bombshell wig, you can skip this step. Be aware however, that your children might have an easier time coping if you look as much like their familiar mom as possible.

Diverting Attention from Hair Loss

You can distract attention from your hair, or lack thereof, by highlighting other features with hats, scarves, wigs, make-up, or jewelry.

Hats and Turbans

A generation ago, women would never dream of appearing in public without a hat. Today's culture is more relaxed, and many women have never worn a hat other than to protect themselves from the cold or sun. But hats make a wonderful personal statement to the world, especially if you lose your hair due to cancer treatment. Some women favor berets, others baseball caps. Some hospital support services provide hand-knitted caps for cancer patients undergoing treatment.

When buying a hat, comfort should be your number one consideration. Hats with soft satin or cotton linings will work well; straw boaters, not so much. If you simply must wear that scratchy headgear, cap liners are available to make them more comfortable.

If you live in a sunny climate, a hat with a wide brim is the best choice for outdoor wear, but you might prefer a beret or close-fitting cloche for indoor wear. Hats must fit correctly, so if you try them before you start treatment, they may not fit once your hair is gone, especially if your hair is very curly or thick. Size adjustment features like adjustable bands or chin straps are a good option. If you have a favorite chapeau that is too big, peel-and-stick hat sizers are available to alter the fit.

Choose a hat color that will cheer you up and that is flattering. Customize your hat by adding a pin you haven't worn recently. If you sew, add a contrasting ribbon trim or sew on a unique button to add panache.

Turbans are another option. They are made of elasticized fabric, so you just pull them on. They look sleek and chic, and also provide warmth. Many turbans are washable, and they are often less expensive than felt hats.

Scarves

Learning to tie a scarf into fashionable head-gear is an art. Silk scarves drape beautifully, but tend to slide. Synthetic scarves may be too hot for comfort. Finding cotton scarves of the right shape and size is your best bet. There are scarves available commercially that include an embedded headband for keeping the scarf in place, and others with built-in bangs.

Wigs

Not every woman chooses to wear a wig, and there are pros and cons associated with this option. Here are some advantages: A wig will hide your hair loss, it can mimic your original hairstyle, and new styles and hair colors can boost morale. The disadvantages are that a wig can be hard to keep in place when there is no existing hair to attach them to, they can be hard to fit if you have a big skull, and they tend to be hot—especially in warm weather. Finally, human hair wigs can be very expensive.

If you think you will want a wig, experts recommend that you pick it out before your chemotherapy begins. Many women choose synthetic wigs because they look and feel good, need minimal upkeep, and cost between $30 to $500—much less than human hair wigs. A wig made of real hair could cost between $800 and $3,000 (or even more), and a real-hair wig requires more upkeep than a synthetic wig.

As with hats, comfort should be your number one consideration when buying a wig. Most wigs are designed as a fashion accessory for women who have hair, so check the scratchiness quotient before you buy.

Choose a wig that is adjustable, as your head size may be smaller after you lose your hair. Keep in mind that your skin color may develop a grayish, greenish, or yellowish cast during chemotherapy. You may want a wig color one shade lighter than your usual hair so there is a less dramatic contrast between hair and skin.

Many health insurance plans will cover all or part of the cost of a wig if the claim includes a health care provider's prescription or letter requesting an "extra-cranial prosthesis" (that's medical code for a wig). Medicare does not cover wigs, but you may be able to claim the cost as a tax deductible medical expense. If you are uninsured or your plan doesn't cover a wig, the American Cancer Society may be able to provide you with one. In addition, some hospitals have specially funded programs to provide female cancer patients with free wigs.

If you can afford it, consider buying more than one wig, and change wigs to suit your mood. Just imagine—no more bad hair days.

Flaunting Hair Loss

If you have a beautifully shaped head and a confident personality, you might choose the bald and proud look. With dramatic earrings and an "I dare you to make a comment" posture, you can carry off the look with verve. Just play Brad Paisley's song "Skin" as inspiration. The lyrics of this song tell how the heroine's boyfriend shaves off his hair before taking her to the prom to support her as she undergoes chemo.

Makeup

Even if you don't ordinarily wear make-up every day, you may want to use makeup to divert attention from thinning or missing lashes and brows and any changes you may experience in skin coloration.

If your eyelashes fall out, they no longer act as a barrier to the eye surface. Eye make-up may cause swelling of the eyelids, as the lashes no longer stop product from contacting the eye surface. You might need hypoallergenic brands until chemotherapy is complete.

You can use eye shadow and subtle eyeliner to make up for the lack of eyelashes or attach false lashes. False eyelashes are available at drug stores, department store beauty counters, and online. There are even lashes edged with sequins for that glam night out.

If your eyebrows thin or disappear, you can learn to draw natural looking brows from department stores beauty consultants or through the Look Good, Feel Better program. False eyebrows are also available.

Experts recommend that you do not get permanent eyeliner or brow tattoos, however. The ink used for this procedure may contain metallic substances that react with magnetic fields. This could interfere with your need for a future MRI [magnetic resonance imaging] scan.

You'll also need to be especially strict about not sharing make-up or skin care products with your friends. Cancer patients are vulnerable to infections, and it is important not to cross contaminate these items.

Skin and Scalp Care

Chemotherapy reduces the amount of oil your glands secrete, so your scalp is likely to feel dry or flaky during treatment if you lose your hair. As your hair grows back, switching to shampoo that is mild and perfume-free may help.

If you don't wear a hat or wig, be careful about sun exposure. Apply a sunscreen with sun protection factor (SPF) of at least 30 on your scalp every time you go outdoors, even when it's cloudy, and especially if your chemotherapy regimen includes fluorouracil (5-FU). Sunscreen users often do not apply enough product, so be sure to read the label and apply the amount recommended.

Support Groups

Other people who have lost their hair and can often give helpful advice about how they have coped. You might connect with someone you meet at the hospital or chemotherapy center. Or, the Wellness Community, for example, offers in-person support groups at 100 locations worldwide.

The American Cancer Society offers a free program nationwide called Look Good, Feel Better to enhance self-esteem for women being treated for cancer. During the LGFB session, participants learn how to draw in eyebrows, apply false eyelashes, and try on various wigs, scarves, and hats. All participants receive a goody bag filled with skin care products and cosmetics that are donated by major manufacturers. Although Look Good, Feel Better is not technically a support group, women do find emotional support from sharing their experiences with each other.

Chapter 54

Complementary and Alternative Medicine (CAM) Therapies Used for the Side Effects of Breast Cancer and Its Treatment

Chapter Contents

Section 54.1

Cancer Survivors More Likely to Use CAM

"Cancer Survivors Are More Likely Than General Population to Use CAM, According to National Survey Analysis," by the National Center for Complementary and Alternative Medicine (NCCAM, www.nccam.nih.gov), part of the National Institutes of Health, March 1, 2011.

A recent analysis of the 2007 National Health Interview Survey revealed that cancer survivors are more likely to use complementary and alternative medicine (CAM) compared with the general population. According to the data published in the [March 2011] *Journal of Cancer Survivorship: Research and Practice,* cancer survivors are also more likely to use CAM based on a recommendation by their health care providers and to talk to their health care providers about their CAM use.

Researchers from the University of Pennsylvania School of Medicine investigated CAM use, reasons and motivations for use, and communication of CAM use with health care providers among 23,393 American adults—1,471 cancer survivors and 21,922 non-cancer controls. The researchers found that 65 percent of cancer survivors have used CAM in their lifetime, and 43 percent used CAM in the past year. In contrast, only 53 percent of the non-cancer respondents used CAM in their lifetime, and 37 percent used CAM in the past year. The most common reasons for which cancer survivors reported using CAM were wellness or general disease prevention (29 percent); enhancement of immune function (11 percent); energy enhancement (11 percent); pain management (6 percent); psychological distress (2 percent); and insomnia (1 percent). Cancer survivors were more likely than the control group to use CAM for wellness and general disease prevention, enhancing immune function, and pain management.

Cancer survivors cited various motivations for using CAM therapies; nearly 15 percent reported using CAM on the advice of a friend, family member, or coworker, while approximately 13 percent used CAM because of a recommendation from a health care provider. Fewer used CAM because conventional medical treatments did not help (5 percent) or because conventional treatments were too expensive (2 percent). Although cancer survivors were more likely than the control group to talk about CAM use with their providers, they disclosed less than a quarter of their CAM use to them.

The authors of the analysis noted that this is the first study that uses a population-based approach to examine the specific motivations of cancer survivors for using CAM therapies, as well as the degree of communication between cancer survivors and their health care providers. Although cancer survivors communicated more about their CAM use than the general population, the authors emphasized the overall need for improving communication between patients and providers about CAM use to help ensure coordinated care.

Reference

Mao JJ, Palmer CS, Healy KE, et al. Complementary and alternative medicine use among cancer survivors: A population-based study. *Journal of Cancer Survivorship: Research and Practice.* 2011;5(1):8–17.

Section 54.2

Hypnosis May Reduce Hot Flashes in Breast Cancer Survivors

From the National Center for Complementary and Alternative Medicine (NCCAM, www.nccam.nih.gov), part of the National Institutes of Health, September 22, 2008.

Hot flashes are a problem for many menopausal women and a common side effect of breast cancer treatment. For many breast cancer survivors, vasomotor symptoms result in discomfort, disrupted sleep, anxiety, and decreased quality of life. Hormonal (estrogen) drugs have been used to treat hot flashes, but because estrogens are associated with an increased risk of breast cancer, they usually are avoided by breast cancer survivors. Since nonhormonal treatments do not work for some women and may have adverse effects, new interventions for hot flashes are needed. Previous research has indicated that hypnosis may be a promising alternative.

In a study published in September 2008, researchers funded by the National Cancer Institute and NCCAM investigated the effects of hypnosis on hot flashes among women with a history of primary breast cancer, no current evidence of detectable disease, and at least 14 hot flashes per week over a 1-month period. Sixty women were assigned to receive either hypnosis (weekly 50-minute sessions, plus instructions for at-home self-hypnosis) or no treatment; 51 women completed the 5-week study.

The women who received hypnosis had a 68-percent reduction in self-reported hot flash frequency/severity and experienced an average of 4.39 fewer hot flashes per day. Compared with controls, they also had significant improvements in self-reported anxiety, depression, interference with daily activities, and sleep.

The researchers concluded that hypnosis appears to reduce perceived hot flashes in breast cancer survivors and may have additional benefits such as improved mood and sleep. They recommend long-term, randomized, placebo-controlled studies to further explore the benefits of hypnosis for breast cancer survivors. The researchers are currently conducting a randomized clinical trial with 200 participants.

Reference

Elkins G, Marcus J, Stearns V et al. Randomized trial of a hypnosis intervention for treatment of hot flashes among breast cancer survivors. *Journal of Clinical Oncology.* Published online September 22, 2008.

Section 54.3

Spirituality in Cancer Care

Excerpted from PDQ® Cancer Information Summary. National Cancer Institute; Bethesda, MD. Spirituality in Cancer Care (PDQ): Patient version. Updated 08/2011. Available at: www.cancer.gov. Accessed March 14, 2012.

Studies have shown that religious and spiritual values are important to Americans. Most American adults say that they believe in God and that their religious beliefs affect how they live their lives. However, people have different ideas about life after death, belief in miracles, and other religious beliefs. Such beliefs may be based on gender, education, and ethnic background.

Many patients with cancer rely on spiritual or religious beliefs and practices to help them cope with their disease. This is called spiritual coping. Many caregivers also rely on spiritual coping. Each person may have different spiritual needs, depending on cultural and religious traditions. For some seriously ill patients, spiritual well-being may affect how much anxiety they feel about death. For others, it may affect what they decide about end-of-life treatments. Some patients and their family caregivers may want doctors to talk about spiritual concerns, but may feel unsure about how to bring up the subject.

Some studies show that doctors' support of spiritual well-being in very ill patients helps improve their quality of life. Health care providers who treat patients coping with cancer are looking at new ways to help them with religious and spiritual concerns. Doctors may ask patients which spiritual issues are important to them during treatment as well as near the end of life. When patients with advanced cancer receive spiritual support from the medical team, they may be more likely to choose hospice care and less aggressive treatment at the end of life.

The terms spirituality and religion are often used in place of each other, but for many people they have different meanings. Religion may be defined as a specific set of beliefs and practices, usually within an organized group. Spirituality may be defined as an individual's sense of peace, purpose, and connection to others, and beliefs about the meaning of life. Spirituality may be found and expressed through an organized

495

religion or in other ways. Patients may think of themselves as spiritual or religious or both.

Serious illnesses like cancer may cause patients or family caregivers to have doubts about their beliefs or religious values and cause much spiritual distress. Some studies show that patients with cancer may feel that they are being punished by God or may have a loss of faith after being diagnosed. Other patients may have mild feelings of spiritual distress when coping with cancer.

Spirituality and Quality of Life

Spiritual and religious well-being may help improve quality of life.

It is not known for sure how spirituality and religion are related to health. Some studies show that spiritual or religious beliefs and practices create a positive mental attitude that may help a patient feel better and improve the well-being of family caregivers. Spiritual and religious well-being may help improve health and quality of life in the following ways:

- Decrease anxiety, depression, anger, and discomfort
- Decrease the sense of isolation (feeling alone) and the risk of suicide
- Decrease alcohol and drug abuse
- Lower blood pressure and the risk of heart disease
- Help the patient adjust to the effects of cancer and its treatment
- Increase the ability to enjoy life during cancer treatment
- Give a feeling of personal growth as a result of living with cancer
- Increase positive feelings, including the following:
  - Hope and optimism
  - Freedom from regret
  - Satisfaction with life
  - A sense of inner peace

Spiritual and religious well-being may also help a patient live longer.

Spiritual distress may also affect health.

Spiritual distress may make it harder for patients to cope with cancer and cancer treatment. Health care providers may encourage patients to meet with experienced spiritual or religious leaders to help deal with their spiritual issues. This may improve their health, quality of life, and ability to cope.

Meeting the Patient's Spiritual and Religious Needs

To help patients with spiritual needs during cancer care, medical staff will listen to the wishes of the patient.

Spirituality and religion are very personal issues. Patients should expect doctors and caregivers to respect their religious and spiritual beliefs and concerns. Patients with cancer who rely on spirituality to cope with the disease should be able to count on the health care team to give them support. This may include giving patients information about people or groups that can help with spiritual or religious needs. Most hospitals have chaplains, but not all outpatient settings do. Patients who do not want to discuss spirituality during cancer care should also be able to count on the health care team to respect their wishes.

Doctors and caregivers will try to respond to their patients' concerns, but may not take part in patients' religious practices or discuss specific religious beliefs.

The health care team will help with a patient's spiritual needs when setting goals and planning treatment.

The health care team may help with a patient's spiritual needs in the following ways:

- Suggest goals and options for care that honor the patient's spiritual and/or religious views

- Support the patient's use of spiritual coping during the illness

- Encourage the patient to speak with his/her religious or spiritual leader

- Refer the patient to a hospital chaplain or support group that can help with spiritual issues during illness

- Refer the patient to other therapies that have been shown to increase spiritual well-being

These include mindfulness relaxation, such as yoga or meditation, or creative arts programs, such as writing, drawing, or music therapy.

Section 54.4

Yoga May Help Women with Breast Cancer Conquer Physical and Emotional Pain

"Yoga helps breast cancer survivors conquer emotional, physical pain,"
by Sharita Forrest, University of Illinois News Bureau, May 26, 2011.
© University of Illinois Board of Trustees. Reprinted with permission.

After breast cancer surgery, increased self-consciousness and perceptions of disfigurement prompt some women to shy away from involvement in group fitness and recreational activities during a time when they might benefit the most physically and emotionally.

However, a [May 2011] study by researchers at the University of Illinois and Indiana University indicates that participating in group yoga sessions can help female breast cancer survivors overcome self-consciousness about their appearance and self-imposed limitations on physical activities after surgery, improving their overall fitness and enhancing their quality of life. The study appeared recently in the *International Journal of Yoga Therapy*.

Participants, who were recruited from a cancer center's breast cancer database, engaged in group sessions of Hatha yoga for 2.5 hours per week and practiced postures/sequences at home three times a week for a total of 90 minutes. Women in the control group attended a traditional light exercise group for 30 minutes each week during which they engaged mainly in seated exercises focused on improving their core and lower-body strength.

At the end of the eight-week study, yoga participants reported substantial psychological benefits—their body images had improved, and they felt freed from the psychological barriers they had constructed that limited their physical activities.

Additionally, their confidence in their attractiveness had been renewed, lowering their concern about dressing to conceal the physical changes produced by the surgery.

Yoga participants also reported numerous physical benefits as well—reduced pain, better muscle tone and sense of balance, greater

498

upper and lower body strength and flexibility, and weight loss. Becoming more physically fit improved other aspects of their lives, the women said. Yoga became a catalyst for engaging in other activities and taking time for themselves.

To be eligible to join the study, women had to be at least nine months post treatment, finished with radiation or chemotherapy, and not awaiting further surgery.

Oncologists at the cancer center suggested the nine-month benchmark because by that time subjects would have gotten beyond the acute stress and side effects associated with the cancer diagnosis and treatment and would have settled into any chronic conditions that might occur.

Participants in the study ranged in age from 33 to 84, with the mean age of the women who completed the study at just over 56. Most were Caucasian, married, worked full time, and rated their health as good or very good.

Although a number of studies have explored the potential benefits of yoga for breast cancer survivors, including its use as a tool in managing pain and fatigue, this is believed to be the first study to examine yoga's impact on the psychological constraints that discourage survivors from participating in leisure and recreational activities.

Hatha yoga is an Indian practice that uses a combination of postures, breathing, and meditation to enhance physical, mental, intellectual, and spiritual well-being. The yoga postures/sequences chosen for the group sessions focused on stretching the chest, improving balance, core, and overall strength and flexibility, and managing stress, and were modified as necessary for participants' individual needs. A certified yoga teacher led the classes and modeled the postures in photographs, which were assembled into a workbook that participants used to perform the routines at home.

"It really was the perfect exercise for this group of women because of the whole mind-body connection, the stretching, and the opening up of the chest," said Kimberly J. Shinew, a professor of recreation, sport, and tourism at Illinois. "Given the scar tissue, particularly in the chest area, that's probably why this was such a beneficial activity for them."

Another important benefit: The sense of community formed by the women in the yoga group, which provided social support.

Most of the participants had not participated in yoga before, and some said they never would have joined a support group "where they'd go and discuss their experiences, but because this was activity based, they could focus on the activity and not the illness or themselves,"

Shinew said. "Something that was certainly confirmed was the whole concept of being with similar others when you exercised. Social comparison theory talks about how we're constantly comparing ourselves to other people. We thought that would be there but we didn't realize how strongly it would come out in the findings."

Although the women who participated in the light exercise group began the study demonstrating better agility on a timed test as measured by how quickly they could rise from a chair unassisted and walk 3 m, there were no significant differences between their group's and the yoga group's performance on that test or any other fitness measures by the end of the study.

Breast cancer is the second most frequently diagnosed cancer (after skin cancer) and the second leading cause of cancer death (after lung cancer) among American women. More than 207,000 new cases were expected to be diagnosed and more than 39,000 American women were expected to die from the disease during 2010, according to the most recent estimates from the National Cancer Institute. However, improved detection and treatment technologies have raised the five-year mean survival rate to 89 percent.

Pei-Chun Hsieh and Marieke Van Puymbroeck, faculty members in the department of recreation, park, and tourism studies at Indiana University at Bloomington, and Arlene Schmid, who holds appointments at Roudebush Veteran Affairs Medical Center, Indianapolis, and in the department of occupational therapy at Indiana University-Purdue University at Indianapolis, were co-authors on the study.

Part Seven

Living with Breast Cancer

Chapter 55

Nutrition and Cancer

Nutrition is a process in which food is taken in and used by the body for growth, to keep the body healthy, and to replace tissue. Good nutrition is important for good health. Eating the right kinds of foods before, during, and after cancer treatment can help the patient feel better and stay stronger. A healthy diet includes eating and drinking enough of the foods and liquids that have the important nutrients (vitamins, minerals, protein, carbohydrates, fat, and water) the body needs.

When the body does not get or cannot absorb the nutrients needed for health, it causes a condition called malnutrition or malnourishment.

Nutrition therapy is used to help cancer patients get the nutrients they need to keep up their body weight and strength, keep body tissue healthy, and fight infection. Eating habits that are good for cancer patients can be very different from the usual healthy eating guidelines.

Healthy eating habits and good nutrition can help patients deal with the effects of cancer and its treatment. Some cancer treatments work better when the patient is well nourished and gets enough calories and protein in the diet. Patients who are well nourished may have a better prognosis (chance of recovery) and quality of life.

Excerpted from PDQ® Cancer Information Summary. National Cancer Institute; Bethesda, MD. Nutrition in Cancer Care (PDQ): Patient version. Updated 12/2011. Available at: www.cancer.gov. Accessed March 20, 2012.

Some tumors make chemicals that change the way the body uses certain nutrients. The body's use of protein, carbohydrates, and fat may be affected, especially by tumors of the stomach or intestines. A patient may seem to be eating enough, but the body may not be able to absorb all the nutrients from the food.

For many patients, the effects of cancer and cancer treatments make it hard to eat well. Cancer treatments that affect nutrition include the following:

- Surgery
- Chemotherapy
- Radiation therapy
- Immunotherapy
- Stem cell transplant

When the head, neck, esophagus, stomach, or intestines are affected by the cancer treatment, it is very hard to take in enough nutrients to stay healthy.

The side effects of cancer and cancer treatment that can affect eating include the following:

- Anorexia (loss of appetite)
- Mouth sores
- Dry mouth
- Trouble swallowing
- Nausea
- Vomiting
- Diarrhea
- Constipation
- Pain
- Depression
- Anxiety

Cancer and cancer treatments may affect taste, smell, appetite, and the ability to eat enough food or absorb the nutrients from food. This can cause malnutrition (a condition caused by a lack of key nutrients). Malnutrition can cause the patient to be weak, tired, and unable to fight infections or get through cancer treatment. Malnutrition may be made worse if the cancer grows or spreads. Eating too little protein and calories is a very common problem for cancer patients. Having enough protein and calories is important for healing, fighting infection, and having enough energy.

Anorexia (the loss of appetite or desire to eat) is a common symptom in people with cancer. Anorexia may occur early in the disease or later, if the cancer grows or spreads. Some patients already have anorexia when they are diagnosed with cancer. Almost all patients who have advanced cancer will have anorexia. Anorexia is the most common cause of malnutrition in cancer patients.

Cachexia is a condition marked by a loss of appetite, weight loss, muscle loss, and general weakness. It is common in patients with tumors of the lung, pancreas, and upper gastrointestinal tract. It is important to watch for and treat cachexia early in cancer treatment because it is hard to correct.

Cancer patients may have anorexia and cachexia at the same time. Weight loss can be caused by eating fewer calories, using more calories, or both.

It is important that cancer symptoms and side effects that affect eating and cause weight loss are treated early. Both nutrition therapy and medicine can help the patient stay at a healthy weight. Medicine may be used for the following:

- To help increase appetite
- To help digest food
- To help the muscles of the stomach and intestines contract (to keep food moving along)
- To prevent or treat nausea and vomiting
- To prevent or treat diarrhea
- To prevent or treat constipation
- To prevent and treat mouth problems (such as dry mouth, infection, pain, and sores)
- To prevent and treat pain

Nutrition Therapy in Cancer Care

Screening and Assessment

Screening is used to look for nutrition risks in a patient who has no symptoms. This can help find out if the patient is likely to become malnourished, so that steps can be taken to prevent it.

505

Assessment checks the nutritional health of the patient and helps to decide if nutrition therapy is needed to correct a problem.

Screening and assessment may include questions about the following:

- Weight changes over the past year

- Changes in the amount and type of food eaten compared to what is usual for the patient

- Problems that have affected eating, such as loss of appetite, nausea, vomiting, diarrhea, constipation, mouth sores, dry mouth, changes in taste and smell, or pain

- Ability to walk and do other activities of daily living (dressing, getting into or out of a bed or chair, taking a bath or shower, and using the toilet)

A physical exam is also done to check the body for general health and signs of disease. The doctor will look for loss of weight, fat, and muscle, and for fluid buildup in the body.

Finding and Treating Nutrition Problems Early

Early nutrition screening and assessment help find problems that may affect how well the patient's body can deal with the effects of cancer treatment. Patients who are underweight or malnourished may not be able to get through treatment as well as a well-nourished patient. Finding and treating nutrition problems early can help the patient gain weight or prevent weight loss, decrease problems with the treatment, and help recovery.

The Healthcare Team of Nutrition Specialists

A nutrition support team will check the patient's nutritional health often during cancer treatment and recovery. The team may include the following specialists:

- Physician

- Nurse

- Registered dietitian

- Social worker

- Psychologist

A patient whose religion doesn't allow eating certain foods may want to talk with a religious advisor about allowing those foods during cancer treatment and recovery.

Main Goals of Nutrition Therapy

The main goals of nutrition therapy for patients in active treatment and recovery are to provide nutrients that are missing, maintain nutritional health, and prevent problems. The health care team will use nutrition therapy to do the following:

- Prevent or treat nutrition problems, including preventing muscle and bone loss

- Decrease side effects of cancer treatment and problems that affect nutrition

- Keep up the patient's strength and energy

- Help the immune system fight infection

- Help the body recover and heal

- Keep up or improve the patient's quality of life

Good nutrition continues to be important for patients who are in remission or whose cancer has been cured.

Types of Nutrition Care

It is best to take in food by mouth whenever possible. Some patients may not be able to take in enough food by mouth because of problems from cancer or cancer treatment. Medicine to increase appetite may be used.

Nutrition support for patients who cannot eat can be given in different ways. A patient who is not able to take in enough food by mouth may be fed using enteral nutrition (through a tube inserted into the stomach or intestines) or parenteral nutrition (infused into the bloodstream). The nutrients are given in liquid formulas that have water, protein, fats, carbohydrates, vitamins, and/or minerals.

Nutrition support can improve a patient's quality of life during cancer treatment, but there are harms that should be considered before making the decision to use it. The patient and health care providers should discuss the harms and benefits of each type of nutrition support.

507

Enteral Nutrition

Enteral nutrition is also called tube feeding.

Enteral nutrition is giving the patient nutrients in liquid form (formula) through a tube that is placed into the stomach or small intestine. The following types of feeding tubes may be used:

- A nasogastric tube is inserted through the nose and down the throat into the stomach or small intestine. This kind of tube is used when enteral nutrition is only needed for a few weeks.

- A gastrostomy tube is inserted into the stomach or a jejunostomy tube is inserted into the small intestine through an opening made on the outside of the abdomen. This kind of tube is usually used for long-term enteral feeding or for patients who cannot use a tube in the nose and throat.

The type of formula used is based on the specific needs of the patient. There are formulas for patients who have special health conditions, such as diabetes. Formula may be given through the tube as a constant drip (continuous feeding) or one to two cups of formula can be given three to six times a day (bolus feeding).

Enteral nutrition is sometimes used when the patient is able to eat small amounts by mouth, but cannot eat enough for health. Nutrients given through a tube feeding add the calories and nutrients needed for health.

Enteral nutrition may continue after the patient leaves the hospital.

If enteral nutrition is to be part of the patient's care after leaving the hospital, the patient and caregiver will be trained to do the nutrition support care at home.

Parenteral Nutrition

Parenteral nutrition carries nutrients directly into the blood stream.

Parenteral nutrition is used when the patient cannot take food by mouth or by enteral feeding. Parenteral feeding does not use the stomach or intestines to digest food. Nutrients are given to the patient directly into the blood, through a catheter (thin tube) inserted into a vein. These nutrients include proteins, fats, vitamins, and minerals.

Parenteral nutrition is used only in patients who need nutrition support for five days or more.

A central venous catheter is placed beneath the skin and into a large vein in the upper chest. The catheter is put in place by a surgeon. This type of catheter is used for long-term parenteral feeding.

A peripheral venous catheter is placed into a vein in the arm. A peripheral venous catheter is put in place by trained medical staff. This type of catheter is usually used for short-term parenteral feeding.

The patient is checked often for infection or bleeding at the place where the catheter enters the body.

Parenteral nutrition support may continue after the patient leaves the hospital. If parenteral nutrition is to be part of the patient's care after leaving the hospital, the patient and caregiver will be trained to do the nutrition support care at home.

Going off parenteral nutrition support needs to be done slowly and is supervised by a medical team. The parenteral feedings are decreased by small amounts over time until they can be stopped, or as the patient is changed over to enteral or oral feeding.

Effects of Cancer Treatment on Nutrition

Surgery and Nutrition

The body needs extra energy and nutrients to heal wounds, fight infection, and recover from surgery. If the patient is malnourished before surgery, it may cause problems during recovery, such as poor healing or infection. For these patients, nutrition care may begin before surgery.

More than half of cancer patients are treated with surgery. Surgery that removes all or part of certain organs can affect a patient's ability to eat and digest food. The following are nutrition problems caused by specific types of surgery:

Surgery to the head and neck may cause problems with the following:

- Chewing
- Swallowing
- Tasting or smelling food
- Making saliva
- Seeing

Surgery that affects the esophagus, stomach, or intestines may keep these organs from working as they should to digest food and absorb nutrients.

All of these can affect the patient's ability to eat normally. Emotional stress about the surgery itself also may affect appetite.

Nutrition therapy can relieve or decrease the side effects of surgery and help cancer patients get the nutrients they need. Nutrition therapy may include the following:

- Nutritional supplement drinks
- Enteral nutrition (feeding liquid through a tube into the stomach or intestines)
- Parenteral nutrition (feeding through a catheter into the bloodstream)
- Medicines to increase appetite

It is common for patients to have pain, tiredness, and/or loss of appetite after surgery. For a short time, some patients may not be able to eat what they usually do because of these symptoms. Following certain tips about food may help. These include the following:

- Stay away from carbonated drinks (such as sodas) and foods that cause gas, such as beans, peas, broccoli, cabbage, Brussels sprouts, green peppers, radishes, and cucumbers.

- Increase calories by frying foods and using gravies, mayonnaise, and salad dressings. Supplements high in calories and protein can also be used.

- Choose high-protein and high-calorie foods to increase energy and help wounds heal. Good choices include eggs, cheese, whole milk, ice cream, nuts, peanut butter, meat, poultry, and fish.

- If constipation is a problem, increase fiber by small amounts and drink lots of water. Good sources of fiber include whole-grain cereals (such as oatmeal and bran), beans, vegetables, fruit, and whole-grain breads.

Chemotherapy and Nutrition

Chemotherapy affects fast-growing cells and is used to treat cancer because cancer cells grow and divide quickly. Healthy cells that normally grow and divide quickly may also be killed. These include cells in the mouth, digestive tract, and hair follicles.

Chemotherapy may cause side effects that cause problems with eating and digestion. When more than one anticancer drug is given, more side effects may occur or they may be more severe. The following side effects are common:

- Loss of appetite
- Inflammation and sores in the mouth
- Changes in the way food tastes
- Feeling full after only a small amount of food
- Nausea
- Vomiting
- Diarrhea
- Constipation

Patients who have side effects from chemotherapy may not be able to eat normally and get all the nutrients they need to restore healthy blood counts between treatments. Nutrition therapy can help relieve these side effects, help patients recover from chemotherapy, prevent delays in treatment, prevent weight loss, and maintain general health. Nutrition therapy may include the following:

- Nutrition supplement drinks between meals
- Enteral nutrition (tube feedings)
- Changes in the diet, such as eating small meals throughout the day

Radiation Therapy and Nutrition

Radiation therapy can kill cancer cells and healthy cells in the treatment area. The amount of damage depends on the following:

- The part of the body that is treated
- The total dose of radiation and how it is given

Radiation therapy to any part of the digestive system often has side effects that cause nutrition problems. Most of the side effects begin a few weeks after radiation therapy begins and go away a few weeks after it is finished. Some side effects can continue for months or years after treatment ends.

The following are some of the more common side effects for radiation therapy to the head and neck:

- Loss of appetite
- Changes in the way food tastes
- Pain when swallowing

- Dry mouth or thick saliva

- Sore mouth and gums

- Narrowing of the upper esophagus, which can cause choking, breathing, and swallowing problems

The following are some of the more common side effects for radiation therapy to the chest:

- Infection of the esophagus

- Trouble swallowing

- Esophageal reflux (a backward flow of the stomach contents into the esophagus)

The following are some of the more common side effects for radiation therapy to the abdomen or pelvis:

- Diarrhea

- Nausea

- Vomiting

- Inflamed intestines or rectum

- A decrease in the amount of nutrients absorbed by the intestines

Radiation therapy may also cause tiredness, which can lead to a decrease in appetite.

Nutrition therapy during radiation treatment can help the patient get enough protein and calories to get through treatment, prevent weight loss, help wound and skin healing, and maintain general health. Nutrition therapy may include the following:

- Nutritional supplement drinks between meals

- Enteral nutrition (tube feedings)

- Changes in the diet, such as eating small meals throughout the day

Biologic Therapy and Nutrition

The side effects of biologic therapy are different for each patient and each type of biologic agent. The following nutrition problems are common:

- Fever

- Nausea

- Vomiting

- Diarrhea

- Loss of appetite

- Tiredness

- Weight gain

The side effects of biologic therapy can cause weight loss and malnutrition if they are not treated. Nutrition therapy can help patients receiving biologic therapy get the nutrients they need to get through treatment, prevent weight loss, and maintain general health.

Nutrition in Cancer Prevention

The American Cancer Society and the American Institute for Cancer Research both have dietary guidelines that may help prevent cancer. Their guidelines are a lot alike and include the following:

- Eat a plant-based diet, with at least five servings of fruit and vegetables a day. Have several servings a day of beans and grain products (such as cereals, breads, and pasta). Eat less meat.

- Eat foods low in fat.

- Eat foods low in salt.

- Get to and stay at a healthy weight.

- Be active for 30 minutes on most days of the week.

- Drink few alcoholic drinks or don't drink at all.

- Prepare and store food safely.

- Do not use tobacco in any form.

The effect of soy on breast cancer and breast cancer prevention is being studied. Study results include the following:

- Some studies show that eating soy may decrease the risk of having breast cancer.

- Taking soy supplements in the form of powders or pills has not been shown to prevent breast cancer.

- Adding soy foods to the diet after being diagnosed with breast cancer has not been shown to keep the breast cancer from coming back.

Soy has substances in it that act like estrogen in the body. Studies were done to find out how soy affects breast cancer in patients who have tumors that need estrogen to grow. Some studies have shown that soy foods are safe for women with breast cancer when eaten in moderate amounts as part of a healthy diet.

If you are a breast cancer survivor be sure to check the most up-to-date information when deciding whether to include soy in your diet.

Chapter 56

Exercise after Cancer

A panel of 13 researchers with expertise in cancer, fitness, obesity, and exercise training is spreading what they believe to be one of the most important messages for cancer patients and survivors: Avoid inactivity.

The panel was convened in 2009 by the American College of Sports Medicine (ACSM) to develop guidelines on exercise and physical activity in patients who are undergoing active treatment for cancer or who have completed treatment.

In addition to promoting the benefits of exercise and physical activity in this group, the panel had another goal in formulating the guidelines, said lead author Dr. Kathryn Schmitz of the University of Pennsylvania's Abramson Cancer Center. "Our hope is that there will be more conversations about the need for formalized exercise programs for patients during and right after treatment—programs that will be the cancer equivalent to cardiac rehab," she said.

The benefits of exercise are well documented in a number of cancers, Dr. Schmitz continued, namely in areas such as fatigue and physical functioning, both of which directly influence quality of life. While survival is the ultimate outcome measure, with an estimated 12 million cancer survivors and growing in the United States, the importance of improving quality of life has grown exponentially.

"Guidelines Urge Exercise for Cancer Patients, Survivors," by the National Cancer Institute (NCI, www.cancer.gov), part of the National Institutes of Health, June 29, 2010.

The evidence linking physical activity with improved quality of life in those undergoing active treatment and those who have completed it "is incredibly strong," said Dr. Rachel Ballard-Barbash of NCI's Division of Cancer Control and Population Sciences.

The most robust evidence is for people who have completed active cancer treatment, noted Dr. Kerry Courneya from the University of Alberta, who has led a number of clinical trials of physical activity in cancer patients. But, he continued, because of differences in study design and other factors, it's difficult to compare findings involving patients under active treatment with findings involving patients who have completed treatment.

Overall, said Dr. Courneya during an education session on exercise and cancer at the recent ASCO annual meeting, "We're finding that patients can do a lot more than we originally thought they could do, even when they're on chemotherapy or radiation therapy."

And that's critical, stressed Dr. Ballard-Barbash. "Even a modest amount of exercise, like brief walks, is beneficial, and we see gains versus doing nothing at all."

Adapt, But Be Realistic

Patients with different cancer types receive different treatments. So the new ACSM guidelines identify considerations that patients/survivors and the fitness professionals working with them should take into account.

In men who have undergone androgen deprivation therapy for prostate cancer, for example, trainers need to be aware of fracture risk and adjust the exercises accordingly. And many women with breast cancer will have had surgery "that can really debilitate the shoulder," said McAllister, so the guidelines encourage the use of exercises to stabilize and strengthen the surrounding muscles.

Dr. Schmitz noted that although the benefits of exercise are clear, "sometimes people are just too sick to exercise," particularly during active treatment. Dr. Ballard-Barbash concurred. "If a patient is finding it difficult to tolerate exercise," she said, "he or she may need to decrease activity for a while, or wait a few days before starting again."

Developing the Guidelines

The guidelines, published in the July 2010 *Medicine & Science in Sports & Exercise*, follow the 2008 release of HHS' Physical Activity Guidelines for Americans. But the panel suggested adaptations for exercise in people with different cancer types based on factors such as common adverse effects of treatment, for example, increased risk of bone fractures and cardiac side effects.

Specific recommendations—including the objectives and goals of a prescription for exercise training—and contraindications for exercise are, however, available only for patients with breast, prostate, colon, gynecologic, and hematologic cancers, since they are the cancers for which the panel felt there was sufficient evidence for such recommendations.

Two of the primary goals of exercise highlighted in the guidelines are improved body image and body composition. In the case of the former, many cancer patients undergo extensive surgery or receive treatments that can alter their physical appearance and radically alter feelings about things such as sexual attractiveness, said Dr. Schmitz. "There's good evidence in the literature that physical activity can improve body image, and that may be one mechanism through which exercise can improve quality of life," she explained.

Body composition changes are common in many cancer patients, but the reasons can vary by cancer site. Some cancers, such as gastrointestinal and head and neck cancers, are typically associated with body wasting (loss of weight and muscle mass), so much so that it can be difficult for some patients to get up out of a chair. In this group, exercises that help build lean muscle are important.

But in breast cancer, where the bulk of the studies on physical activity have been performed, the systemic treatments patients often receive can lead to significant weight gain. In those patients, exercise "that is more useful for controlling body weight and losing fat, getting back to a healthy BMI," will be more important, Dr. Schmitz said.

The guidelines also make note of the suggestive evidence—but by no means definitive evidence—in breast and colorectal cancer that regular exercise after treatment improves progression-free and overall survival. As the data continue to emerge in this area, a prescription for exercise could be "an adjunct to curative care," said Dr. Schmitz.

But Dr. Courneya acknowledged that the jury is still out on survival, calling the data "exciting" but "still experimental."

Putting Exercise into Action

There are numerous issues to address before physical activity becomes proactively integrated into treatment or survivorship plans, including insurance coverage of exercise training; educating oncologists, other clinicians, and patients about the benefits of exercise; and expanding the ranks of fitness professionals who understand the issues and needs faced by cancer patients and survivors.

From her perspective, said Marilyn McAllister, a trainer from Boise, ID, who often works with breast cancer survivors in her own studio and at a local hospital, the environment around exercise and cancer is improving, but more progress needs to be made. In her experience, physicians often are "too swamped" dealing with day-to-day patient care issues to learn about or discuss exercise with their patients. "And patients, when they first start treatment, are just overwhelmed with information, so handing them a piece of paper with information about yoga or strength training isn't very helpful."

Several initiatives are under way to expand the supply of fitness professionals with cancer-specific training. ACSM and the American Cancer Society (ACS) have a certification program for trainers who want to work with cancer patients and survivors, and Dr. Schmitz helped ACSM develop a new, six-session cancer exercise trainer certification Webinar. In addition, the Lance Armstrong Foundation has partnered with the YMCA to help train fitness staff at YMCAs across the country to work with and meet the needs of cancer survivors.

Helping any of her clients improve their fitness is gratifying, said McAllister, an ACSM/ACS-certified cancer trainer, but working with cancer patients and survivors offers some unique rewards. "Everybody benefits from exercise, but it can be so dramatic in cancer patients," she said. "It doesn't take much training to produce big results in their lives."

Chapter 57

Breast Cancer and Your Emotions: Tips for Coping

Having breast cancer affects you in many different ways. For example, treatments may change the way you look and how you feel about yourself and your body. The demands of treatment may also affect your personal relationships or make it difficult to manage your usual activities and responsibilities. Fortunately, these are challenges you do not have to face alone.

Here are some tips for coping with the difficult emotions that may come up with breast cancer:

Share your feelings: Talking about your emotions might be hard, but it can comfort you and the people who care about you. When you tell someone whom you love what you're feeling, you give that person a chance to support you. You also give your relationship with that person a chance to grow.

Be specific: When reaching out to others, be specific about the kind of support you need. Saying something like, "It would be helpful if you could shop for groceries this week," or "Can you please drive me to my next appointment?" gives people a clear way to help. This approach cuts down on frustration and reassures your family and friends that they are being helpful.

"Breast Cancer: Coping with Your Changing Feelings," reprinted with permission of www.cancercare.org and Cancer Care, Inc. © 2011. For more information about Cancer*care*'s free, professional support services for people facing cancer, visit the website or call 800-813-HOPE (4673).

Take steps to look and feel your best: Many women feel uncomfortable with their appearance after having surgery or chemotherapy. If you had breast surgery or are experiencing hair loss and changes in your physical appearance, learn about options available, such as breast prostheses and wigs. Give yourself time to adjust to changes, and try different solutions until you find what makes you feel most comfortable.

Let yourself feel loved and cared for: After a lumpectomy or mastectomy, a woman may find that regular activities, such as dressing, undressing, bathing, or being intimate with her partner or spouse, give rise to complex emotions. Some women feel so different that they stop taking care of their emotional and physical needs. For example, a woman may distance herself emotionally from her partner. You can make other choices, such as choosing to remain close with your partner or spouse. Everyone deserves to feel loved and cared for.

Talk to your spouse or partner about the physical closeness you need: Share how you feel about your body, and talk about what you think or worry that your partner is feeling. Whatever your needs are—whether you feel a need for physical affection, or if you are not yet interested in being physically intimate—let your partner know. Your partner is most likely waiting for your signal to know what to do, how to act, and what you need.

Discuss your concerns with your doctor or nurse: If you feel you have lost the desire to be physically intimate, bring it up with your doctor or nurse. These health care professionals can help you understand physical changes that may be causing these feelings. They can also suggest ways to increase your interest in physical intimacy and make appropriate referrals if needed.

Get help for lymphedema: Lymphedema is a painful swelling, usually in an arm or leg, which happens when the body's lymphatic fluid fails to circulate properly and builds up in the soft tissue instead. There are several ways to manage lymphedema. Your doctor or nurse can give you tips to prevent and reduce the swelling.

Learn more about breast cancer: Having accurate information helps you to make the choices that are right for you. Turn to trustworthy sources for reliable information about breast cancer. The National Cancer Information Service (800-4-CANCER) is an excellent source of medical information. So are CancerCare's Connect Education Workshops and publications, which provide the latest cancer information from leading experts.

Seek support: Joining a support group gives you a chance to talk about your feelings and learn from other women going through similar situations. Cancer*Care*'s support groups are led by professional oncology social workers and available in person, online, and over the telephone. We also offer individual counseling. Speaking one on one with an oncology social worker can help you develop strategies for coping with some of the more complex emotions and concerns you may be facing.

Chapter 58

Talking to Family and Loved Ones about Your Cancer

Family Matters

Families are not all alike. Your family may include a spouse (husband or wife), children, and parents. Or maybe you think of your partner or close friends as your family.

Cancer affects the whole family, not just the person with the disease. How are the people in your family dealing with your cancer? Maybe they are afraid or angry, just like you.

When you first find out you have cancer and are going through treatments, day-to-day routines may change for everyone. For example, someone in your family may need to take time off work to drive you to treatments. You may need help with chores and errands.

How your family reacts to your cancer may depend a lot on how you've faced hard times in the past.

Some families find it easy to talk about cancer. They may easily share their feelings about the changes that cancer brings to their lives. Other families find it harder to talk about cancer. The people in these families may be used to solving problems alone and not want to talk about their feelings.

Families that have gone through divorce or had other losses may have even more trouble talking about cancer.

Excerpted from "Taking Time: Support for People with Cancer," by the National Cancer Institute (NCI, www.cancer.gov), part of the National Institutes of Health, January 19, 2011.

If your family is having trouble talking about feelings, think about getting some help. Your doctor or nurse can refer you to a counselor who can help people in your family talk about what cancer means to them. Many families find that, even though it can be hard to do, they feel close to each other when they deal with cancer together.

Changes to Your Roles in the Family

When someone in a family has cancer, everyone takes on new roles and responsibilities. For example, a child may be asked to do more chores or a spouse or partner may need to help pay bills, shop, or do yard work. Family members sometimes have trouble adjusting to these new roles.

Adjusting to Your New Situation

Many families have trouble getting used to the role changes that may be required when a loved one has cancer.

Money: Cancer can reduce the amount of money your family has to spend or save. If you're not able to work, someone else in your family may feel that he or she needs to get a job. You and your family may need to learn more about health insurance and find out what will be covered and what you need to pay for. Most people find it stressful to keep up with money matters.

Living arrangements: People with cancer sometimes need to change where they live or whom they live with. Now that you have cancer, you may need to move in with someone else to get the care you need. This can be hard because you may feel that you are losing your independence, at least for a little while. Or, you may need to travel far from home for treatment. If you have to be away from home for treatments take a few little things from home with you. This way, there will be something familiar even in a strange place.

Daily activities: You may need help with duties such as paying bills, cooking meals, or coaching your children's teams. Asking others to do these things for you can be hard.

Developing a Plan

Even when others offer to help, it's important to let people know that you can still do some things for yourself. As much as you're able, keep up with your normal routine by making decisions, doing household chores, and working on hobbies that you enjoy.

Asking for help is not a sign of weakness. Think about hiring someone or asking for a volunteer. You might be able to find a volunteer through groups in your community.

Paid help or volunteers may be able to help with the following:

- Physical care, such as bathing or dressing

- Household chores, such as cleaning or food shopping

- Skilled care, such as giving you special feedings or medications

Just as you need time for yourself, your family members also need time to rest, have fun, and take care of their other duties. Respite care is a way people can get the time they need. In respite care, someone comes to your home and takes care of you while your family member goes out for a while. Let your doctor or social worker know if you want to learn more about respite care.

Spouses and Partners

Your husband, wife, or partner may feel just as scared by cancer as you do. You both may feel anxious, helpless, or afraid. You may find it hard to be taken care of by someone you love.

People react to cancer in different ways. Some cannot accept that cancer is a serious illness. Others try too hard to be "perfect" caregivers. And some people refuse to talk about cancer. For most people, thinking about the future is scary.

It helps if you and the people close to you can talk about your fears and concerns. You may want to meet with a counselor who can help both of you talk about these feelings.

Sharing Information

Including your spouse or partner in treatment decisions is important. You can meet with your doctor together and learn about your type of cancer. You might want to find out about common symptoms, treatment choices, and their side effects. This information will help both of you plan for the future.

Your spouse or partner will also need to know how to help take care of your body and your feelings. And, even though it's not easy, both of you should think about the future and make plans in case you don't survive your cancer. You may find it helpful to meet with a financial planner or a lawyer.

525

Staying Close

Everyone needs to feel needed and loved. You may have always been the "strong one" in your family, but now is the time to let your spouse or partner help you. This can be as simple as letting the other person fluff your pillow, bring you a cool drink, or read to you.

Feeling sexually close to your partner is also important. You may not be interested in sex when you're in treatment because you feel tired, sick to your stomach, or in pain. But when your treatment is over, you may feel like having sex again. Until then, you and your spouse or partner may need to find new ways to show that you care about each other. This can include touching, holding, hugging, and cuddling.

Time Away

Your spouse or partner needs to keep a sense of balance in his or her life. He or she needs time to take care of personal chores and errands. Your partner will also need time to sort through his or her own feelings about cancer. And most importantly, everyone needs time to rest. If you don't want to be alone when your loved one is away, think about getting respite care or asking a friend to stay with you.

Children

Even though your children will be sad and upset when they learn about your cancer, do not pretend that everything is OK. Even very young children can sense when something is wrong. They will see that you don't feel well or aren't spending as much time with them as you used to. They may notice that you have a lot of visitors and phone calls or that you need to be away from home for treatment and doctor's visits.

Children as young as 18 months old begin to think about and understand what is going on around them. It is important to be honest and tell your children that you are sick and the doctors are working to make you better. Telling them the truth is better than letting them imagine the worst. Give your children time to ask questions and express their feelings. And if they ask questions that you can't answer, let them know that you will find out the answers for them.

When you talk with your children, use words and terms they can understand. For example, say "doctor" instead of "oncologist" or "medicine" instead of "chemotherapy." Tell your children how much you love them and suggest ways they can help with your care. Share books about cancer that are written for children. Your doctor, nurse, or social worker can suggest good ones for your child.

Let other adults in your children's lives know about your cancer. This includes teachers, neighbors, coaches, or other relatives who can spend extra time with them. These other adults may be able to take your children to their activities, as well as listen to their feelings and concerns. Your doctor or nurse can also help by talking with your children and answering their questions. Or you can ask them if there's a child-life specialist on staff. This is a person who can help children understand medical issues and also offer psychological and emotional support.

Children can react to cancer in many different ways. For example, they may experience the following:

- Be confused, scared, or lonely
- Feel guilty and think that something they did or said caused your cancer
- Feel angry when they are asked to be quiet or do more chores around the house
- Miss the amount of attention they are used to getting
- Regress and behave as they did when they were much younger
- Get into trouble at school or at home
- Be clingy and afraid to leave the house

Teenagers and a Parent's Cancer

Teens are at a time in their lives when they are trying to break away and be independent from their parents. When a parent has cancer, breaking away can be hard for them to do. They may become angry, act out, or get into trouble.

Try to get your teens to talk about their feelings. Tell them as much as they want to know about your cancer. Ask them for their opinions and, if possible, let them help you make decisions.

Teens may want to talk with other people in their lives. Friends can be a great source of support, especially those who also have serious illness in their family. Other family members, teachers, coaches, and spiritual leaders can also help. Encourage your teenage children to talk about their fears and feelings with people they trust and feel close to. Some towns even have support groups for teens whose parents have cancer. Also, ask your social worker about internet resources for this group. Many have online chats and forums for support.

Adult Children

Your relationship with your adult children may change now that you have cancer. You may do the following:

- Ask them to take on new duties, such as making health care decisions, paying bills, or taking care of the house.

- Ask them to explain some of the information you've received from your doctor or to go with you to doctor's visits so they can also hear what the doctors are telling you.

- Rely on them for emotional support. For instance, you may ask them to act as "go-betweens" with friends or other family members.

- Want them to spend a lot of time with you. This can be hard, especially if they have jobs or young families of their own.

- Find it hard to receive—rather than give—comfort and support from them.

- Feel awkward when they help with your physical care, such as feeding or bathing.

It is important to talk about cancer with your adult children, even if they get upset or worry about you. Include them when talking about your treatment. Let them know your thoughts and wishes. They should be prepared in case you don't recover from your cancer.

Even adult children worry that their parents will die. When they learn that you have cancer, adult children may realize how important you are to them. They may feel guilty if they haven't been close with you. They may feel bad if they cannot spend a lot of time with you because they live far away or have other duties. Some of these feelings may make it harder to talk to your adult children. If you have trouble talking with your adult children, ask your doctor or nurse to suggest a counselor you can all talk with.

Make the most of the time you have with your adult children. Talk about how much you mean to each other. Express all your feelings—not just love but also anxiety, sadness, and anger. Don't worry about saying the wrong thing. It's better to share your feelings rather than hide them.

Cancer Risk for the Children of People Who Have Cancer

Now that you have cancer, your children may wonder about their chance of getting it as well. A higher risk for some types of cancer is passed from parent to child. However, this is not the case for every type. And everyone's body is different. If concerned, however, children should talk with a doctor about their risk of getting cancer.

Testing for certain genes can be a way to find out if a person is at higher risk of getting cancer. Although some genetic tests can be helpful, they don't always give people the kinds of answers they are seeking. Talk to your doctor if you or someone in your family wants to learn more about genetic changes that increase cancer risk. He or she can refer you to a person who is specially trained in this area. These experts can help you think through your choices and answer your questions.

Parents

Since people are living much longer these days, many people with cancer may also be caring for their aging parents. For example, you may help your parents with their shopping or take them to doctor. Your aging parents may even live with you.

You have to decide how much to tell your parents about your cancer. Your decision may depend on how well your parents can understand and cope with the news. If your parents are in good health, think about talking with them about your disease.

Now that you have cancer, you may need extra help caring for your parents. You may need help only while you are in treatment. Or you may need to make long-term changes in your parents' care. Talk with your family members, friends, health professionals, and community agencies to see how they can help.

Close Friends

Once friends learn of your cancer, they may begin to worry. Some will ask you to tell them ways to help. Others will wonder how they can help but may not know how to ask. You can help your friends cope with the news by letting them help you in some way. Think about the things your friends do well and don't mind doing. Make a list of things you think you might need. This way, when they ask you how they can be of help, you'll be able to share your list of needs and allow them to pick something they're willing to do.

Your sample list of needs might include the following:

- Babysit on days that I go to treatment.

- Prepare frozen meals for my "down days."

- Put my name on the prayer list at my place of worship.

- Bring me a few books from the library when you go.

- Visit for tea or coffee when you can.

- Let others know that it is alright to call or visit me (or let others know that I'm not ready for visitors just yet).

Sharing Your Feelings about Cancer

Friends and Family Have Feelings about Your Cancer

Just as you have strong feelings about cancer, your family or friends will react to it as well. For instance, your friends or family may do the following:

- Hide or deny their sad feelings

- Find someone to blame for your cancer

- Change the subject when someone talks about cancer

- Act mad for no real reason

- Make jokes about cancer

- Pretend to be cheerful all the time

- Avoid talking about your cancer

- Stay away from you, or keep their visits short

Finding a Good Listener

It can be hard to talk about how it feels to have cancer. But talking can help, even though it's hard to do. Many people find that they feel better when they share their thoughts and feelings with their close family and friends.

Friends and family members may not always know what to say to you. Sometimes they can help by just being good listeners. They don't always need to give you advice or tell you what they think. They simply need to show that they care and are concerned about you.

You might find it helpful to talk about your feelings with people who aren't family or friends. Instead, you might want to meet in a support group with others who have cancer or talk with a counselor.

Choosing a Good Time to Talk

Some people need time before they can talk about their feelings. If you aren't ready, you might say, "I don't feel like talking about my cancer right now. Maybe I will later." And sometimes when you want to talk, your family and friends may not be ready to listen.

It's often hard for other people to know when to talk about cancer. Sometimes people send a signal when they want to talk. They might do the following:

- Bring up the subject of cancer
- Talk about things that have to do with cancer, such as a newspaper story about a new cancer treatment that they just read
- Spend more time with you
- Act nervous or make jokes that aren't very funny

You can help people feel more comfortable by asking them what they think or how they feel. Sometimes people can't put their feelings into words. Sometimes, they just want to hug each other or cry together.

Expressing Anger

Many people feel angry or frustrated when they deal with cancer. You might find that you get mad or upset with the people you depend on. You may get upset with small things that never bothered you before.

People can't always express their feelings. Anger sometimes shows up as actions instead of words. You may find that you yell a lot at the kids or the dog. You might slam doors.

Try to figure out why you are angry. Maybe you're afraid of the cancer or are worried about money. You might even be angry about your treatment.

Be True to Your Feelings

Some people pretend to be cheerful, even when they're not. They think that they won't feel sad or angry if they act cheerful. Or they want to seem as if they're able to handle the cancer themselves. Also, your family and friends may not want to upset you and will act as if nothing is bothering them. You may even think that being cheerful may help your cancer go away.

When you have cancer, you have many reasons to be upset. "Down days" are to be expected. You don't have to pretend to be cheerful when you're not. This can keep you from getting the help you need. Be honest and talk about all your feelings, not just the positive ones.

Sharing without Talking

For many, it's hard to talk about being sick. Others feel that cancer is a personal or private matter and find it hard to talk openly about it. If talking is hard for you, think about other ways to share your feelings. For instance, you may find it helpful to write about your feelings. This might be a good time to start a journal or diary if you don't already have one. Writing about your feelings is a good way to sort through them and a good way to begin to deal with them. All you need to get started is something to write with and something to write on.

Journals can be personal or shared. People can use a journal as a way of 'talking' to each other. If you find it hard to talk to someone near to you about your cancer try starting a shared journal. Leave a booklet or pad in a private place that both of you select. When you need to share, write in it and return it to the private place. Your loved one will do the same. Both of you will be able to know how the other is feeling without having to speak aloud.

If you have e-mail, this can also be a good way to share without talking.

People Helping People

No one needs to face cancer alone. When people with cancer seek and receive help from others, they often find it easier to cope.

You may find it hard to ask for or accept help. After all, you are used to taking care of yourself. Maybe you think that asking for help is a sign of weakness. Or perhaps you do not want to let others know that some things are hard for you to do. All these feelings are normal.

People feel good when they help others. However, your friends may not know what to say or how to act when they're with you. Some people may even avoid you. But they may feel more at ease when you ask them something specific, like to cook a meal or pick up your children after school. There are many ways that family, friends, other people who have cancer, spiritual or religious leaders, and health care providers can help. In turn, there are also ways you can help and support your caregivers.

Family and Friends

Family and friends can support you in many ways. But, they may wait for you to give them hints or ideas about what to do. Someone who is not sure if you want company may call "just to see how things are going." When someone says, "Let me know if there is anything I can do," be honest. For example, tell this person if you need help with an errand or a ride to the doctor's office.

Family members and friends can also do the following:

- Keep you company, give you a hug, or hold your hand
- Listen as you talk about your hopes and fears
- Help with rides, meals, errands, or household chores
- Go with you to doctor's visits or treatment sessions
- Tell other friends and family members ways they can help

Other People Who Have Cancer

Even though your family and friends help, you may also want to meet people who have cancer now or have had it in the past. Often, you can talk with them about things you can't discuss with others. People with cancer understand how you feel and can do the following:

- Talk with you about what to expect
- Tell you how they cope with cancer and live a normal life
- Help you learn ways to enjoy each day
- Give you hope for the future

Let your doctor or nurse know that you want to meet other people with cancer. You can also meet other people with cancer in the hospital, at your doctor's office, or through a cancer support group.

Support Groups

Cancer support groups are meetings for people with cancer and those touched by cancer. They can be in person, by phone, or on the internet. These groups allow you and your loved ones to talk with others facing the same problems. Some support groups have a lecture as well as time to talk. Almost all groups have a leader who runs the meeting. The leader can be someone with cancer or a counselor or social worker.

You may think that a support group is not right for you. Maybe you think that a group won't help or that you don't want to talk with others about your feelings. Or perhaps you're afraid that the meetings will make you sad or depressed.

Support groups may not be for everyone. Some people choose to find support in other ways. But many people find them very helpful. People in the groups often do the following:

- Talk about what it's like to have cancer

- Help each other feel better, more hopeful, and not so alone

- Learn about what's new in cancer treatment

- Share tips about ways to cope with cancer

Types of Support Groups

Some groups focus on all kinds of cancer. Others talk about just one kind, such as a group for women with breast cancer or a group for men with prostate cancer.

Groups can be open to everyone or just for people of a certain age, sex, culture, or religion. For instance, some groups are just for teens or young children.

Some groups talk about all aspects of cancer. Others focus on only one or two topics such as treatment choices or self-esteem.

Therapy groups focus on feelings such as sadness and grief. Mental health professionals often lead these types of groups.

In some groups, people with cancer meet in one support group and their loved ones meet in another. This way, people can say what they really think and feel and not worry about hurting someone's feelings.

In other groups, patients and families meet together. People often find that meeting in these groups is a good way for each to learn what the other is going through.

Telephone support groups are where everyone dials in to a phone line and are linked together to talk. They can share and talk to others with similar experiences from all over the country. There is usually little or no charge.

Online support groups are "meetings" that take place by computer. People meet through chat rooms, listservs, or moderated discussion groups and talk with each other over e-mail. People often like online support groups because they can take part in them any time of the day or night. They're also good for people who can't travel to meetings. The biggest problem with online groups is that you can't be sure if what you learn is correct. Always talk with your doctor about cancer information you learn from the internet.

If you have a choice of support groups, visit a few and see what they are like. See which ones make sense for you. Although many groups are free, some charge a small fee. Find out if your health insurance pays for support groups.

Where to Find a Support Group

Many hospitals, cancer centers, community groups, and schools offer cancer support groups. Here are some ways to find groups near you:

- Call your local hospital and ask about its cancer support programs.

- Ask your social worker to suggest groups.

- Do an online search for groups.

- Look in the health section of your local newspaper for a listing of cancer support groups.

Chapter 59

Breast Cancer and Work

Chapter Contents

Section 59.1

Cancer in the Workplace and the Americans with Disabilities Act

Excerpted from "Questions and Answers About Cancer in the Workplace and the Americans with Disabilities Act (ADA)," by the U.S. Equal Employment Opportunity Commission (EEOC, www.eeoc .gov), January 19, 2011.

The Americans with Disabilities Act (ADA) is a federal law that prohibits discrimination against individuals with disabilities. Title I of the ADA covers employment by private employers with 15 or more employees as well as state and local government employers. The Rehabilitation Act provides the same protections related to federal employment. In addition, most states have their own laws prohibiting employment discrimination on the basis of disability. Some of these state laws apply to smaller employers and may provide protections in addition to those available under the ADA.

When is cancer a disability under the ADA?

Cancer is a disability under the ADA when it or its side effects substantially limit(s) one or more of a person's major life activities.

Example: Following a lumpectomy and radiation for aggressive breast cancer, a computer sales representative experienced extreme nausea and constant fatigue for six months. She continued to work during her treatment, although she frequently had to come in later in the morning, work later in the evening to make up the time, and take breaks when she experienced nausea and vomiting. She was too exhausted when she came home to cook, shop, or do household chores and had to rely almost exclusively on her husband and children to do these tasks. This individual's cancer is a disability because it substantially limits her ability to care for herself.

Example: A telephone repairman with an advanced form of testicular cancer has chemotherapy and surgery that render him sterile. He is an individual with a disability under the ADA because he is substantially limited in the major life activity of reproduction.

Even when the cancer itself does not substantially limit any major life activity (such as when it is diagnosed and treated early), it can lead to the occurrence of other impairments that may be disabilities. For example, sometimes depression may develop as a result of the cancer, the treatment for it, or both. Where the condition lasts long enough (i.e., for more than several months) and substantially limits a major life activity, such as interacting with others, sleeping, or eating, it is a disability within the meaning of the ADA.

Cancer also may be a disability because it was substantially limiting some time in the past.

Example: A company president was hospitalized for 30 days immediately following his diagnosis of blood cancer. Because his treatment, which included chemotherapy and a bone marrow transplant, weakened his immune system he was unable to care for himself for six months and had to avoid interactions with almost everyone except his doctors, nurses, and immediate family members. This individual has a record of a disability.

Finally, cancer is a disability when it does not significantly affect a person's major life activities, but the employer treats the individual as if it does.

Example: An individual with a facial scar from surgery to treat skin cancer applies to be an airline customer service representative. The interviewer refuses to consider him for the position because she fears that his scar will make customers uncomfortable. In basing her decision not to hire on the presumed negative reactions of customers, the interviewer is regarding the applicant as substantially limited in working in any job that involves interacting with the public.

Example: After making a job offer, an employer learns that an applicant's genetic profile reveals an increased susceptibility to colon cancer. Although the applicant does not currently have and may never in fact develop colon cancer, the employer withdraws the job offer solely based on concerns about productivity, insurance costs, and attendance. The employer is treating the applicant as if he has a disability.

Under the ADA, the determination of whether an individual currently has, has a record of, or is regarded as having a disability is made on a case-by-case basis.

The ADA requires employers to provide adjustments or modifications to enable people with disabilities to enjoy equal employment opportunities unless doing so would be an undue hardship (i.e., a significant difficulty or expense). Accommodations vary depending on the needs of an individual with a disability. Not all employees with cancer will need an accommodation or require the same accommodations, and most of the accommodations a person with cancer might need will involve little or no cost. An employer must provide a reasonable accommodation that is needed because of the limitations caused by the cancer itself, the side effects of medication or treatment for the cancer, or both. For example, an employer may have to accommodate an employee who is unable to work while she is undergoing chemotherapy or who has depression as a result of cancer, the treatment for it, or both. An employer, however, has no obligation to monitor an employee's medical treatment or ensure that he is receiving appropriate treatment.

What types of reasonable accommodations may employees with cancer need?

Some employees with cancer may need one or more of the following accommodations:

- Leave for doctors' appointments and/or to seek or recuperate from treatment
- Periodic breaks or a private area to rest or to take medication
- Adjustments to a work schedule

Example: An engineer working independently on a long-term project has to undergo radiation for cancer every weekday morning for the next eight weeks. The employer should consider whether it could provide a flexible schedule (e.g., allow him to come in later or work part-time) to accommodate his treatment.

- Permission to work at home
- Modification of office temperature
- Permission to use work telephone to call doctors
- Reallocation or redistribution of marginal tasks to another employee

Example: A janitor, who had a leg amputated to cure bone cancer, can perform all of his essential job functions without accommodation but has difficulty climbing into the attic to occasionally change the building's air filter. The employer likely can reallocate this marginal function to one of the other janitors.

Example: As a result of lymphedema from her mastectomy, a truck driver for a courier service no longer can lift anything heavier than 10 pounds and, therefore, informs her employer that she is unable to do her current job, which requires her to load and unload packages weighing up to 70 pounds. The employer must consider whether a vacant position exists for which the driver is qualified and to which she can be reassigned as a reasonable accommodation, absent undue hardship. The vacant position must be equivalent in terms of pay and status to the original job, or as close as possible if no equivalent position exists. The position need not be a promotion, although the employee should be able to compete for any promotion for which she is eligible. The employer also does not have to "bump" another employee to create a vacancy.

Some employees with cancer may need accommodations other than the ones listed in the preceding text. The employer, therefore, should discuss with the employee her particular limitations and whether there is anything the employer can do to enable her to work. For example, an employer might explore the possibility of providing certain equipment (e.g., a chair or stool to help with fatigue), a temporary transfer, or changes in how work is performed (e.g., altering when or how a function is done to help with concentration problems).

How does an employee with cancer request a reasonable accommodation?

There are no "magic words" that a person has to use when requesting a reasonable accommodation. A person simply has to tell the employer that she needs an adjustment or change at work because of her cancer.

Example: A nurse tells her supervisor that she is having trouble working 12 hours a day because of medical treatments she is undergoing for breast cancer. This is a request for reasonable accommodation.

A request for reasonable accommodation also can come from a family member, friend, health professional, or other representative on behalf of a person with cancer.

May an employer request documentation when an employee who has cancer needs a reasonable accommodation?

Yes. An employer may request reasonable documentation where a disability or the need for reasonable accommodation is not obvious. An employer, however, is entitled only to documentation sufficient to establish that the employee's cancer is a disability and that explains why an accommodation is needed. A request for an employee's entire medical record, for example, would be inappropriate, as it likely would include information about conditions other than the employee's cancer.

541

Example: An employee asks for leave to receive treatment for colon cancer. His oncologist provides a letter indicating that treatment of the condition will require surgery to remove a portion of the large intestines, along with chemotherapy and radiation. The employee will be totally unable to work for the next six months and, even after the cancer has been treated and the employee can return to work, he will have to use a colostomy bag for the rest of his life for waste elimination. The oncologist's letter concludes that, although he hopes the employee will be able to return to a fairly normal lifestyle following his treatments, he will need to remain under close medical supervision for five years to detect and prevent any recurrence. The doctor's letter is sufficient to demonstrate that the employee has a disability and needs the reasonable accommodation of leave. If, after returning to work, the employee makes a subsequent accommodation request related to his colon cancer and the need for accommodation is not obvious, the employer may ask for documentation (e.g., a doctor's note) demonstrating why the accommodation is needed but may not ask for documentation establishing that the employee's colon cancer is a disability.

Does an employer have to grant every request for a reasonable accommodation?

No. An employer does not have to provide an accommodation that would result in "undue hardship." Undue hardship means that providing the reasonable accommodation would result in significant difficulty or expense. However, if a requested accommodation is too difficult or expensive, an employer should determine whether there is another easier or less costly accommodation that would meet the employee's needs.

An employer also is not required to provide the reasonable accommodation that an individual wants but, rather, may choose among reasonable accommodations as long as the chosen accommodation is effective. If more than one accommodation is effective, the employee's preference should be given primary consideration.

May an employer be required to provide more than one accommodation for the same employee with cancer?

Yes. The duty to provide a reasonable accommodation is an ongoing one. Although some employees with cancer may require only one reasonable accommodation, others may need more than one. For example, an employee with cancer may require leave for surgery and subsequent recovery but may be able to return to work on a part-time or modified schedule while receiving chemotherapy. An employer must consider each request for a reasonable accommodation and determine whether it would be effective and whether providing it would pose an undue hardship.

Is an employer required to remove one or more of a job's essential functions to accommodate an employee with cancer?

No. An employer never has to reallocate essential functions as a reasonable accommodation but can do so if it wishes. In fact, it may be mutually beneficial to the employer and employee to remove an essential function that the employee is unable to do, at least on a temporary basis, because of limitations caused by the cancer, its treatment, and/ or side effects.

Example: A doctor becomes too fatigued from cancer treatments to perform surgery, but she still is able to conduct surgical consults and perform her research and teaching duties. Her employer may temporarily remove her from the surgery schedule, rather than placing her on leave, while allowing her to continue performing her other duties.

May an employer automatically deny a request for leave from someone with cancer because the employee cannot specify an exact date of return?

No. Granting leave to an employee who is unable to provide a fixed date of return may be a reasonable accommodation. Although many types of cancer can be successfully treated—and often cured—the treatment and severity of side effects often are unpredictable and do not permit exact timetables. An employee requesting leave because of cancer, therefore, may be able to provide only an approximate date of return (e.g., "in six to eight weeks," "in about three months"). In such situations, or in situations in which a return date must be postponed because of unforeseen medical developments, employees should stay in regular communication with their employers to inform them of their progress and discuss the need for continued leave beyond what originally was granted. The employer also has the right to require that the employee provide periodic updates on his condition and possible date of return. After receiving these updates, the employer may reevaluate whether continued leave constitutes an undue hardship.

Section 59.2

Your Rights after a Mastectomy

Excerpted from the U.S. Department of Labor (www.dol.gov),
October 2009.

If you have had a mastectomy or expect to have one, you may be entitled to special rights under the Women's Health and Cancer Rights Act of 1998 (WHCRA).

The following text clarifies your basic WHCRA rights. Under WHCRA, if your group health plan covers mastectomies, the plan must provide certain reconstructive surgery and other post-mastectomy benefits.

Your health plan or issuer is required to provide you with a notice of your rights under WHCRA when you enroll in the health plan, and then once each year.

The following information provides answers to frequently asked questions about WHCRA.

I've been diagnosed with breast cancer and plan to have a mastectomy. How will WHCRA affect my benefits?

Under WHCRA, group health plans, insurance companies, and health maintenance organizations (HMOs) offering mastectomy coverage also must provide coverage for certain services relating to the mastectomy in a manner determined in consultation with your attending physician and you. This required coverage includes all stages of reconstruction of the breast on which the mastectomy was performed, surgery and reconstruction of the other breast to produce a symmetrical appearance, prostheses, and treatment of physical complications of the mastectomy, including lymphedema.

I have not been diagnosed with cancer. However, due to other medical reasons I must undergo a mastectomy. Does WHCRA apply to me?

Yes, if your group health plan covers mastectomies and you are receiving benefits in connection with a mastectomy. Despite its name, nothing in the law limits WHCRA rights to cancer patients.

Does WHCRA require all group health plans, insurance companies, and HMOs to provide reconstructive surgery benefits?

Generally, group health plans, as well as their insurance companies and HMOs, that provide coverage for medical and surgical benefits with respect to a mastectomy must comply with WHCRA.

However, if your coverage is provided by a "church plan" or "governmental plan," check with your plan administrator. Certain plans that are church plans or governmental plans may not be subject to this law.

May group health plans, insurance companies, or HMOs impose deductibles or coinsurance requirements on the coverage specified in WHCRA?

Yes, but only if the deductibles and coinsurance are consistent with those established for other benefits under the plan or coverage.

I just changed jobs and am enrolled under my new employer's plan. I underwent a mastectomy and chemotherapy treatment under my previous employer's plan. Now I want reconstructive surgery. Under WHCRA, is my new employer's plan required to cover my reconstructive surgery?

If your new employer's plan provides coverage for mastectomies and if you are receiving benefits under the plan that are related to your mastectomy, then your new employer's plan generally will be required to cover reconstructive surgery if you request it. In addition, your new employer's plan generally is required to cover the other benefits specified in WHCRA. It does not matter that your mastectomy was not covered by your new employer's plan.

However, a group health plan may limit benefits relating to a health condition that was present before your enrollment date in your current employer's plan through a preexisting condition exclusion. A Federal law known as the Health Insurance Portability and Accountability Act of 1996 (HIPAA) limits the circumstances under which a preexisting condition exclusion may be applied.

Specifically, HIPAA provides that a plan may impose a preexisting condition exclusion only if:

- the exclusion relates to a condition (whether physical or mental) for which medical advice, diagnosis, care, or treatment was recommended or received within the six-month period ending on your enrollment date;

- the exclusion extends no more than 12 months (or 18 months in the case of a late enrollee in the new plan) after the enrollment date; and

- the preexisting condition exclusion period is reduced by the days of prior creditable coverage (if any, which is defined in HIPAA as most health coverage).

The plan also must provide you with written notification of the existence and terms of any preexisting condition exclusion under the plan and of your rights to demonstrate prior creditable coverage.

My employer's group health plan provides coverage through an insurance company. Following my mastectomy, my employer changed insurance companies. The new insurance company is refusing to cover my reconstructive surgery. Does WHCRA provide me with any protections?

Yes, as long as the new insurance company provides coverage for mastectomies, you are receiving benefits under the plan related to your mastectomy, and you elect to have reconstructive surgery. If these conditions apply, the new insurance company is required to provide coverage for breast reconstruction as well as the other benefits required under WHCRA. It does not matter that your mastectomy was not covered by the new insurance company.

I understand that my group health plan is required to provide me with a notice of my rights under WHCRA when I enroll in the plan. What information can I expect to find in this notice?

Plans must provide a notice to all employees when they enroll in the health plan describing the benefits that WHCRA requires the plan and its insurance companies or HMOs to cover. These benefits include coverage of all stages of reconstruction of the breast on which the mastectomy was performed, surgery and reconstruction of the other breast to produce a symmetrical appearance, prostheses, and treatment of physical complications of the mastectomy, including lymphedema.

The enrollment notice also must state that for the covered employee or their family member who is receiving mastectomy-related benefits, coverage will be provided in a manner determined in consultation with the attending physician and the patient.

Finally, the enrollment notice must describe any deductibles and coinsurance limitations that apply to the coverage specified under WHCRA. Deductibles and coinsurance limitations may be imposed only if they are consistent with those established for other benefits under the plan or coverage.

What can I expect to find in the annual WHCRA notice from my health plan?

Your annual notice should describe the four categories of coverage required under WHCRA and information on how to obtain a detailed description of the mastectomy-related benefits available under your plan. For example, an annual notice might look something like this:

"Do you know that your plan, as required by the Women's Health and Cancer Rights Act of 1998, provides benefits for mastectomy-related services including all stages of reconstruction and surgery to achieve symmetry between the breasts, prostheses, and complications resulting from a mastectomy, including lymphedema? Call your plan administrator [phone number here] for more information."

Your annual notice may be the same notice provided when you enrolled in the plan if it contains the information described above.

My state requires health insurance issuers to cover the benefits required by WHCRA and also requires health insurance issuers to cover minimum hospital stays in connection with a mastectomy (which is not required by WHCRA). If I have a mastectomy and breast reconstruction, am I also entitled to the minimum hospital stay?

If your employer's group health plan provides coverage through an insurance company or HMO, you are entitled to the minimum hospital stay required by the state law. Many state laws provide more protections than WHCRA. Those additional protections apply to coverage provided by an insurance company or HMO (known as "insured" coverage).

If your employer's plan does not provide coverage through an insurance company or HMO (in other words, your employer "self-insures" your coverage), then the state law does not apply. In that case, only the federal law, WHCRA, applies, and it does not require minimum hospital stays.

547

To find out if your group health coverage is "insured" or "self-insured," check your health plan's Summary Plan Description or contact your plan administrator.

If your coverage is "insured" and you want to know if you have additional state law protections, check with your state insurance department.

My health coverage is through an individual policy, not through an employer. What rights, if any, do I have under WHCRA?

Health insurance companies and HMOs are generally required to provide WHCRA benefits to individual policies, too. These requirements are generally within the jurisdiction of the state insurance department.

Chapter 60

Purchasing Breast Prostheses and Post-Mastectomy Bras

What is a breast prosthesis?

A breast prosthesis or breast form is an artificial breast that is used after a surgery in which the breast has been altered or removed. Whether the loss of the breast is permanent or temporary, a breast form can be worn to simulate the natural breast and body shape. Full breasts and partial breasts, known as equalizers, can be purchased to balance the appearance depending on what type of surgical procedure was performed. These forms come in a variety of materials (usually silicone, foam, or fiberfill) and they can be worn inside a bra or attached to the body with a special adhesive.

Why would I need a breast prosthesis?

Many women who have been treated for breast cancer have had a surgery that leads to an alteration in their physical appearance. Sometimes these alterations are permanent; they may be temporary if reconstruction is scheduled for a later time. The common types of surgeries include:

- lumpectomy—removal of a breast tumor and some of the breast;

- modified/simple mastectomy—removal of the breast tissue;
- radical mastectomy—surgical removal of breast tissue and underlying muscle.

A silicone breast prosthesis is weighted and simulates the natural breast. One of its advantages is that it helps your body be symmetrical again and remain in balance. When the body is out of balance following a surgery of this kind, other muscle-skeletal problems can develop. Back, neck, and shoulder problems are common as well as a tendency for one shoulder to drop downward and inward while the other rises up. Women also often report that the bra rides up or moves around if there is no weighted breast form on one side of the bra.

What are the advantages of having a breast prosthesis?

Wearing a breast prosthesis is a personal choice. Many women want to wear one because they want to wear the same clothing that they wore prior to the surgery and they want to look symmetrical. There are other advantages to having a breast prosthesis.

It can:

- give you warmth;
- protect your chest and scars;
- help balance your posture;
- keep your bra from shifting or riding up;
- help prevent problems with curvature of the spine, shoulder drop, and muscular pain in the neck and back.

What is a mastectomy bra?

Special bras are made that have pockets to hold the prosthesis. There are many attractive bras that come in varying colors (e.g., white, ivory, black, and nude/beige) that can be fitted at the time of the prosthesis. New products are always becoming available (in different shapes, weights, etc.) so it is a good idea to visit a store to see if there have been any advances since your last fitting.

How soon after surgery can a breast form be worn?

It is a good idea to consult your physician. It varies for each woman depending on her surgery and healing. Most women will be able to wear a prosthesis (breast form) within two to eight weeks after her surgery. Camisoles that have soft attachable prostheses can be worn immediately after surgery until the surgical site is healed.

How do you obtain these products?

You can go to a special store that fits breast prostheses and bras and provides other services. Unlike some lingerie or department stores, these stores cater to the needs of individuals with breast cancer. There are many different brands of prostheses. The most important concern is finding one that is comfortable and fits your body. An expert certified breast prosthesis fitters can fit the bra and prosthesis. You may schedule an appointment for your fitting. The first fitting usually takes about an hour.

How are these products paid for?

You may purchase the prostheses yourself; however, it is a good idea to check your medical insurance before doing this to find out if they will cover the price, how frequently they will replace the prosthesis, and what kind of authorizations are needed.

Many insurance companies will pay for all or part of a new prosthesis every two years and two to three bras every six months to a year. Most insurance plans will determine these things based on medical necessity, but some will have more strict guidelines. You will not know until you ask. For example, patients with Medicare will receive what is medically necessary, which for many patients is a new prosthesis every two years and two bras every six months. However, if a woman's weight changes during this time, her existing breast may change size and this could mean that she needs a new prosthesis or bras to accommodate this change.

When selecting a location to purchase a breast prosthesis, try to determine if the location will bill your insurance, whether your insurance will pay for it at that location, and how much of the balance you could be responsible for after the insurance pays. Sometimes the payments are difficult to know prior to submitting the charge. Many stores will bill you for the balance once the insurance company or insurance companies have paid their portion and determined the patient's portion.

Some stores ask you to pay in advance and then seek reimbursement from your insurance. Since prostheses have a wide range of prices, it is a good idea to find out as much as possible in advance. You need to play an active role in determining what is allowed by your insurance or medical group so that you can receive the best value as well as the best fit and comfort.

Do I need a prescription?

A doctor usually writes a prescription for a breast form, and some insurance companies require a special authorization just like they do for specialists or other medical procedures referred from a primary care doctor. A typical prescription for a breast prosthesis and bras would say the following: "Breast prosthesis for (right, left, or bilateral) and (quantity) prosthetic bras for (diagnosis)."

Please note that if there has been a recent change in your body that requires a new prosthesis such as weight gain for weight loss, your doctor should include this information on the prescription. Any information that supports the medical necessity of the prosthesis at this point in time will help your insurance plan to understand what you need and why. This will facilitate more rapid authorization and or payment processing by your insurance plan.

How much does a breast form (prosthesis) or mastectomy bra cost?

There are many different kinds of breast forms, and the prices vary. A high priced breast form does not insure good quality or a good fit. A proper fitting in our store is the best way to find a good fit that meets your budget. Here is the range of prices that you can expect:

- Silicone prostheses: $215–$350

- Non-silicone prostheses: $40–$80

- Equalizers and enhancers: $80–$225

- Postreconstructive/surgical bras: $36

- Postsurgical camisoles: $65–$80

- Mastectomy bras: $36–$65

Chapter 61

Insurance and Paying for Breast Cancer Treatment

Health Insurance Reform and Breast Cancer

Rising health care costs and inadequate coverage burden many Americans. Alarmingly, those Americans most likely to fall through the cracks are also those who need care the most. Breast cancer patients face great uncertainty in the current health care system. Women diagnosed with breast cancer, whether insured or not, face significant and sometimes devastating hurdles to receiving timely, affordable treatment.

Breast cancer is the second leading type of cancer among women. The disease will affect one in eight American women during their lifetime, with treatment costs totaling $7 billion in 2007. Older women are more likely to develop breast cancer, as well as women who are obese and those who have a history of cancer in their family. This year alone, an estimated 192,370 American women will be diagnosed with breast cancer and 40,170 will die from the disease, making it the second leading cause of cancer deaths in women.

The affordability of treatment is often a concern for women diagnosed with breast cancer. Rising health care costs have left a growing number of Americans either uninsured or with less meaningful

This chapter contains text excerpted from "Health Insurance Reform and Breast Cancer: Making the Health Care System Work for Women," by the U.S. Department of Health and Human Services (HHS, www.healthreform.gov), 2009, and "Clinical Trials and Insurance Coverage," by the National Cancer Institute (NCI, www.cancer.gov), part of the National Institutes of Health, May 8, 2009.

coverage than they need and deserve. The results of a recent survey estimated that 72 million, or 41 percent, of nonelderly adults have accumulated medical debt or had difficulty paying medical bills in the past year—and 61 percent of those experiencing difficulty paying medical bills had insurance.

Problem: Breast cancer patients have high and potentially ruinous out-of-pocket health care costs.

With each passing year, women face increasingly high deductibles, copayments, and other cost-sharing requirements, forcing them to make difficult decisions to make ends meet. Women affected by breast cancer are particularly susceptible to these rising costs. Breast cancer patients with employer-based insurance had total out-of-pocket costs averaging $6,250 in 2007, higher than out-of-pocket spending for patients with asthma, diabetes, chronic obstructive pulmonary disease (COPD), or high blood pressure.

In addition to rising deductibles, copayments, and coinsurance, health insurance plans often contain annual and lifetime benefit caps, particularly in the nongroup insurance market. Because breast cancer treatment is costly and long-term, patients are more likely to surpass these benefit caps, leaving them essentially uninsured. In one recent national survey, 10 percent of all cancer patients reported that they reached a benefit limit in their insurance policy and were forced to seek alternative insurance coverage or pay the remainder of their treatment out-of-pocket.

Jamie Drzewicki, Florida: Jamie reached her employer-sponsored insurance plan's $100,000 annual limit after she was diagnosed with breast cancer. As a result, she amassed about $75,000 in unpaid medical bills. Her hospital eventually forgave $40,000 of her debt, but about $30,000 in debt remains. The medical debt caused significant stress for Jamie, who received many calls from collection agencies. "I am a hard worker and now I am making decisions between paying for my groceries and paying off some of my bills," she says. "I stress about my bills, my job, my cancer."

Problem: Too few women have access to stable, employer-based coverage.

Women are less likely than men to be employed full-time (52 percent versus 73 percent), making them less likely to be eligible for employer-based health benefits. Most women not covered directly through an employer are covered through a spouse (41 percent), while smaller proportions purchase insurance directly through the individual market (5 percent), or are insured through public programs (10 percent). Notably, 38 percent of these women remain uninsured. Such a piecemeal framework for obtaining health insurance can create uncertainty and anxiety for women already fighting a life-threatening disease like breast cancer.

Difficulty finding and maintaining employer-based coverage is especially pronounced for older women, who are more likely to develop conditions like breast cancer. Women are twice as likely as men to get employer-sponsored insurance through their spouse, but this coverage becomes unstable for older women as their spouses may go on Medicare. This can lead to a loss of coverage at a time when older women need it most.

Compounding these difficulties with employer-based coverage, breast cancer is also a physically and emotionally taxing disease, oftentimes precipitating an inability to work. Almost 20 percent of families experiencing any cancer reported that the cancer caused someone in the household to lose a job, change jobs, or work fewer hours.

When employer-sponsored insurance is lost, limited protections exist to ensure families can find adequate coverage. Through COBRA coverage, breast cancer patients can usually continue their employer-sponsored insurance coverage for an average of 18 months by paying the full premiums themselves (with no employer contribution). Through the Health Insurance Portability and Accountability Act (HIPAA), breast cancer patients who previously had employer-based coverage can be protected in finding new employer-based and sometimes individual coverage, but this is subject to several conditions, including at least 18 months of prior uninterrupted group coverage.

Problem: Insurance discrimination based on pre-existing conditions prevent breast cancer patients from accessing necessary treatment in the health care system.

In 45 states across the United States, when a person with a health condition such as breast cancer tries to buy health insurance through the individual insurance market, insurance companies can charge higher premiums, exclude coverage for certain conditions, or even deny coverage altogether because of the pre-existing medical condition. Women are doubly affected by discrimination in the insurance market, particularly in their child-bearing years, when a 22-year-old woman can be charged one and a half times the premium of a 22-year-old man.

Because of this, breast cancer patients, even when in remission, are unlikely to find meaningful insurance coverage in the individual insurance market. A full 11 percent of individuals with any cancer said they could not obtain health coverage because of their illness.

The stress, costs, and uncertainty in maintaining coverage can lead people with chronic conditions like breast cancer to stay in a job they would otherwise leave in order to maintain health benefits—a phenomenon called "job lock." This inability to change jobs has been estimated to cost $3.7 billion in forgone wages in a year.

Joni Lownsdale, Illinois: Joni completed her treatments for stage I breast cancer in 2007 and is insured through her state's high-risk pool. She pays $556 per month for coverage with a $500 deductible and a $1,500 out-of-pocket maximum. She and her husband are self-employed. They have two daughters and spend approximately 14 percent of their income on health insurance premiums and other medical expenses. They try to limit their family's doctor visits in order to save money. "It is frustrating to me," Joni says. "I am at low risk for recurrence, but because I have this cancer diagnosis on my chart, I am uninsurable."

In addition to the inability to find meaningful coverage, if an individual is diagnosed with an expensive condition like breast cancer while covered by a nongroup plan, some insurance companies will review her initial health status questionnaire for errors. In most states' individual insurance markets, insurance companies can retroactively cancel the entire policy if any condition was missed—even if the medical condition is unrelated, or if the person was not aware of the condition at the time. This practice is called rescission.

Problem: Breast cancer prevention and early treatment are underemphasized.

Women who receive recommended mammograms for breast cancer increase their chances for survival and significantly decrease the projected cost of treatment. In recent decades, the size of breast tumors at diagnosis has decreased as mammograms have become more prevalent. However, many effective prevention measures that help with the early detection of cancer are not used often enough. One in five women aged 50 and above have not received a mammogram in the past two years.

Uninsured women in the United States are less likely to receive these vital preventive screenings than women with insurance. A woman who was uninsured for more than 12 months was half as likely to get a mammogram in the past 2 years than a woman who had continuous insurance. As a result, uninsured women with breast cancer are significantly more likely than insured women to be diagnosed with a larger tumor or more advanced cancer. Women without insurance are also more likely to experience a 90 day delay between diagnosis and treatment (23 percent versus 3 percent) and are more likely to receive a mastectomy (37 percent versus 26 percent). And while they are more likely to initiate chemotherapy than insured women, they are less likely to complete it.

Even for women with insurance, cost can be a deterrent to obtaining recommended screenings. Among Medicare beneficiaries, women with insurance plans that required a copayment for a mammogram were significantly less likely to obtain the mammogram than those beneficiaries whose insurance covered the full cost (69 percent versus 78 percent).

In 2009, 40,170 women will lose their lives to breast cancer. It is estimated that 4,000 breast cancer deaths could be prevented just by increasing the percentage of women who receive recommended breast cancer screenings to 90 percent.

Problem: Low-income and minority communities are hit particularly hard by breast cancer.

Treating illnesses is a costly and stressful ordeal, and many minority and low-income women are disproportionately affected by breast cancer. African-American women have a lower risk of developing breast cancer than White women, but once they develop the disease, they have a higher rate of dying from it. African-American women experience five-year survival rates of 78 percent compared to 90 percent for White women.

This is due in part to disparities in prevention. Women with less than a high school education, who are racial or ethnic minorities, who are low-income, and who are recent immigrants are all less likely to have had a recent mammogram. Low-income women have had greater declines in mammography usage in recent years compared with higher-income women.

Disparities also exist in treatment. Studies have demonstrated that Black and Hispanic women with early-stage breast cancer who undergo surgical treatment are less likely than White women to consult oncologists and receive recommended follow-up radiation and/or chemotherapies. A recent study showed that Spanish-speaking Latina women were six times more likely than White women to become dissatisfied with or regret their decisions regarding breast cancer treatment. African-American women were twice as likely to have regrets about their treatment as Whites.

557

Clinical Trials and Insurance Coverage

As you think about taking part in a clinical trial, you will face the issue of how to cover the costs of care. Even if you have health insurance, your plan may not cover all of the costs related to receiving treatment in a clinical trial. This is because some health insurance companies define clinical trials as "experimental."

What are the costs involved in treatment clinical trials?

There are two types of costs associated with a clinical trial: patient care costs and research costs.

Patient care costs fall into two groups. Routine care costs are those related to treating your cancer, whether you are in a trial or receiving standard therapy. These costs include the following:

- Doctor visits
- Hospital stays
- Lab tests
- X-rays and scans

These costs are often covered by health insurance.

Extra care costs are those related to taking part in a clinical trial. These costs might include extra tests that you need as part of the trial, but not as part of your routine care. These costs are not always covered by health insurance.

Research costs are those related to conducting the trial. Examples include the following:

- Research doctor and nurse time
- Analysis of results
- Clinical tests performed purely for research purposes

These costs are often covered by the organization sponsoring the trial.

How can you get your health insurance to cover a clinical trial?

There are several steps you can follow to deal with insurance coverage issues when deciding to enter a clinical trial. Here are some things to try:

- Work closely with your doctor. Ask your doctor if there is someone on his or her staff who can help with health insurance issues. This person might be a financial counselor or research coordinator. Or, this person might work in the hospital's patient finance department.

- Work closely with the research coordinator or research nurse. Ask the research coordinator or nurse if other patients have had problems getting their health insurance companies to cover their costs. If so, you might ask the research coordinator or nurse for help in sending information to your health insurance company that explains why this clinical trial would be appropriate for you. This package might include the following:

  - Medical journal articles that show patient benefits from the treatment that is being tested

  - A letter of medical necessity

  - Letters from researchers that explain the clinical trial

  - Support letters from patient advocacy groups

- Work with your health insurance company. If your doctor does not have a staff person to help with insurance issues, call the customer service number on the back of your health insurance card.

- Ask to speak to the benefit plan department.

- Ask if your health insurance plan covers routine patient care in clinical trial. If your health insurance covers routine patient care in a clinical trial, ask if an authorization is required. An authorization means the health insurance company will review information about the clinical trial before deciding to cover it. If your health insurance company requires an authorization, ask the name and contact information of the person you are talking and what information you need to provide. Examples might include copies of your medical records, a letter from your doctor, and a copy of the consent form for the trial.

If an authorization is not required, you don't have to do anything else. But, it is a good idea to request a letter from your health insurance company that states an authorization is not needed for you to take part in a clinical trial.

Understand the costs related to the trial. Ask your doctor or the trial's contact person about the costs that must be covered by you or your health insurance.

Work closely with your employer's benefits manager. This person may be able to help you work with your health insurance company.

Give your health insurance company a deadline. Ask the hospital or cancer center to set a target date for when you should start treatment. This can help to ensure that coverage decisions are made promptly.

What should you do if your claim is denied after you begin taking part in a trial?

If your claim is denied, contact the research coordinator or nurse for the clinical trial. He or she will know how to appeal your health insurance company's decision. If your treatment in the trial is taking place in your doctor's office, ask the office billing manager for help.

You can also read your health insurance policy to find out what steps you can follow to make an appeal. Ask your doctor to help you. It might help if he or she contacts the medical director of your health plan.

How do health insurers decide to cover clinical trial costs?

Health insurance companies consider certain factors when deciding if they will cover the costs of clinical trials. Some of the factors in your favor may include whether the following are true:

- You live in a state that requires coverage for clinical trials. Some states have laws or special agreements that require health insurance companies to pay for routine care you receive in a clinical trial.

- Language in your health insurance policy allows coverage of routine patient care in a clinical trial.

- The trial is medically necessary. This is often decided on a case-by-case basis.

- The trial is a phase III trial. A health insurance company may be willing to cover a phase III trial because the treatments have already been successful with a number of people.

- The routine care costs of the trial are about the same as the routine care costs for standard therapy.

- There is no standard therapy for your type and stage of cancer.

- The trial is sponsored by the National Institutes of Health or one of the groups it supports.

What should you do if you have Medicare?

Medicare will pay for routine costs in most treatment clinical trials that are funded by federal agencies, such as the National Institutes of Health.

Chapter 62

Caregiving for Someone with Breast Cancer

What Does Someone with Breast Cancer Expect, Want, and Need from a Caregiver?

From the moment a loved one delivers the news of a breast cancer diagnosis, a host of questions arise about how your family is going to cope with everything that needs to be done in the days and months ahead. The role of caregiver can encompass a huge variety of responsibilities, large and small, and deciding who's going to do what is a process you and your family need to tackle together. Start by sitting down with everyone involved and making a list of everything that needs doing, so you can prioritize which ones you should focus on.

To get you started, here are some of the most common responsibilities that can come under the "caregiver" job description.

Helping with Physical Needs

- Communicating and coordinating with primary care physician, oncologist, and other medical staff
- Obtaining and helping organize medications, equipment, and other supplies

"Defining Your Role as a Breast Cancer Caregiver," reprinted with permission from http://www.caring.com/articles/breast-cancer-caregiver. © 2012 Caring, Inc. (www.caring.com). All rights reserved.

- Managing pain, nausea, vomiting, constipation, diarrhea, and other symptoms

- Handling grocery shopping and cooking, helping with eating and cleaning up

- Taking care of cleaning, laundry, and other household tasks

- Driving to and from appointments and running other errands

Helping with Emotional Issues

- Supporting and dealing with issues such as depression and anxiety

- Finding and coordinating membership in a support group or other supportive therapy

- Being available to talk through sadness, fear, and other emotional issues that arise

- Supporting her relationship with her spouse or partner

Helping with Financial Issues

- Paying bills

- Getting answers to medical insurance coverage questions

- Handling other insurance issues

- Planning long-term financial issues

Supporting Her Social Life

- Helping coordinate visits with friends, family, support staff, and other community members so she doesn't become isolated

- Communicating with family and friends about her status and needs

- Helping her continue with favorite activities and hobbies

What to Watch out For

One caveat: It's important to recognize, from the very beginning, the dangers of caregiver burnout. There's no way you can take on all aspects of caregiving alone, and if you try, you're bound to grow frustrated and discouraged pretty quickly. Keep in mind that breast cancer treatment takes time, and you're at the beginning of a long and difficult journey. If you use up all your reserves of time, energy, and support at the beginning, during the "crisis" phase, you might not have enough stamina to hang in there during the prolonged phase of care management.

Your role will constantly change as you and the person in your care evaluate what she can do and what she needs you or someone else to do for her. "It will be a constant evolution as she goes through periods of helplessness and then through times of feeling empowered," says Bonnie Bajorek Daneker, author of *The Compassionate Caregiver's Guide to Caring for Someone with Cancer.* "You'll find you're constantly trying to balance between these two stances. You always have to adjust, depending on how she's feeling."

For example, Daneker says, it's common for cancer patients to feel strong and capable during periods between chemotherapy treatments, and then extremely fatigued and emotional during and right after treatment. Or you may find that the steroids often prescribed during chemo give the person in your care a short-lived energy boost that lasts for a day or two before dissipating, at which point the fatigue hits. "As a caregiver, you have to be so in tune with what the patient wants and needs," Daneker says. "It's important to be flexible and highly communicative to deal with the constant changes."

What Are You Able and Willing to Do, and What Can't You Do?

Becoming a caregiver for someone with breast cancer may be a role you choose, or it may feel like a role that's been thrust on you. After all, it's not easy for you—or anyone—to accept the idea that a serious illness has entered your life. You may struggle with denial and acceptance just as the person in your care is struggling with these issues.

By stepping into the role of caregiver, you're offering the incredible gift of having someone to turn to in a difficult time. It's important, though, to try to be as realistic as possible about what's needed, and about your own limitations, right from the get-go.

Start by accepting the fact that caring for someone with breast cancer is a very big job. Practical considerations such as whether you live nearby or at a distance, how much time you have available, how many other responsibilities you have on your plate (children? work?), and how comfortable you are dealing with certain situations will play a role in which aspects of caregiving you take on, and which you choose to delegate to professionals, family, and friends.

563

Talk as openly as possible with everyone involved about both your strengths and limitations as a caregiver, and explain what you're able to take on, and what you've asked others to do. You might say something like, "As you know, my job doesn't make it easy for me to take time off during the day, so I'm going to come to your oncology appointments, but Bob and Betty are going to take turns driving you to your chemo appointments."

One huge challenge you'll likely encounter is how to support and encourage her optimism and will to fight the cancer while absorbing information that can at times be frightening and discouraging. You may find yourself torn, for example, between wanting to say positive and encouraging things while still helping her face the reality of a less-than-positive prognosis.

Establishing Clear Lines of Communication

Talk with other caregivers, and you'll quickly learn that one of the hardest parts of being in this role is dealing with guilt, anxiety, and the constant feeling that you aren't doing enough. (That's why it's essential to let yourself off the hook: You're doing all you can, and that's good enough.) To help protect yourself—and other involved—from these feelings, you're going to need to set limits for yourself. And the key to doing this is clear communication.

You may, for instance, need to explain a little more than you ever have before about your job—what your responsibilities entail, when you can get away, and when you can't. You may need to set some limits around your own family time, such as asking family not to call past a certain point in the evening unless it's an emergency, or setting up a phone tree so that calls about some issues come to you, and others are directed to your siblings or to family friends.

Establishing Clear Expectations

Another way to establish limits is to set clear expectations with everyone involved, especially the person with cancer. What can she expect your help with, and what's beyond the scope of what you can provide? Explain that while you're going to be the "point person" for caregiving, others will help you make sure everything gets done.

Using the list you made together of all the things she needs help with, focus on working together to assemble a reliable team of helpers to get it all accomplished. If you have siblings, set up a communications system that enables you to delegate tasks to them. Even those who live at a distance can take on a set of obligations. For example, you might give your sister on the opposite coast the job of dealing with medical insurance, or your brother could take over financial planning questions.

If you don't know all of your loved one's friends and neighbors, don't be shy about asking. Remind her about her bowling league, her church community, and any support network available, and ask how to get in touch with these folks.

Friends, neighbors, and other members of her community will ask how they can help, and when they do, suggest that they pitch in with cooking, cleaning, driving, and other household needs—then choose a specific task and assign it.

Ensuring That the System Works

To make everything run smoothly, you'll want to get your siblings, other family members, and other potential members of your caregiving team on the same page. What you especially want to avoid is the "Call me syndrome," where every problem that arises—and there will be lots of them—triggers a call to you. Protect yourself from becoming a communications hub by making clear who's doing what. You might say, "Sarah's handling insurance, so call her when you have questions about what's covered." If there's a friend or neighbor you can put in charge of coordinating driving for errands and routine appointments, then ask your family to call that person directly, and only call you when it's an appointment or errand that involves you. If it's hard for your loved one to keep it all straight, you might type up a list of responsibilities and contact numbers and tape it to the wall by the phone.

Another key to avoiding feeling overwhelmed is to marshal professional resources so that every issue that arises doesn't land on your plate. You might, for instance, need to discuss expectations about cooking, cleaning, and other household tasks. Perhaps there's money available to hire someone to clean once a week, or to call a handyman—rather than you—when routine maintenance issues crop up.

One thing you'll probably start to realize fairly quickly is that there aren't any hard-and-fast rules for how involved or take-charge you'll need to be. There will be times when you'll be asked to step in and make key decisions, and other times when your role will be to simply listen and offer your emotional support.

Part Eight

Additional Help
and Information

Chapter 63

Glossary of Breast Cancer Terms

abnormal: Not normal. An abnormal lesion or growth may be cancer, premalignant (likely to become cancer), or benign (not cancer).

adjuvant therapy: Additional cancer treatment given after the primary treatment to lower the risk that the cancer will come back. Adjuvant therapy may include chemotherapy, radiation therapy, hormone therapy, targeted therapy, or biological therapy.

areola: The area of dark-colored skin on the breast that surrounds the nipple.

aromatase inhibitor: A drug that prevents the formation of estradiol, a female hormone, by interfering with an aromatase enzyme. Aromatase inhibitors are used as a type of hormone therapy for postmenopausal women who have hormone-dependent breast cancer.

benign breast disease: A common condition marked by benign (not cancer) changes in breast tissue. These changes may include irregular lumps or cysts, breast discomfort, sensitive nipples, and itching. These symptoms may change throughout the menstrual cycle and usually stop after menopause.

benign: Not cancerous. Benign tumors may grow larger but do not spread to other parts of the body. Also called nonmalignant.

Definitions in this chapter were compiled from documents published by the National Cancer Institute (NCI, www.cancer.gov), part of the National Institutes of Health.

biopsy: The removal of cells or tissues for examination by a pathologist. The pathologist may study the tissue under a microscope or perform other tests on the cells or tissue.

breast cancer gene 1 (BRCA1): A gene on chromosome 17 that normally helps to suppress cell growth. A person who inherits certain mutations (changes) in a BRCA1 gene has a higher risk of getting breast, ovarian, prostate, and other types of cancer.

breast cancer gene 2 (BRCA2): A gene on chromosome 13 that normally helps to suppress cell growth. A person who inherits certain mutations (changes) in a BRCA2 gene has a higher risk of getting breast, ovarian, prostate, and other types of cancer.

breast cancer: Cancer that forms in tissues of the breast, usually the ducts (tubes that carry milk to the nipple) and lobules (glands that make milk). It occurs in both men and women, although male breast cancer is rare.

breast carcinoma in situ: There are two types of breast carcinoma in situ: Ductal carcinoma in situ (DCIS) and lobular carcinoma in situ (LCIS). DCIS is a noninvasive condition in which abnormal cells are found in the lining of a breast duct (a tube that carries milk to the nipple). The abnormal cells have not spread outside the duct to other tissues in the breast. In some cases, DCIS may become invasive cancer and spread to other tissues, although it is not known how to predict which lesions will become invasive cancer. LCIS is a condition in which abnormal cells are found in the lobules (small sections of tissue involved with making milk) of the breast. This condition seldom becomes invasive cancer; however, having LCIS in one breast increases the risk of developing breast cancer in either breast. Also called stage 0 breast carcinoma in situ.

breast density: Describes the relative amount of different tissues present in the breast. A dense breast has less fat than glandular and connective tissue. Mammogram films of breasts with higher density are harder to read and interpret than those of less dense breasts.

breast duct: A thin tube in the breast that carries milk from the breast lobules to the nipple. Also called milk duct.

breast implant: A silicone gel-filled or saline-filled sac placed under the chest muscle to restore breast shape.

breast lobe: A section of the breast that contains the lobules (the glands that make milk).

breast reconstruction: Surgery to rebuild the shape of the breast after a mastectomy.

breast self-exam: An exam by a woman of her breasts to check for lumps or other changes.

breast: Glandular organ located on the chest. The breast is made up of connective tissue, fat, and breast tissue that contains the glands that can make milk. Also called mammary gland.

breast-conserving surgery: An operation to remove the breast cancer but not the breast itself.

calcification: Deposits of calcium in the tissues.

carcinoma: Cancer that begins in the skin or in tissues that line or cover internal organs.

clinical breast exam (CBE): A physical exam of the breast performed by a health care provider to check for lumps or other changes.

clinical trial: A type of research study that tests how well new medical approaches work in people. These studies test new methods of screening, prevention, diagnosis, or treatment of a disease. Also called clinical study.

curative surgery: An operation to remove cancerous tissue.

diethylstilbestrol (DES): A synthetic form of the hormone estrogen that was prescribed to pregnant women between about 1940 and 1971 because it was thought to prevent miscarriages. Diethylstilbestrol may increase the risk of uterine, ovarian, or breast cancer in women who took it. It also has been linked to an increased risk of clear cell carcinoma of the vagina or cervix in daughters exposed to diethylstilbestrol before birth.

digital mammography: The use of a computer, rather than x-ray film, to create a picture of the breast.

early-stage breast cancer: Breast cancer that has not spread beyond the breast or the axillary lymph nodes. This includes ductal carcinoma in situ and stage I, stage IIA, stage IIB, and stage IIIA breast cancers.

estrogen receptor negative (ER-): Describes cells that do not have a protein to which the hormone estrogen will bind. Cancer cells that are ER- do not need estrogen to grow, and usually do not stop growing when treated with hormones that block estrogen from binding.

estrogen receptor positive (ER+): Describes cells that have a receptor protein that binds the hormone estrogen. Cancer cells that are ER+ may need estrogen to grow, and may stop growing or die when treated with substances that block the binding and actions of estrogen.

estrogen receptor: A protein found inside the cells of the female reproductive tissue, some other types of tissue, and some cancer cells. The hormone estrogen will bind to the receptors inside the cells and may cause the cells to grow. Also called estrogen receptor.

genetic susceptibility: An inherited increase in the risk of developing a disease. Also called genetic predisposition.

genetic testing: Analyzing deoxyribonucleic acid (DNA) to look for a genetic alteration that may indicate an increased risk for developing a specific disease or disorder.

grade: A description of a tumor based on how abnormal the cancer cells look under a microscope and how quickly the tumor is likely to grow and spread. Grading systems are different for each type of cancer.

hormone receptor: A cell protein that binds a specific hormone. The hormone receptor may be on the surface of the cell or inside the cell. Many changes take place in a cell after a hormone binds to its receptor.

hormone replacement therapy (HRT): Hormones (estrogen, progesterone, or both) given to women after menopause to replace the hormones no longer produced by the ovaries.

human epidermal growth factor receptor 2 (HER2/neu): A protein involved in normal cell growth. It is found on some types of cancer cells, including breast and ovarian. Cancer cells removed from the body may be tested for the presence of HER2/neu to help decide the best type of treatment.

inflammatory breast cancer: A type of breast cancer in which the breast looks red and swollen and feels warm. The skin of the breast may also show the pitted appearance called peau d'orange (like the skin of an orange). The redness and warmth occur because the cancer cells block the lymph vessels in the skin.

invasive breast cancer: Cancer that has spread from where it started in the breast into surrounding, healthy tissue. Most invasive breast cancers start in the ducts (tubes that carry milk from the lobules to the nipple). Invasive breast cancer can spread to other parts of the body through the blood and lymph systems. Also called infiltrating breast cancer.

laser surgery: A surgical procedure that uses the cutting power of a laser beam to make bloodless cuts in tissue or to remove a surface lesion such as a tumor.

lumpectomy: Surgery to remove abnormal tissue or cancer from the breast and a small amount of normal tissue around it. It is a type of breast-sparing surgery.

lymphatic system: The tissues and organs that produce, store, and carry white blood cells that fight infections and other diseases. This system includes the bone marrow, spleen, thymus, lymph nodes, and lymphatic vessels (a network of thin tubes that carry lymph and white blood cells). Lymphatic vessels branch, like blood vessels, into all the tissues of the body.

lymphedema: A condition in which extra lymph fluid builds up in tissues and causes swelling. It may occur in an arm or leg if lymph vessels are blocked, damaged, or removed by surgery.

mammary: Having to do with the breast.

mastectomy: Surgery to remove the breast (or as much of the breast tissue as possible).

medullary breast carcinoma: A rare type of breast cancer that often can be treated successfully. It is marked by lymphocytes (a type of white blood cell) in and around the tumor that can be seen when viewed under a microscope.

metastasize: To spread from one part of the body to another. When cancer cells metastasize and form secondary tumors, the cells in the metastatic tumor are like those in the original (primary) tumor.

neoadjuvant therapy: Treatment given as a first step to shrink a tumor before the main treatment, which is usually surgery, is given. Examples of neoadjuvant therapy include chemotherapy, radiation therapy, and hormone therapy. It is a type of induction therapy.

oncologist: A doctor who specializes in treating cancer. Some oncologists specialize in a particular type of cancer treatment. For example, a radiation oncologist specializes in treating cancer with radiation.

oophorectomy: Surgery to remove one or both ovaries.

Paget disease of the nipple: A form of breast cancer in which the tumor grows from ducts beneath the nipple onto the surface of the nipple.

prophylactic mastectomy: Surgery to reduce the risk of developing breast cancer by removing one or both breasts before disease develops. Also called preventive mastectomy.

reconstructive surgery: Surgery that is done to reshape or rebuild (reconstruct) a part of the body changed by previous surgery.

recurrence: Cancer that has recurred (come back), usually after a period of time during which the cancer could not be detected. The cancer may come back to the same place as the original (primary) tumor or to another place in the body.

staging: Performing exams and tests to learn the extent of the cancer within the body, especially whether the disease has spread from the original site to other parts of the body. It is important to know the stage of the disease in order to plan the best treatment.

tamoxifen: A drug used to treat certain types of breast cancer in women and men. It is also used to prevent breast cancer in women who have had ductal carcinoma in situ (abnormal cells in the ducts of the breast) and in women who are at a high risk of developing breast cancer.

triple-negative breast cancer: Describes breast cancer cells that do not have estrogen receptors, progesterone receptors, or large amounts of HER2/neu protein.

Chapter 64

Directory of Organizations That Offer Information and Financial Assistance to People with Breast Cancer

Government Agencies That Provide Information about Breast Cancer

Agency for Healthcare Research and Quality
Office of Communications and Knowledge Transfer
540 Gaither Road, Suite 2000
Rockville, MD 20850
Phone: 301-427-1104
Website: www.ahrq.gov

Resources in this chapter were compiled from several sources deemed reliable; all contact information was verified and updated in March 2012. The information under the heading "Find a Breast Cancer Screening Provider If You Are Uninsured or Underinsured," is from "Find a Screening Provider Near You," by the National Breast and Cervical Cancer Early Detection Program (NBCCEDP), part of the Centers for Disease Control and Prevention (CDC, www.cdc.gov/cancer/nbccedp), May 25, 2011.

Centers for Disease Control and Prevention
1600 Clifton Road
Atlanta, GA 30333
Toll-Free: 800-CDC-INFO
(800-232-4636)
Toll-Free TTY: 888-232-6348
Phone: 404-639-3311
Website: www.cdc.gov
E-mail: cdcinfo@cdc.gov

Federal Trade Commission
600 Pennsylvania Avenue NW
Washington, DC 20580
Phone: 202-326-2222
Website: www.ftc.gov
E-mail: webmaster@ftc.gov

575

Healthfinder®
National Health Information
Center
PO Box 1133
Washington, DC 20013-1133
Toll-Free: 800-336-4797
Phone: 301-565-4167
Fax: 301-984-4256
Website: www.healthfinder.gov
E-mail: healthfinder@nhic.org

National Cancer Institute
NCI Office of Communications
and Education
Public Inquiries Office
6116 Executive Boulevard
Suite 300
Bethesda, MD 20892-8322
Toll-Free: 800-4-CANCER
(800-422-6237)
Toll-Free TTY: 800-332-8615
Website: www.cancer.gov
E-mail:
cancergovstaff@mail.nih.gov

National Center for Complementary and Alternative Medicine
National Institutes of Health
NCCAM Clearinghouse
PO Box 7923
Gaithersburg, MD 20898-7923
Toll-Free: 888-644-6226
Toll-Free TTY: 866-464-3615
Toll-Free Fax: 866-464-3616
Website: www.nccam.nih.gov
E-mail: info@nccam.nih.gov

National Center for Health Statistics
3311 Toledo Road
Hyattsville, MD 20782
Toll-Free: 800-CDC-INFO
(800-232-4636)
Website: www.cdc.gov/nchs
E-mail: cdcinfo@cdc.gov

National Institute on Aging
Building 31, Room 5C27
31 Center Drive, MSC 2292
Bethesda, MD 20892
Toll-Free: 800-222-2225
Toll-Free TTY: 800-222-4225
Phone: 301-496-1752
Fax: 301-496-1072
Website: www.nia.nih.gov
E-mail: niaic@nia.nih.gov

National Institutes of Health
9000 Rockville Pike
Bethesda, Maryland 20892
Phone: 301-496-4000
TTY: 301-402-9612
Website: www.nih.gov
E-mail: NIHinfo@od.nih.gov

National Women's Health Information Center
Office on Women's Health
200 Independence Avenue SW
Room 712E
Washington DC 20201
Toll-Free: 800-994-9662
Toll-Free TDD: 888-220-5446
Phone: 202-690-7650
Fax: 202-205-2631
Website: www.womenshealth.gov

Sister Study
Toll-Free: 877-4SISTER
(877-474-7837)
TTY: 866-TTY-4SIS
(866-889-4747)
Website: www.sisterstudy.org
E-mail:
postmaster@sisterstudy.org

U.S. Department of Health and Human Services
200 Independence Avenue SW
Washington, DC 20201
Toll-Free: 877-696-6775
Website: www.hhs.gov

U.S. Food and Drug Administration
10903 New Hampshire Avenue
Silver Spring, MD 20993
Toll-Free: 888-INFO-FDA
(888-463-6332)
Website: www.fda.gov

U.S. National Library of Medicine
8600 Rockville Pike
Bethesda, MD 20894
Toll-Free: 888-FIND-NLM
(888-346-3656)
Toll-Free TDD: 800-735-2258
Phone: 301-594-5983
Fax: 301-402-1384
Website: www.nlm.nih.gov
E-mail: custserv@nlm.nih.gov

Private Agencies That Provide Information about Breast Cancer

Advanced Breast Cancer Community
Website:
www.advancedbreastcancer
community.org
E-mail: help@advanced
breastcancercommunity.org

African American Breast Cancer Alliance
PO Box 8981
Minneapolis, MN 55408
Phone: 612-825-3675
Fax: 612-827-2977
Website: www.aabcainc.org
E-mail: aabca@aabcainc.org

American Cancer Society
250 Williams Street NW
Atlanta, GA 30303
Toll-Free: 800-227-2345
Toll-Free TTY: 866-228-4327
Website: www.cancer.org

American College of Radiology
1891 Preston White Drive
Reston, VA 20191
Toll-Free: 800-227-5463
Phone: 703-648-8900
Website: www.acr.org
E-mail: info@acr.org

American Institute for Cancer Research
1759 R Street NW
Washington, DC 20009
Toll-Free: 800-843-8114
Phone: 202-328-7744
Fax: 202-328-7226
Website: www.aicr.org
E-mail: aicrweb@aicr.org

American Medical Association
515 North State Street
Chicago, IL 60654
Toll-Free: 800-621-8335
Website: www.ama-assn.org

American Society for Clinical Oncology
2318 Mill Road
Suite 800
Alexandria, VA 22314
Toll-Free: 888-651-3038
Phone: 571-483-1780
Fax: 571-366-9537
Website: www.cancer.net
E-mail: contactus@cancer.net

American Society for Radiation Oncology
8280 Willow Oaks Corporate Drive
Suite 500
Fairfax, VA 22031
Toll-Free: 800-962-7876
Phone: 703-502-1550
Fax: 703-502-7852
Website: www.astro.org

American Society of Plastic and Reconstructive Surgeons
444 East Algonquin Road
Arlington Heights, IL 60005
Phone: 847-228-9900
Website: www.plasticsurgery.org

Association of Cancer Online Resources
173 Duane Street, Suite 3A
New York NY 10013-3334
Phone: 212-226-5525
Website: www.acor.org
E-mail: feedback@acor.org

Avon Foundation Breast Center
Website:
www.hopkinsmedicine.org/avon_foundation_breast_center

Breast Cancer Care
5-13 Great Suffolk Street
London SE1 0NS
United Kingdom
Website:
www.breastcancercare.org.uk
E-mail:
info@breastcancercare.org.uk

Breast Cancer Research Foundation
60 East 56th Street, 8th Floor
New York, NY 10022
Toll-Free: 866-FIND-A-CURE
(866-346-3228)
Phone: 646-497-2600
Fax: 646-497-0890
Website: www.bcrfcure.org
E-mail: bcrf@bcrfcure.org

Breast Cancer Society, Inc.
6859 East Rembrandt Avenue
Suite 128
Mesa, AZ 85212
Toll-Free: 888-470-7909
Fax: 480-659-9807
Website:
www.breastcancersociety.org
E-mail:
info@breastcancersociety.org

BreastCancerTrials.org
3450 California Street
San Francisco, CA 94118
Phone: 415-476-5777
Website:
www.breastcancertrials.org

Breastcancer.org
7 East Lancaster Avenue
3rd Floor
Ardmore, PA 19003
Phone: 610-642-6550
Website: www.breastcancer.org

Cancer and Careers
Website:
www.cancerandcareers.org
E-mail:
cancerandcareers@cew.org

Cancer Support Community
1050 17th Street NW
Suite 500
Washington, DC 20036
Toll-Free: 888-793-9355
Phone: 202-659-9709
Website: www.cancer
supportcommunity.org
E-mail: help@cancersupport
community.org

CancerCare
275 Seventh Avenue
New York, NY 10001
Toll-Free: 800-813-HOPE
(800-813-4673)
Phone: 212-712-8400
Fax: 212-712-8495
Website: www.cancercare.org
E-mail: info@cancercare.org

CancerConnect.com
491 North Main Street
Suite 200
PO Box 2581
Ketchum, ID 83340
Website: www.cancerconnect.com
E-mail:
info@cancerconsultants.com

Caring.com
2600 South El Camino Real
Suite 300
San Mateo, CA 94403
Website: www.caring.com

Cleveland Clinic
9500 Euclid Avenue
Cleveland, OH 44195
Toll-Free: 800-223-2273
Toll-Free: 866-588-2264
(Info Line)
Phone: 216-636-5860 (Info Line)
TTY: 216-444-0261
Website: my.clevelandclinic.org

579

Coalition of Cancer Cooperative Groups
1818 Market Street
Suite 1100
Philadelphia, PA 19103
Toll-Free: 877-520-4457
Fax: 215-789-3655
Website:
www.cancertrialshelp.org
E-mail:
info@CancerTrialsHelp.org

College of American Pathologists
325 Waukegan Road
Northfield, IL 60093-2750
Toll-Free: 800-323-4040
Phone: 847-832-7000
Fax: 847-832-8000
Website: www.cap.org

Facing Our Risk of Cancer Empowered (FORCE)
16057 Tampa Palms Boulevard W
PMB #373
Tampa, FL 33647
Toll-Free: 866-288-RISK
(866-288-7475)
Toll-Free Helpline:
866-824-RISK (866-824-7475)
Fax: 954-827-2200
Website: www.facingourrisk.org
E-mail: info@facingourrisk.org

Family Caregiver Alliance
785 Market Street, Suite 750
San Francisco, CA 94103
Toll-Free: 800-445-8106
Phone: 415-434-3388
Website: www.caregiver.org
E-mail: info@caregiver.org

Imaginis
25 East Court Street, Suite 301
Greenville, SC 29601
Phone: 864-209-1139
Website: www.imaginis.com
E-mail: learnmore@imaginis.com

Inflammatory Breast Cancer Research Foundation
Toll-Free: 877-786-7422
Website: www.ibcresearch.org
E-mail: information@
mail.ibcresearch.org

International Agency for Research on Cancer
150 Cours Albert Thomas
69372 Lyon CEDEX 08
France
Tel: 33 04 72 73 84 85
Fax: 33 04 72 73 85 75
Website: www.iarc.fr

Susan G. Komen for the Cure
5005 LBJ Freeway, Suite 250
Dallas, TX 75244
Toll-Free: 877 GO KOMEN
(877-465-6636)
Website: ww5.komen.org

Lab Tests Online
American Association for
Clinical Chemistry
1850 K Street NW, Suite 625
Washington, DC 20006
Toll-Free: 800-892-1400
Fax: 202-887-5093
Website: www.labtestsonline.org

Living Beyond Breast Cancer
354 West Lancaster Avenue
Suite 224
Haverford, PA 19041
Phone: 610-645-4567
Phone: 484-708-1550
Fax: 610-645-4573
Website: www.lbbc.org
E-mail: mail@lbbc.org

Lymph Notes
Website: www.lymphnotes.com

Men Against Breast Cancer
PO Box 150
Adamstown, MD 21710-0150
Toll-Free: 866-547-MABC
(866-547-6222)
Fax: 301-874-8657
Website: www.menagainst
breastcancer.org
E-mail: info@menagainstbreast
cancer.org

Metastatic Breast Cancer Network
PO Box 1449
New York, NY 10159
Toll-Free: 888-500-0370
Website: www.mbcnetwork.org
E-mail: mbcn@mbcn.org

Mothers Supporting Daughters with Breast Cancer
25235 Fox Chase Drive
Chestertown, MD 21620
Phone: 410-778-1982
Fax: 410-778-1411
Website:
www.mothersdaughters.org
E-mail: msdbc@verizon.net

National Breast Cancer Coalition
1101 17th Street NW, Suite 1300
Washington, DC 20036
Toll-Free: 800-622-2838
Phone: 202-296-7477
Fax: 202-265-6854
Website: www.breastcancer
deadline2020.org

National Breast Cancer Foundation, Inc.
2600 Network Boulevard
Suite 300
Frisco, TX 75034
Website:
www.nationalbreastcancer.org

National Coalition for Cancer Survivorship
1010 Wayne Avenue, Suite 770
Silver Spring, MD 20910
Toll-Free: 877-NCCS-YES
(877-622-7937)
Phone: 301-650-9127
Website:
www.canceradvocacy.org
E-mail: info@canceradvocacy.org

National Comprehensive Cancer Network
275 Commerce Drive, Suite 300
Fort Washington, PA 19034
Phone: 215-690-0300
Fax: 215-690-0280
Website: www.nccn.org

National Hospice and Palliative Care Organization
1731 King Street, Suite 100
Alexandria, VA 22314
Toll-Free: 800-658-8898
Phone: 703-837-1500
Fax: 703-837-1233
Website: www.nhpco.org
E-mail: nhpco_info@nhpco.org

National Lymphedema Network
116 New Montgomery Street
Suite 235
San Francisco, CA 94105
Toll-Free: 800-541-3259
Phone: 415-908-3681
Fax: 415-908-3813
Website: www.lymphnet.org
E-mail: nln@lymphnet.org

National Society of Genetic Counselors
401 North Michigan Avenue
22nd Floor
Chicago, IL 60611
Phone: 312-321-6834
Website: www.nsgc.org
E-mail: nsgc@nsgc.org

OncoLink
The Perelman Center for Advanced Medicine
3400 Civic Center Boulevard
Suite 2338
Philadelphia, PA 19104
Phone: 215-349-8895
Fax: 215-349-5445
Website: www.oncolink.org
E-mail: hampshire@uphs.upenn.edu

SHARE: Self Help for Women with Breast or Ovarian Cancer
1501 Broadway, Suite 704A
New York, NY 10036
Toll-Free: 866-891-2392
Phone: 212-719-0364
Phone: 212-382-2111
E-mail: info@sharecancersupport.org
Website: www.sharecancersupport.org

Sharsheret: Your Jewish Community Facing Breast Cancer
1086 Teaneck Road, Suite 3A
Teaneck, NJ 07666
Toll-Free: 866-474-2774
Phone: 201-833-2341
Fax: 201-837-5025
Website: www.sharsheret.org
E-mail: info@sharsheret.org

Sisters Network Inc.
2922 Rosedale Street
Houston, TX 77004
Toll-Free: 866-781-1808
Phone: 713-781-0255
Fax: 713-780-8998
Website:
www.sistersnetworkinc.org
E-mail:
infonet@sistersnetworkinc.org

Society of Interventional Radiology
3975 Fair Ridge Drive
Suite 400 North
Fairfax, VA 22033
Toll-Free: 800-488-7284
Phone: 703-691-1805
Fax: 703-691-1855
Website: www.sirweb.org

Society of Nuclear Medicine
1850 Samuel Morse Drive
Reston, VA 20190
Telephone: 703-708-9000
Fax: 703-708-9015
Website: www.snm.org
E-mail: feedback@snm.org

Tigerlily Foundation
11654 Plaza America Drive #725
Reston, VA 20190
Toll-Free: 888-580-6253
Fax: 703-663-9844
Website:
www.tigerlilyfoundation.org
E-mail:
info@tigerlilyfoundation.org

Triple Negative Breast Cancer Foundation
PO Box 204
Norwood, NJ 07648
Toll-Free: 877-880-8622
Phone: 646-942-0242
Website:
www.tnbcfoundation.org
E-mail: info@tnbcfoundation.org

Well Spouse Foundation
63 West Main Street, Suite H
Freehold, NJ 07728
Toll-Free: 800-838-0879
Phone: 732-577-8899
Fax: 732-577-8644
Website: www.wellspouse.org
E-mail: info@wellspouse.org

Y-ME National Breast Cancer Organization
135 South LaSalle Street
Suite 2000
Chicago, IL 60603
Toll-Free: 800-221-2141
Phone: 312-986-8338
Fax: 312-294-8597
Website: www.y-me.org
E-mail: info@y-me.org

Young Survival Coalition
61 Broadway, Suite 2235
New York, NY 10006
Toll-Free: 877-972-1011
Website: www.youngsurvival.org

Financial Resources for People with Breast Cancer

The following government departments provide financial and income assistance programs for people with cancer:

Department of Health and Human Services
Toll-Free: 877-696-6775
Website: www.hhs.gov

Medicare and Medicaid
Toll-Free: 877-267-2323
Website: www.cms.hhs.gov

National Breast and Cervical Cancer Early Detection Program
Toll-Free: 800-CDC-INFO (800-232-4636)
Website: www.cdc.gov/cancer/nbccedp

Social Security
Toll-Free: 800-772-1213
Website: www.ssa.gov

U.S. Administration on Aging
Toll-Free: 800-677-1116
Website: www.eldercare.gov

The following private organizations provide financial assistance to people with breast cancer:

American Cancer Society
Toll-Free: 800-227-2345
Website: www.cancer.org/Treatment/SupportProgramsServices

The American Cancer Society offers programs for cancer patients to help pay the costs of transportation, treatment, lodging, and other expenses.

CancerCare Co-Payment Assistance Foundation
Toll-Free: 866-55-COPAY (866-552-6729)
Website: www.cancercarecopay.org

This organization offers help to those who cannot afford their insurance copayments for cancer care.

Fertile Hope

Toll-Free: 866-965-7205 (LIVESTRONG Survivor Care)
Website: www.fertilehope.org/financial-assistance/index.cfm

This organization provides financial help to people with cancer whose insurance will not cover fertility treatment.

NeedyMeds

Website: www.needymeds.org

This website collects information about patient assistance programs for medications and medical supplies sponsored by government agencies, nonprofit organizations, and pharmaceutical companies.

Partnership for Prescription Assistance

Toll-Free 888-4PPA-NOW (888-477-2669)
Website: www.pparx.org

This organization assists patients who do not have coverage for prescription medications to receive free or low-cost medications.

Patient Advocate Foundation

Toll-Free: 800-532-5274
Website: www.patientadvocate.org

This organization assists patients with medical debt, access to insurance issues, and job retention.

Find a Breast Cancer Screening Provider If You Are Uninsured or Underinsured

The National Breast and Cervical Cancer Early Detection Program (NBCCEDP) provides breast and cervical cancer screenings and diagnostic services to low-income, uninsured, and underinsured women across the United States.

To search for free and low-cost screenings in your state, use the interactive map at apps.nccd.cdc.gov/dcpc_Programs/default.aspx?NPID=1 to find local contacts for breast and cervical cancer screening.

What services does the NBCCEDP provide?

The NBCCEDP programs offer the following services for eligible women in your area:

- Clinical breast examinations

- Mammograms
- Pap tests
- Pelvic examinations
- Diagnostic testing if results are abnormal
- Referrals to treatment

Who should get breast and cervical cancer screenings?

All women are at risk for breast and cervical cancer, but regular screenings can prevent or detect these diseases early. The U.S. Preventive Services Task Force has established the following guidelines for screening, but you should discuss with your health care provider how often you should get screened.

- Breast cancer: Women between 50 and 74 years old should get mammograms every two years. Those under 50 should talk with their provider about when they should be screened.
- Cervical cancer: Women should get their first Pap test within three years of the first time they have sex or at age 21 (whichever happens first) and continue screening at least every three years.

Are you eligible for free or low-cost screenings?

You may be eligible for free or low-cost screenings if you meet these qualifications:

- You are between 40 and 64 years of age for breast cancer screening.
- You are between 18 and 64 years of age for cervical cancer screening.
- You have no insurance, or your insurance does not cover screening exams.
- Your yearly income is at or below 250% of the federal poverty level.

Index

Index

Page numbers followed by 'n' indicate a footnote. Page numbers in *italics* indicate a table or illustration.

breast cancer, *continued*
  treatment side effects
    overview 417–33
  see also inflammatory
    breast cancer; invasive
    breast cancer; medullary
    breast carcinoma
"Breast Cancer and the Environment:
  Questions and Answers" (National
  Academy of Sciences) 131n
Breast Cancer Care
  contact information 578
  medullary breast carcinoma
    publication 91n
"Breast Cancer: Coping with
  Your Changing Feelings"
  (Cancer Care, Inc.) 519n
breast cancer gene 1 *see* BRCA1
breast cancer gene 2 *see* BRCA2
Breastcancer.org,
  contact information 579
"Breast Cancer Prevention (PDQ):
  Patient version" (NCI) 178n
"Breast Cancer Recurrence"
  (Cleveland Clinic) 400n
Breast Cancer Research Foundation,
  contact information 578
Breast Cancer Risk Assessment
  Tool (BCRAT), invasive breast
  cancer 82–84
breast cancer screening
  breast implants 204–6
  described 19–21
  overview 196–200
  see also breast self-examination;
    clinical breast examination;
    mammograms
"Breast Cancer Screening (PDQ):
  Patient version" (NCI) 196n
Breast Cancer Society, Inc., contact
  information 579
"Breast Cancer - Step 2:
  Which Risk Factors May
  Apply to You?" (NCI) 113n
"Breast Cancer - Step 3:
  Take Action" (NCI) 113n
"Breast Cancer Treatment and
  Pregnancy (PDQ): Patient
  version" (NCI) 379n

BreastCancerTrials.org,
  contact information 579
breast carcinoma in situ, defined 570
breast changes
  benign 13–16
  described 5–7
breast-conserving surgery
  breast cancer 23–24
  defined 571
  described 312
breast density
  breast cancer risk 115, 117, 211
  defined 570
breast ducts
  defined 570
  described 4, 17
breastfeeding
  breast cancer treatments 380
  flaxseed 376, 378
  mastitis 14
breast implants
  breast cancer screening 204–6
  defined 570
  mammograms 7, 214
  reconstruction surgery 313
  reconstructive procedures 327–30
breast lobes
  defined 570
  described 4, 17
"Breast lump removal"
  (A.D.A.M., Inc.) 318n
"Breast MRI scan"
  (A.D.A.M., Inc.) 226n
breast prostheses, overview 549–52
breast reconstruction
  defined 571
  described 30–31, 190, 290, 313
  implants 327–30
  medullary breast carcinoma 92
  natural tissue 331–34
"Breast reconstruction - implants"
  (A.D.A.M., Inc.) 331n
"Breast reconstruction - natural
  tissue" (A.D.A.M., Inc.) 327n
breasts
  defined 571
  depicted 4
  described 17
  overview 3–11

"Pathology Reports" (NCI) 257n
pathology reports,
    overview 257–60, 290–96
Patient Advocate Foundation,
    contact information 585
patient-controlled analgesia (PCA),
    pain management 465
patient education, fatigue 445
Paxil (paroxetine), hot flashes 142
peau d'orange
    described 572
    inflammatory breast cancer 96
pegfilgrastim, infection risks 452
personalized treatment plan,
    described 287
Petitti, Diana 202, 204
PET scan, metastatic cancer 398
Peutz-Jeghers syndrome 49
photodynamic therapy,
    described 322
physical inactivity,
    breast cancer risk 115,
    118, 121, 212
physical interventions, pain
    management 466–67
physicians, overview 275–79
post-mastectomy bras, overview
    549–52
pregabalin, hot flashes 142
pregnancy
    breast cancer treatments 379–83
    breast changes 14
    flaxseed 376, 378
    tamoxifen 356
"Preventive Mastectomy" (NCI) 187n
primary therapy, described 301
Pristiq (desvenlafaxine),
    hot flashes 142
"Probability of Breast Cancer in
    American Women" (NCI) 59n
procedural pain management 473
progesterone, hormone
    replacement therapy 137
progesterone receptors, medullary
    breast carcinoma 93–94
    see also triple negative breast cancer
progestin
    hormone replacement therapy 137
    uterine cancer 43

prognostic indicators,
    recurrent breast cancer 401
prophylactic mastectomy
    breast cancer prevention 182–83
    defined 574
    genetic testing 17
    lobular carcinoma in situ 77
    overview 187–90
prophylactic oophorectomy
    breast cancer prevention 183
    overview 191
protective factors, breast cancer
    178–84
Prozac (fluoxetine), hot flashes 142
psychological factors,
    sexual function 478–79
psychostimulant medications,
    fatigue 442
PTEN gene
    described 49
    genetic counseling 169
    recent research 67

Q

quality of life, spirituality 495–97
"Questions and Answers about CAM
    and Cancer Treatment" (NCI) 362n
"Questions and Answers About
    Cancer in the Workplace and
    the Americans with Disabilities
    Act (ADA)" (EEOC) 538n

R

racial factor
    breast cancer risk 115
    breast cancer statistics 61–62
    invasive breast cancer 81–84
    triple negative breast cancer 106
radiation exposure
    breast cancer risk factor 52, 114,
    120, 180
    male breast cancer 386
    mammograms 210
radiation oncology, described 276
radiation therapy
    adjuvant therapy 303
    breast cancer treatment 25–26
    diet and nutrition 511–12

604

Health Reference Series

Adolescent Health Sourcebook, 3rd Edition

Adult Health Concerns Sourcebook

AIDS Sourcebook, 5th Edition

Alcoholism Sourcebook, 3rd Edition

Allergies Sourcebook, 4th Edition

Alzheimer Disease Sourcebook, 5th Edition

Arthritis Sourcebook, 3rd Edition

Asthma Sourcebook, 3rd Edition

Attention Deficit Disorder Sourcebook

Autism & Pervasive Developmental Disorders Sourcebook, 2nd Edition

Back & Neck Sourcebook, 2nd Edition

Blood & Circulatory Disorders Sourcebook, 3rd Edition

Brain Disorders Sourcebook, 3rd Edition

Breast Cancer Sourcebook, 4th Edition

Breastfeeding Sourcebook

Burns Sourcebook

Cancer Sourcebook for Women, 4th Edition

Cancer Sourcebook, 6th Edition

Cancer Survivorship Sourcebook

Cardiovascular Disorders Sourcebook, 4th Edition

Caregiving Sourcebook

Child Abuse Sourcebook, 2nd Edition

Childhood Diseases & Disorders Sourcebook, 3rd Edition

Colds, Flu & Other Common Ailments Sourcebook

Communication Disorders Sourcebook

Complementary & Alternative Medicine Sourcebook, 4th Edition

Congenital Disorders Sourcebook, 2nd Edition

Contagious Diseases Sourcebook, 2nd Edition

Cosmetic & Reconstructive Surgery Sourcebook, 2nd Edition

Death & Dying Sourcebook, 2nd Edition

Dental Care & Oral Health Sourcebook, 4th Edition

Depression Sourcebook, 3rd Edition

Dermatological Disorders Sourcebook, 2nd Edition

Diabetes Sourcebook, 5th Edition

Diet & Nutrition Sourcebook, 4th Edition

Digestive Diseases & Disorder Sourcebook

Disabilities Sourcebook, 2nd Edition

Disease Management Sourcebook

Domestic Violence Sourcebook, 4th Edition

Drug Abuse Sourcebook, 3rd Edition

Ear, Nose & Throat Disorders Sourcebook, 2nd Edition

Eating Disorders Sourcebook, 3rd Edition

Emergency Medical Services Sourcebook

Endocrine & Metabolic Disorders Sourcebook, 2nd Edition

Environmental Health Sourcebook, 3rd Edition

Ethnic Diseases Sourcebook

Eye Care Sourcebook, 4th Edition

Family Planning Sourcebook

Fitness & Exercise Sourcebook, 4th Edition

Food Safety Sourcebook

Forensic Medicine Sourcebook

Gastrointestinal Diseases & Disorders Sourcebook, 2nd Edition

Genetic Disorders Sourcebook, 4th Edition

Head Trauma Sourcebook

Headache Sourcebook

Health Insurance Sourcebook

Healthy Aging Sourcebook

Healthy Children Sourcebook

Healthy Heart Sourcebook for Women

Hepatitis Sourcebook

Household Safety Sourcebook

Hypertension Sourcebook

Immune System Disorders Sourcebook, 2nd Edition

Infant & Toddler Health Sourcebook

Infectious Diseases Sourcebook